Cardiac Anesthesia and Postoperative Care in the 21st Century

Marc Vives · Alberto Hernandez
Editors

Cardiac Anesthesia and Postoperative Care in the 21st Century

Springer

Editors
Marc Vives
Hospital Universitari de Girona
Girona, Spain

University of Girona
Girona, Spain

Alberto Hernandez
Bellvitge University Hospital
Barcelona, Spain

University of Barcelona
Barcelona, Spain

ISBN 978-3-030-79720-1 ISBN 978-3-030-79721-8 (eBook)
https://doi.org/10.1007/978-3-030-79721-8

This Springer imprint is published by the registered company Springer Nature Switzerland AG
The registered company address is: Gewerbestrasse 11, 6330 Cham, Switzerland

Foreword

Over the last decade, cardiac anesthesiologists have seen a huge advancement of interventions and procedures to treat cardiovascular diseases requiring their critical care experience be brought outside the theater. More and more fragile patients are offered transcatheter procedures, more and more procedures are performed without cardiopulmonary bypass, and more and more patients undergo interventions with unprotected airways. A big change for the cardiac anesthesiologist is in terms of organization, risks, communication. But a great opportunity to strengthen the presence in the heart team and to be considered an active member whose competencies are essential from the preoperative phase up to the postoperative care.

I'm honored to preface this volume dedicated to cardiac anesthesia and postoperative care. The content truly covers every aspect of the complex and difficult management of the cardiac patient. Experts from major institutions, whose excellence and reputation in the field are highly recognized, have provided comprehensive chapters where both the junior and the senior will find the basis and the advanced information needed to cope with the difficult everyday scenario of cardiac anesthesia and postoperative care.

This book aims to allow the readers to plumb the theory and to provide them with the practical issues that experts believe will improve the care of our patients.

I congratulate Marc Vives and Alberto Hernandez for making this project happen.

Pisa, Italy Fabio Guarracino

Aknowledgements

This book is dedicated to our parents, for their love and support, and also to all my trainers who taught me with generosity.

Contents

Intraoperative Management

Postoperative Care

About the Editors

Marc Vives is currently working as a cardiac anesthetist at Hospital Universitari de Girona Dr Josep Trueta. In 2010, he completed his Ph.D. on Acute Kidney Injury after cardiac surgery at University of Navarra. In 2011, he completed a clinical fellowship in Cardiac Anesthesia & Cardiac Critical Care at Hammersmith Hospital, London, UK. In 2012, he completed a clinical fellowship in Cardiothoracic Anesthesia and Transplantation/Mechanical Support and Cardiothoracic Critical Care at Harefield Hospital, London, UK. In 2013, he completed a clinical fellowship in Cardiovascular Anesthesia, Cardiac Critical Care & Perioperative Echocardiography, at Toronto General Hospital, Canada. He is the EACTA Representative Council for Spain and an active Board member of the Educational Committee (from CPB Subcommittee) at the European Association of Cardiothoracic Anesthesia and Intensive Care (EACTAIC). He has published around 30 papers in peer-reviewed journals. He is review editor at Journal of Cardiothoracic and Vascular Anesthesia.

Alberto Hernandez is currently the Director of Anesthesia & Perioperative Medicine at Policlinica Ibiza Hospital. He has a wide experience as a cardiac anesthetist. He worked in the UK and gained experience in top cardiac hospitals, like Royal Brompton Hospital, St George´s Hospital, Hammersmith Hospital, and Wythenshawe Hospital. Based in Barcelona at Hospital Universitario Belllvitge, he did his Ph.D. on 3D Transesophageal Echocardiography for mitral valve repair at the Autonomous University of Barcelona. He is also an active member of the European Association of Cardiothoracic Anaesthesiology and Intensive Care (EACTAIC) and currently is the ICU delegate for the Educational committee.

Basic Concepts

Anatomy and Functionality of the Heart

Alberto Hernandez, Robert H. Anderson, and Diane E. Spicer

Introduction

The heart is a fascinating organ both anatomically and functionally. Cardiac anatomy is complex. Its understanding, nonetheless, is essential for cardiac surgeons, cardiac anesthesiologists, and intensivists. The heart is an incredibly hard-working organ. Each minute, it pushes about 5 L of blood into the aorta to provide oxygenated blood to different parts of the body. From a purely anatomical point of view, the cardiac pump is a muscle, histologically striated, but functionally the myocardium behaves like smooth muscle, since its functioning is involuntary. The heart has its own irrigation system, provided by the coronary arteries, and it is made up by four cavities, two atriums and two ventricles. The chambers have very different functional characteristics, despite being part of the same structure. If we would follow the traditional anatomical approach for this chapter, our account of cardiac anatomy would be fundamentally incorrect. Teaching anatomy in medical schools is still based on cadaveric dissection, but this approach is obsolete. It has led to a misinterpreted notion of heart anatomy. In this chapter, we provide a contemporary view of cardiac anatomy.

A. Hernandez (✉)
Department of Anaesthesia and Intensive Care, Policlínica Ibiza Hospital, Ibiza, Spain

R. H. Anderson
Biosciences Institute, Newcastle University, Newcastle-Upon-Tyne, UK

D. E. Spicer
Heart Institute, Johns Hopkins All Children's Hospital, St. Petersburg, Florida, USA

M. Vives and A. Hernandez (eds.), *Cardiac Anesthesia and Postoperative Care in the 21st Century*, https://doi.org/10.1007/978-3-030-79721-8_1

The Need for an Attitudinal Approach

The cardiac components are not always described according to the position they occupy within the body. For clinicians, that is obviously less than satisfactory. The traditional approach to cardiac anatomy has its origins in the dissection room. Anatomists typically isolate the heart when examining it outside the thoracic cavity. They then describe it using the so-called "Valentine" approach. Once the heart is removed from the donor, and examined as sitting on its apex, it is studied in an inappropriate manner when compared to its orientation during life. This can lead to confusion, and for clinicians an incorrect understanding of the true location of cardiac components. Techniques based on modern cardiac imaging now provide accurate three-dimensional reconstructions of the cardiac components. These datasets are able to enhance the quality of anatomical knowledge. They show unequivocally that non-attitudinal description of the heart is incorrect.

The basic rules of human anatomy state that all bodily parts should be described as viewed in the so-called anatomical position. This means that the heart also should be described as it is positioned within the thorax. It is unfortunate, therefore, that the "Valentine" approach (Fig. 1 left) remains the standard for current teaching, and continues to retain its currency for most medical practitioners, including cardiologists. As emphasised above, the advent of three-dimensional techniques for

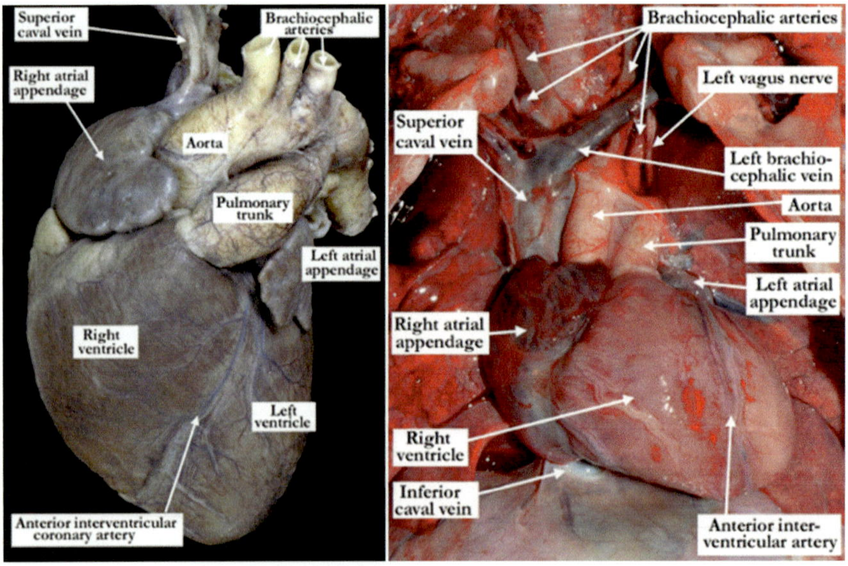

Fig. 1 The left panel demonstrates the so-called 'Valentine' position with the apex of the heart pointing downward. The diaphragmatic aspect is now facing posterior and much more of the left ventricle is seen anteriorly than when the heart is in anatomic position as in the right panel. In anatomic position the anterior most surface of the heart is composed of the right atrium and ventricle

imaging show that the "Valentine" nomenclature is wrong. The heart occupies the middle part of the mediastinum, but its long axis is markedly skewed relative to the long axis of body, extending obliquely in both posteroanterior and right-left directions (Fig. 1). It is the attitudinally appropriate approach that should now be used when describing the spatial relationships of the chambers and the other cardiac components.

Problems with Non-attitudinal Description

Attitudinally incorrect nomenclature, which is still usually used for description of the coronary arteries, myocardial segmentation, and the cardiac valves with their papillary muscles, can lead to important mistakes in clinical practice. At least two glaring problems persist in the nomenclature used to describe the coronary arteries. First, the so-called anterior descending artery follows the so-called "anterior" interventricular groove. In reality, the groove is positioned superiorly and to the left, and is positioned only slightly anterior. More importantly, the artery commonly called the "posterior" descending artery is neither posteriorly located, nor does it markedly descend. The current description of myocardial segmentation also needs to be addressed. It is a step in the right direction that the American Heart Association recently changed its recommended terminology to accept that inferior infarcts are, indeed, the consequence of obstruction in the inferior interventricular artery.

Regarding the valves, the terms commonly used to describe the leaflets of the tricuspid and mitral valves are attitudinally incorrect. The leaflets of the tricuspid valve are typically considered to be anterior, posterior, and septal. In reality, the leaflets are positioned anterosuperiorly, inferiorly, and septally. Similar problems exist for the mitral valve, although the terms used to describe it are a bit closer to reality than those currently used for the tricuspid valve. The two leaflets of the mitral valve are commonly described as being anterior and posterior. The leaflets, however, are not strictly anterior nor posterior. Based on attitudinally appropriate terms, it would be better to define them as being antero-superior and postero-inferior. It is better still to describe them as being aortic and mural, which is less dependent on orientation, and also technically correct.

The Location of the Cardiac Chambers Within the Cardiac Silhouette

When illustrated using the "Valentine" approach, the atrial chambers are shown inappropriately directly above the ventricles, with the right-sided structures placed as though truly right-sided relative to their allegedly left-sided counterparts. The so-called right heart chambers, however, are not strictly to the right, nor are the allegedly left chambers strictly to the left. It is the superior and inferior walls of the left ventricular cone, as seen in attitudinally appropriate orientation, that are equivalent to those currently described as being anterior and posterior by those using the "Valentine" approach. The inappropriate use of "posterior" in this regard has been recognized recently when accounting for the inferior wall of the left ventricle by those using echocardiography. The real position of the heart within the thorax during life is now evident from the images provided either with magnetic resonance or computed tomography.

The Cardiac Chambers

The Morphologically Right Atrium

The morphologically right atrial chamber possesses, a venous component, a triangular appendage, a vestibule supporting the tricuspid valve, and a small part of the body. The body is a small remnant of the developmental "building block" present initially within the linear heart tube that becomes committed to the definitive right atrium. The venous component receives systemic venous drainage from the superior caval vein at its roof, and the inferior caval vein in its floor. (Fig. 2a)

It also receives most of the blood from the heart itself, which drains through the coronary sinus. The orifice of the inferior caval vein is guarded by the Eustachian valve. This valve is usually a triangular flap, but sometimes may be more extensive and aneurysmal, or may take the form of a Chiari network.

Forming the border between the smooth venous component and the appendage is a prominent muscle bundle called the terminal crest, or crista terminalis. The location of the crest is marked externally by the terminal groove. This area is important for the interventional electrophysiologist because the sinus node is found within the groove at the superior cavoatrial junction. The terminal crest can be the origin of many focal atrial tachycardias, and is also a barrier to conduction in isthmus dependent atrial flutter. The right edge of the cardiac silhouette is formed entirely by the right atrial appendage, which is lined by the characteristic pectinate muscles. The phenotypic feature of the morphologically right atrium is that the pectinate muscles extend round the vestibule so as to reach to the so-called cardiac crux. In comparison to the left atrium, the right atrium has thinner walls. Hence, it dilates more easily given the same degree of pressure overload.

Its inferior paraseptal region contains the triangle of Koch, which is defined by the mouth of the coronary sinus, the hinge of the septal leaflet of the tricuspid valve, and the tendon of Todaro, a tendinous structure connecting the valve of the inferior

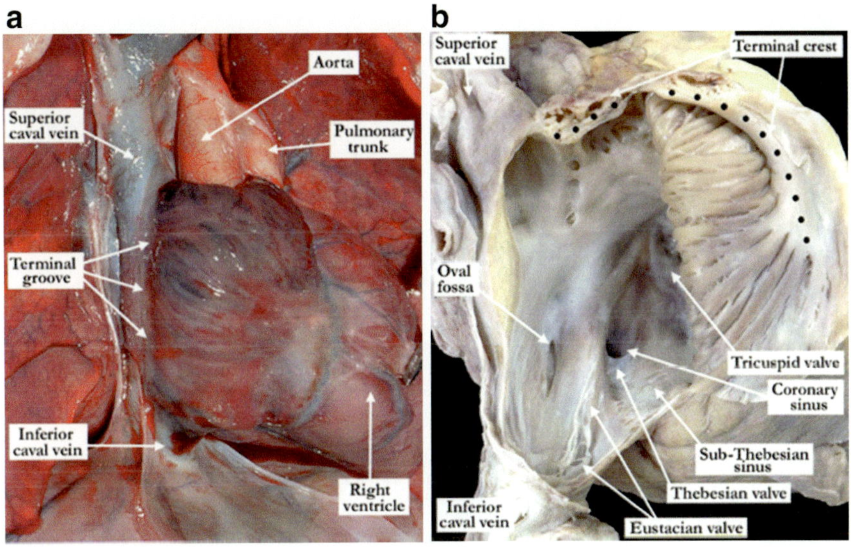

Fig. 2 **a** This in-situ, right anterolateral view of the morphologically right atrium shows the superior caval vein draining to the roof of the atrium and the inferior caval vein at its floor. Along the length of the venous sinus is the terminal groove. The appendage has a blunt triangular tip and the parallel pectinate muscles are appreciated over the entire anterior aspect. **b** The morphologically right atrium has been opened along the terminal groove, as shown in Fig. 2, and folded forward to expose the terminal crest (black dots). The pectinate muscles extend from the terminal crest and around the right atrioventricular junction. Note the fenestrations or Chiari malformation of the Eustachian valve. The atrial vestibule is the thin, smooth area between the pectinate muscles and the hinge point of the tricuspid valve (see Fig. 4)

caval vein (Eustachian valve) to the central fibrous body. The triangle is the anatomical landmark to the atrioventricular node. When considered in attitudinally appropriate fashion, the apex of the triangle points superiorly. (Fig. 3)

The right atrium is separated from the left atrium by the septum, made up by the floor of the oval fossa and its anterior buttress. Interatrial communications are among the most common of congenital heart malformations. Defects of the oval fossa, or "ostium secundum" defects, are located within the true septum, and hence within the oval fossa. Persistent patency of the oval foramen is more frequent. This is a tunnel-like passageway between the free edge of the overlapping flap valve, representing the true septum, and the muscular rims of the fossa, which are mostly folds. Other defects, such as the superior and inferior sinus venosus defects, the coronary sinus defects, and the ostium primum defects, all lie outside the area of the true septum.

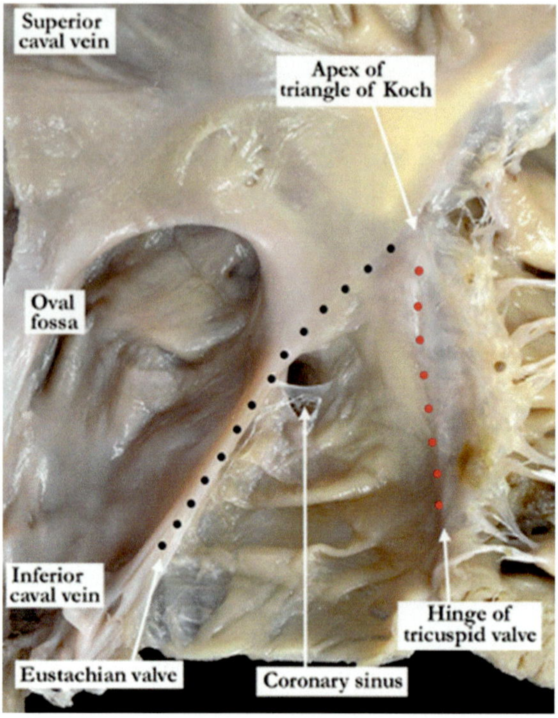

Fig. 3 The triangle of Koch is formed by the tendon of Todaro (black dots) and the hinge point of the tricuspid valve (red dots). At the base of the triangle is the coronary sinus with its ápex in superior position and marking the site of the atrioventricular node. Note the pectinate muscles extending to the crux of the heart and within the sub-Thebesian sinus

Tricuspid Valve

In functional anatomy, the tricuspid valve, which is supported by the right atrial vestibule, consists not only of leaflets, but also the supporting tendinous cords, papillary muscles, and ventricular musculature. Hence, the valve is better considered as forming a junctional atrioventricular complex. In the normal heart, the hinge of the septal leaflet of the valve is located slightly closer to the apex than the leaflet of the mitral valve. The so-called displacement index between the hinges is calculated by dividing the linear distance between their septal insertions by the body surface area of the patient. Excessive apical displacement of the valve, present with the displacement index is greater than 8 mm/m^2, is indicative of Ebstein's malformation. The valve has three leaflets, positioned antero-superiorly, inferiorly, and septally. The antero-superior leaflet is the largest leaflet, with the inferior leaflet usually being the smallest of the three. The septal leaflet is located leftward and posteriorly within the right atrioventricular junction. The supporting papillary muscles are positioned anteriorly, inferiorly, and septally, respectively. The septal muscle is particularly characteristic, and is also known as Lancisi's muscle, or the medial papillary muscle (Fig. 4).

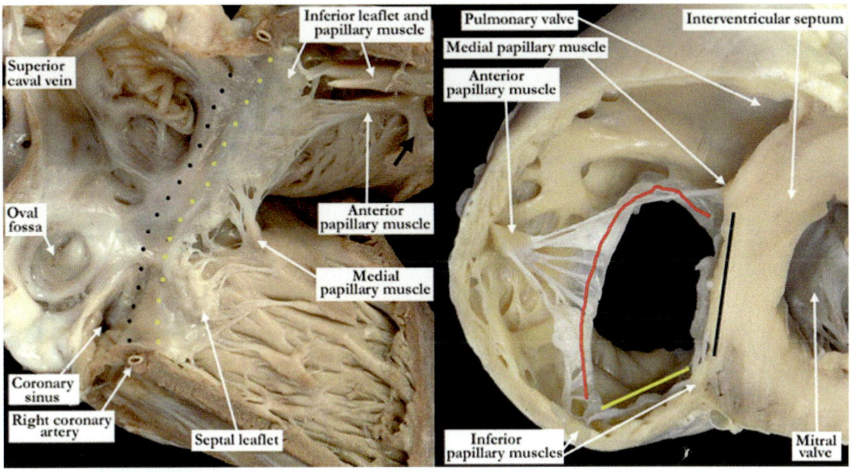

Fig. 4 The left panel shows the opened tricuspid valve and its relationship with the right atrial vestibule with the black dots marking the extent of the pectinate muscles and the yellow dots the hinge of the tricuspid valve. The leaflets and their supporting papillary muscles are also apparent with the inferior leaflet and papillary muscle at the top of the image secondary to the right atrioventricular wall being folded open and lifted away from the diaphragmatic aspect. The black arrow marks the moderator band. The right panel is a short axis apical view of the right ventricle and tricuspid valve. The septal leaflet (black line) lies against the interventricular septum, the inferior leaflet (yellow line) lies along the inferior or diaphragmatic aspect, and the largest of the three, the anterior superior leaflet (red line) is along the free wall. The support to the inferior leaflet can vary and in this specimen there are two supporting papillary muscles

Morphologically Right Ventricle

The right ventricle is positioned anteriorly and to the right of the left ventricle. It forms the inferior cardiac border, lying nearly horizontal to the diaphragm, having an acute angle between its inferior and anterior walls. The inferior surface is flat, with the pericardium adjoined to the central tendon and a muscular portion of the diaphragm. The ventricle is best analysed in tripartite fashion, with the inlet component surrounding and supporting the tricuspid valvar junctional complex as described above. The apical part is coarsely trabeculated. It is the coarse trabeculations that are the phenotypic feature of the ventricle. One of the trabeculations is prominent, and is called the septomarginal trabeculation or septal band. A series of septoparietal trabeculations arise from the septal band with the most inferior connecting with the base of the anterior papillary muscle. It was named the "moderator" band in the belief that it would act as a protective mechanism to resist ventricular over distension, although there is no evidence to support this notion. Echocardiographers use the structure as a marker of the right ventricle. It has also been mistaken for an apical thrombus. Another characteristic feature is the long infundibulum, the distal part of which is a free-standing muscular sleeve. This lifts the leaflets of the pulmonary valve away from the base of the ventricular cone. It is the presence of the free-standing infundibular sleeve that permits the entirety of the pulmonary root to be removed and used as an aortic autograft in the Ross procedure. The pulmonary root itself is located anteriorly and leftward relative to the aortic root. Having exited through the pulmonary valve, the blood passes from the right ventricle into the pulmonary trunk, which runs in the transverse plane before bifurcating at the margins of the pericardial cavity into the right and left pulmonary arteries. The right ventricle becomes hypertrophied in the settings of pulmonary hypertension or pulmonary stenosis, and can suffer loss of function and become dilated in the setting of ischemic heart disease. It is a traditional destination for placement of pacemaker leads. These can be anchored at the apex, in the outflow tract and, more recently, on the ventricular septum. (Fig. 5)

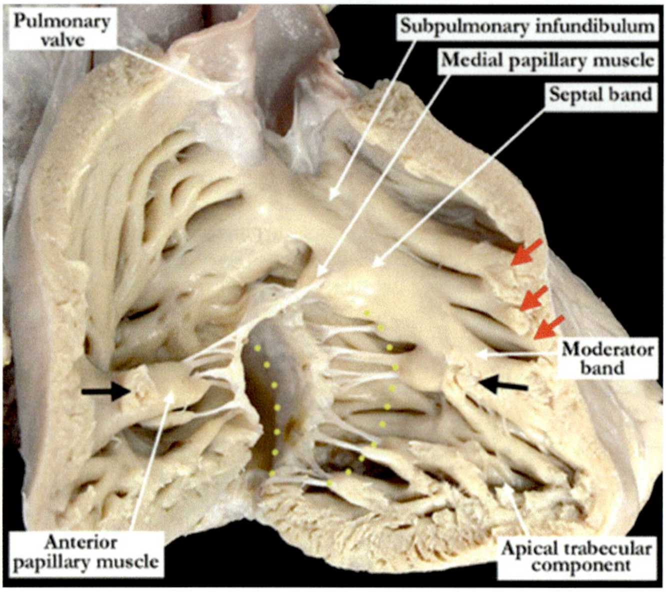

Fig. 5 The right ventricle has been opened in clam-shell fashion and shown in attitudinally appropriate position. The inlet is marked by the yellow dots, extending from hinge of the tricupsid valve to the distal extent of the tendinous cords. There is a coarse apical trabecular component which is the morphologic determinate of the right ventricle. The septal band is a prominent trabeculation with a caudal arm giving rise to the medial papillary muscle and the cephalic arm extending upward to become part of the subpulmonary infundibulum. The septal band gives rise to the septoparietal trabeculations (red arrows) and the moderator band (black arrows). The moderator band extends between the septal and free walls of the ventricle and joins the base of the anterior papillary muscle. The pulmonary valve lies within the outlet component and is supported by the subpulmonary infundibulm which is a circumferential, free-standing, musclar sleeve lifting the valve off of the right ventricular base

The Morphologically Left Atrium

Like its morphologically right partner, the left atrium possesses part of the body derived from the primary heart tube. Indeed, the larger part of the body is destined to form the basis of the left atrium. Also like its right-sided counterpart, it then possesses a venous component, a small and fingerlike appendage, and a vestibule, which supports the mitral valve. The pectinate muscles are confined within the tubular appendage, with this feature serving to distinguish the chamber phenotypically. The appendage frequently acts as a nidus for formation of thrombus. The atrial chamber receives its venous drainage from the pulmonary veins, which are positioned superiorly rather than posteriorly. The veins, usually four in number, show significant variability in their dimensions, shape, and patterns of branching. The septal surface is dominated by the flap valve of the oval fossa, which is derived from the primary atrial septum. (Fig. 6a+b)

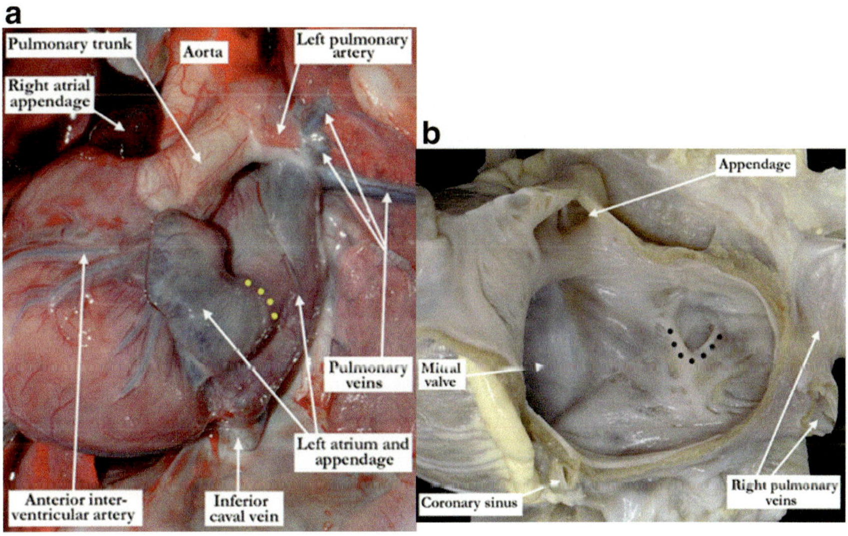

Fig. 6 **a** In this in-situ view, the apex of the heart has been lifted toward the right demonstrating the outward appearance of the morphologically left atrial appendage. The appendage is tubular or finger-like, often with scalloped edges, and a narrow junction (yellow dots) with the body of the atrium. The left pulmonary veins are seen entering the atrium superiorly. **b** The opened, morphologically left atrium shows the narrow junction of the atrial appendage with the pectinate muscles confined to the appendage. The walls of the left atrium are smooth with focal, trabeculations usually associated with the flap valve or the atrial septum. The typical horseshoe appearance (black dots) is easily appreciated

Mitral Valve

The mitral valve, like the tricuspid valve, is best analysed in terms of an atrioventricular junctional complex, made up of the left atrial wall, the atrioventricular junction, the leaflets, the tendinous cords, and the papillary muscles. All parts need to work in harmony to ensure normal function. The valve has two leaflets, which close along a solitary zone of apposition. It is the ends of the solitary zone of apposition that are usually described as the commissures. The aortic leaflet of the valve guards one-third of the valvar orifice. It is deep, whereas the mural leaflet, which guards two-thirds of the circumference, is shallower. The commissures are located supero-laterally and infero-septally. The mural leaflet is typically described as possessing three major scallops, named P1, P2, and P3, although there are also commissural leaflets at the ends of the zone of apposition. The aortic leaflet does not have formal scallops, but its parts are named A1, A2, and A3 based on their adjacent positions to the mural scallops. The papillary muscles are located directly beneath the commissures. Hence, they too are positioned ínfero-septally and supero-laterally, although currently they are usually incorrectly described as being "postero-medial" and "antero-lateral". Their correct positioning is important when considering repair in the setting of functional mitral regurgitation. Restrictive mitral annuloplasty leads to their progressive displacement, which may cause valvar incompetence and potential failure of the annuloplasty. In fact, functional mitral regurgitation is frequently a disease of the ventricular myocardium and subvalvar apparatus, as opposed to the leaflets and orifice. The aim of surgery, therefore, is not just to place a ring, but to contemplate approximation or elevation of the papillary muscles, as well as commissural plication and fixture of the tendinous cords. The aim is to alleviate tethering forces and ventricular geometric distortions that contribute to failure of the repair. Nowadays, transcatheter repair is becoming increasingly popular. Interventionists using this approach gain access to the valve through the inferior caval vein and cross through the oval fossa. This route has been shown to be safer when compared to the apical approach, which is typically used for replacement of the valve, and for transcatheter neocordal implantation. (Fig. 7)

Morphologically Left Ventricle

The left ventricle, when assessed attitudinally, is the inferior ventricle. The majority of its free wall lies on the diaphragm, which is of course inferior to the heart. Since the so-called "posterior descending artery" traverses this surface, both the groove and artery should now be named as being inferior. Fortunately, for those using computed tomography, imagers now correctly describe the diaphragmatic portion of the left ventricle as being inferior. Infarction of the wall previously considered to be "posterior" is now, according to the consensus document of the American Heart Association, properly recognized as involving the inferobasal segment of the

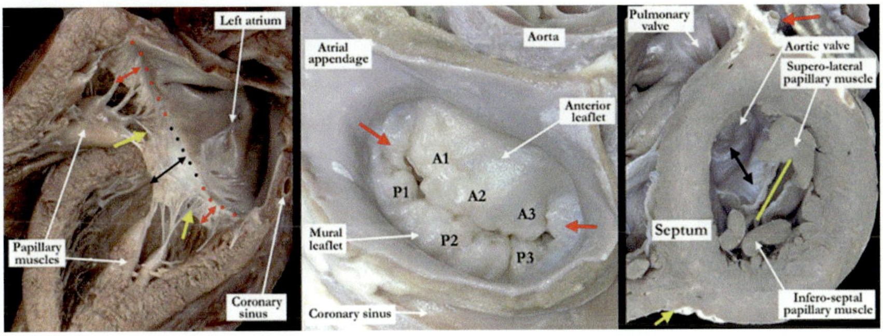

Fig. 7 The left panel shows the opened left atrioventricular junction and its inlet component. Note the smooth left atrial vestibule and the coronary sinus within the left atrioventricular groove. The mitral valve has no attachments to the ventricular septum and is entirely supported by papillary muscles. The anterior or aortic leaflet (black dots) makes up about 1/3 or the overall circumference and is a deep or broad leaflet (doublé headed black arrow). The mural leaflet makes up the remaining 2/3 of the circumference (red dots) and is a shallow leaflet (doublé headed red arrows). When closed, there is a solitary zone of apposition with the commissures demononstrated by yellow arrows in the opened position. The middle panel shows the closed mitral valve from the atrial aspect. It demonstrates the solitary zone of apposition with the characteristic scallops associated with both the mural (P) and anterior leaflet (A). The commisural leaflets are marked with the red arrows. The right panel is a short axis apical view of the left ventricle showing the solitary zone of apposition (yellow line) and the papillary muscles that support the leaflets. The doublé headed black arrow marks the area of fibrous continuity between the mitral and aortic valves. The mitral valve has no attachments to the interventricular septum. The red arrow marks the anterior interventricular artery and the yellow arrow the inferior interventricular artery along the diaphragmatic aspect

inferior wall, with the electrocardiographic vector headed towards V_3. Even the so-called "anterior interventricular groove" has been challenged. It does not lie truly anterior, but rather it lies more superior, anterior, and to the left. Thus, the groove, and the artery within it, are more correctly described as being antero-superior".

Like its right partner, the morphologically left ventricle has an inlet portion surrounding the mitral valvar apparatus (see Fig. 7 left panel), an apical trabecular component containing fine trabeculations, and an outlet portion leading to the aortic valve. As with the right ventricle, it is the nature of the apical trabeculations that provide the best phenotypic recognition. (Fig. 8)

The left ventricle is conical, with the right ventricle wrapping round it in banana-like fashion. When seen in short axis, therefore, the left ventricle is circular in cross section. It also has a much thicker wall than the right ventricle. (Fig. 9)

The wall, however, is very thin at the apex, where it is no more than 1 to 2 mm thick. When the heart is viewed from the anterior aspect, most of the left ventricle is hidden by the right ventricle. The ventricular septum is muscular, except for a small fibrous portion immediately beneath the aortic valve. If crossed by the hinge of the septal leaflet of the tricuspid valve, the fibrous part, usually described as the membranous septum, can have interventricular and atrioventricular components. The atrioventricular component, together with the right fibrous trigone, form the

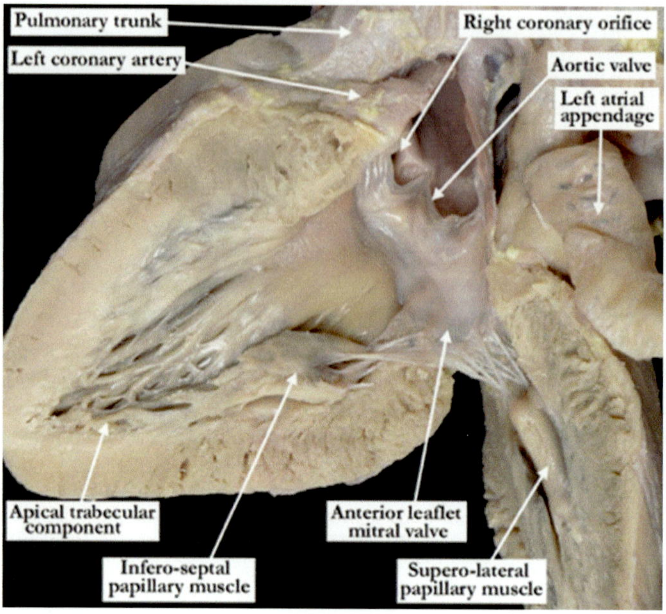

Fig. 8 The left ventricle has been opened in clam-shell fashion and is shown in attitudinally appropriate position. There are fine trabeculations at the apex which are the morphologic determinate for the left ventricle. The septal surface typically becomes smooth toward the outlet component which supports the aortic valve

central fibrous body. The atrioventricular conduction bundle penetrates the septal component of the fibrous body, extending into the subaortic outflow tract and branching on the crest of the muscular septum. (Fig. 10)

As emphasised, it is the fine, criss-crossing pattern of the apical trabeculations that distinguish the left from the right ventricle. Occasionally, fine muscular strands, or so-called false tendons, extend from the septum to the papillary muscles and the parietal wall. Echocardiographers may mistake such false tendons for ruptured tendinous cords or vegetations. The outlet portion is smooth, and bordered posteriorly by fibrous continuity between the leaflets of the aortic and mitral valves.

Aortic Root

The aortic root has become of increasing importance with the development of transcatheter or transapical and percutaneous sutureless replacement of the aortic valve. It is essential, therefore, to have a full understanding of its anatomy. As with the atrioventricular valves, the aortic root can be considered to constitute a valvar complex, but now a ventrículo-arterial complex. The root is made up of the sinuses of Valsalva, the semilunar valve leaflets, and the sinutubular junction. Beyond the

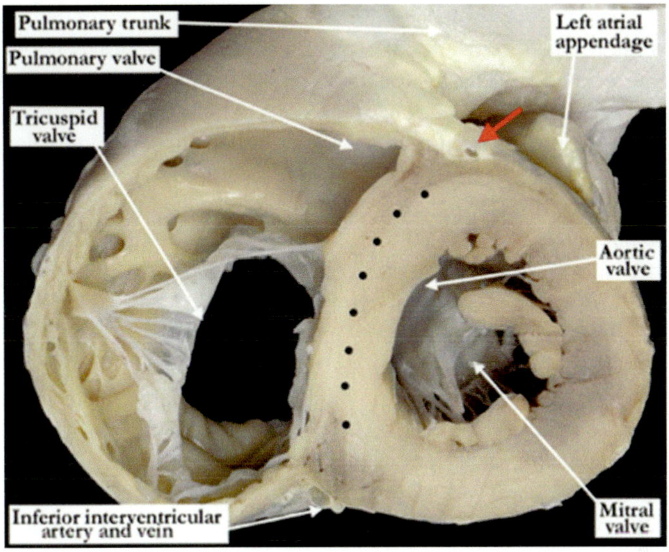

Fig. 9 This short axis, apical view of both ventricles is shown in anatomical position. The right ventricular outflow tract wraps around the outlet component of the left ventricle. The left ventricle has a circular appearance and is much thicker than the right ventricle. The interventricular septum is marked with black dots and the anterior interventricular artery with a red arrow

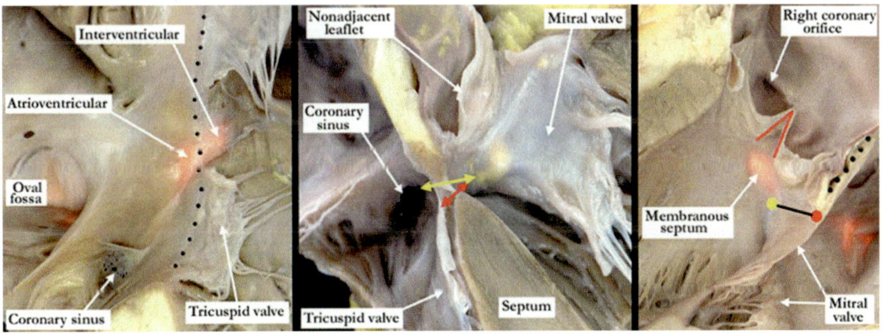

Fig. 10 The left panel shows the membranous septum from the right with a portion of the tricuspid valve removed. The membranous septum is photographed with a back light which easily demonstrates where the hinge line (black dots) of the tricuspid valve separates it into the atrioventricular and interventricular components. The middle panel is a close up, four chamber view demonstrating the atrioventricular (double headed yellow arrow) and the interventricular (double headed red arrow) components of the membranous septum. The right panel shows the left ventricular side of the membranous septum which was photographed with a back light. The membranous septum lies beneath the interleaflet triangle (red lines) between the right and non-coronary leaflets. The right (yellow dot) and left (red dot) fibrous trigones lie on either aspect of the fibrous continuity (black line) between the mitral and aortic valves. The junction between the membranous septum and the right fibrous trigone form the central fibrous body. The black dots mark the transverse sinus

sinutubular junction, the root becomes the intrapericardial ascending aorta. The entrance to the root is often called the "annulus". In reality, this is no more than a virtual plane, created by joining together the basal attachments of the semilunar hinges. It has no anatomical counterpart. The semilunar leaflets meet together peripherally at the circumference of the sinutubular junction. Competency of the root is maintained by its different components working in harmony.

The aortic valve normally has three leaflets. Two of the leaflets are supported by the sinuses that give rise to the coronary arteries, The third sinus does not usually give rise to a coronary artery, and hence is described as the non-coronary leaflet. Very rarely, it can give rise to a coronary artery. Then, recognizing its posterior location, it can be distinguished as the non-adjacent sinus. The leaflets themselves are formed with a fibrous core and an endothelial lining. The fibrous core is thickened at the free edge of the leaflet, especially centrally, where it is known as the nodule of Arantius. When performing echocardiography, it is important not to confuse the nodule with a vegetation. The right coronary leaflet is visualized lower than are the left coronary and the non-coronary leaflets. It, and the left coronary leaflet, are supported by the myocardium of the ventricular septum at their base. (Fig. 11)

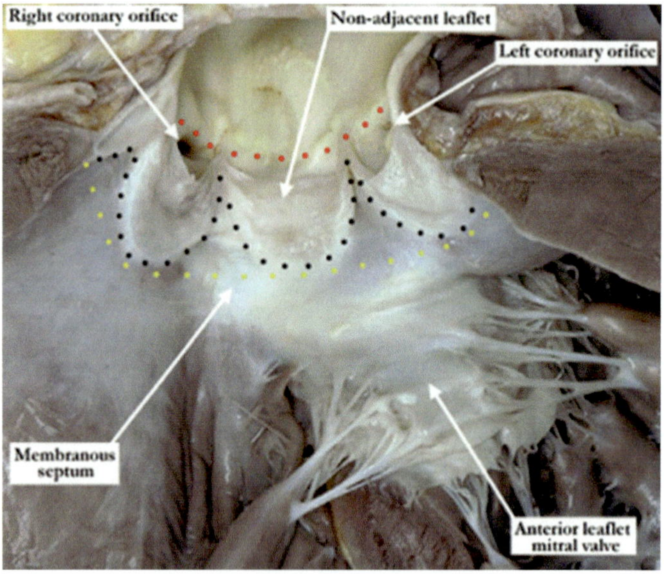

Fig. 11 The opened aortic valve is supported by both muscle and fibrous tissue. The leaflets are marked by the black dots with the right coronary leaflet and the majority of the left coronary leaflet supported by muscle. Typically a portion of the left coronary leaflet and the entire non-coronary leaflet are supported by fibrous tissue or the area of aorta to mitral valve fibrous continuity. Note the membranous septum beneath the interleaflet triangle between the right and non-coronary leaflets. The semilunar leaflets attach at their most distal extent at the sinutubular junction (red dots). At the basal attachments of the valvar leaflets, the yellow dots mark the so-called echocardiographic 'annulus'

The Coronary Circulation

The coronary circulation consists of arterial perfusion and its venous drainage. The venous flow occurs during diastole and systole, and can be considered in terms of its greater and smaller components. The greater cardiac venous system is comprised of the coronary sinus and its tributaries. The smaller part is comprised of the anterior cardiac veins, which drain directly to the cavity of the right atrium. There is also a minimal cardiac venous system, made up of the Thebesian vessels, which drain directly into the atrial or ventricular cavities through tiny orifices.

The coronary sinus is the largest cardiac venous structure. It is a continuation of the great cardiac vein, becoming the sinus at the union of the great vein with the oblique vein of the left atrium, the latter also known as the vein of Marshall. The union of the veins is usually marked by the presence of the valve of Vieussens. The coronary sinus also receives the middle cardiac vein, better described as the inferior interventricular vein. It originates near the apex and occupies the inferior atrioventricular groove. Also draining into the coronary sinus is the small cardiac vein, which runs within the right atrioventricular groove. (Fig. 12)

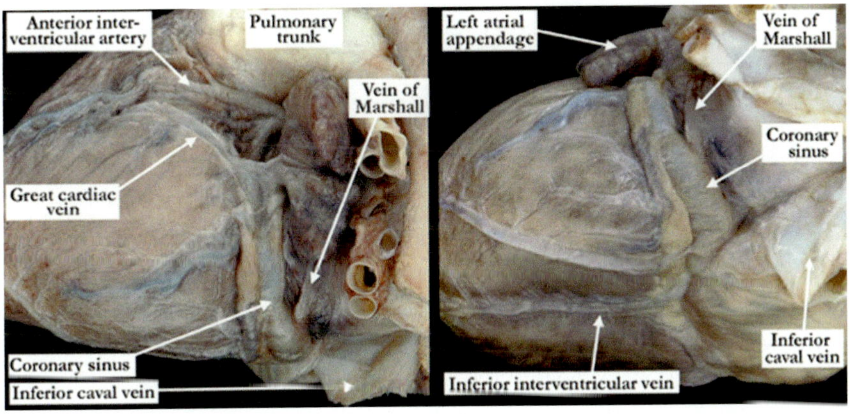

Fig. 12 The left panel shows the posterior aspect of the heart in attitudinal orientation and with the left atrial appendage pulled off of the atrioventricular groove. The great cardiac vein lies nearly parallel with the anterior interventricular artery and extends to join the coronary sinus within the left atrioventricular groove. The coronary sinus continues toward the diaphragmatic aspect where it will drain to the right atrium. Note the close approximation to the inferior caval vein. The right panel is the same heart as is shown in the left panel, but rotated to show the diaphragmatic surface. Here, the inferior interventricular vein extends from the apex to join the coronary sinus just as it enters the right atrium. In both panels, note that several venous tributaries extend over the free wall of the left ventricle and join the coronary sinus

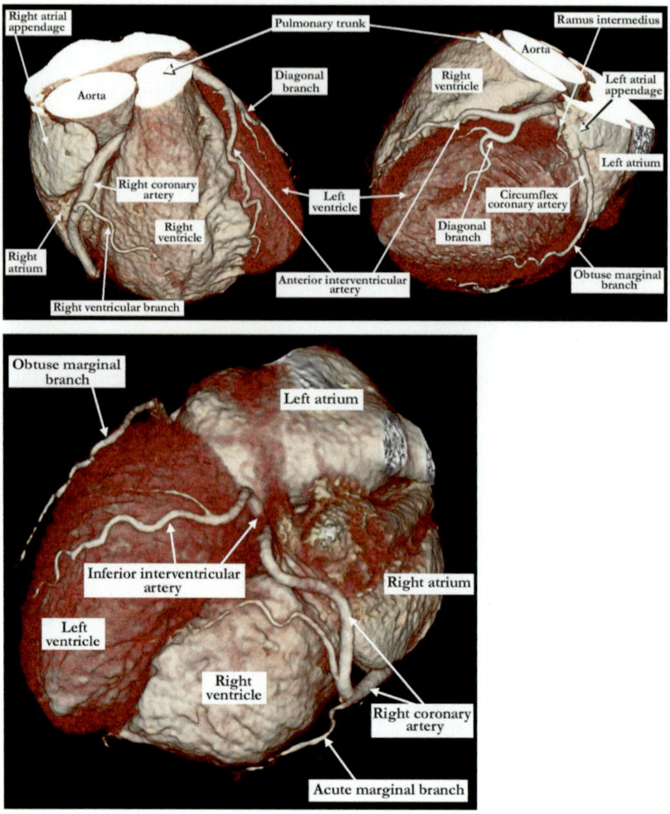

Fig. 13 Cardiac CT Angiography performed with AIDR 3D (Canon medical system) showing the coronary arteries from an attitudinally appropriate approach

Knowledge of the anatomy of the coronary sinus is important because of its relevance in electrophysiologic procedures, such as left ventricular pacing, and mapping and ablation of arrhythmias. It is important during cardiac surgical procedures for administration of retrograde cardioplegia. It traverses the left atrioventricular groove, opening into the septal vestibular area of the right atrium. Cardiac anesthesiologists should be aware that the coronary sinus is always absent in hearts with isomerism of the right atrial appendages. It can also be difficult, on occasion, to place a cannula in the coronary sinus due to a large Thebesian valve. This maneuver may be impossible should the valve be atretic. The use of transesophageal echocardiography, therefore, is mandatory to guide placement of the retrograde cannula in the coronary sinus during cardiac surgery.

The Coronary Arteries

The coronary arteries are the first branches of the aortic root. Although there are three aortic valvar sinuses, the coronary arteries take origin only from the two that are adjacent to the pulmonary root.

The left coronary artery, which arises from the left coronary aortic sinus, has but a short main stem. It divides almost immediately into two major arteries of nearly equal diameter, the anterior interventricular artery, usually described as the left anterior descending artery, and the circumflex artery. In some patients, the main stem also gives rise to a third intermediate artery. The right coronary artery, having taken its origin from the right coronary aortic sinus, encircles the orifice of the tricuspid valve. In nine-tenths of individuals, it gives rise to the inferior interventricular artery, which usually continues beyond the crux to supply the diaphragmatic wall of the left ventricle. This arrangement is known as right coronary arterial dominance. In the remaining tenth of the population, it is the circumflex artery that is dominant, and which gives rise to the inferior interventricular artery. The circumflex and right coronary arteries occupy the atrioventricular grooves, while the anterior interventricular artery occupies the anterior interventricular groove.

The Pericardium

The fibrous pericardium, which encloses the heart, has within it a double layered sac, the serous pericardium. The outer layer lines the fibrous pericardium, while the inner layer coats the outer surface of the heart as the epicardium. The layers are continuous as two cuffs, one around the aorta and pulmonary trunk, and the other around the veins. Two recesses are found within the pericardial cavity. The first, named the transverse sinus (Fig. 14), lies between the posterior aspect of the arterial trunks and the anterior aspect of the atrial chambers.

The other, the oblique sinus (Fig. 15), is behind the left atrium. It is limited by the right pulmonary veins and the caval veins to the right side, and the left pulmonary veins to the left side.

Significant extracardiac structures are directly related to the pericardium. The right phrenic nerve descends along the right superior caval vein and continues its descent immediately in front of the right pulmonary veins in the lung hilium before reaching the diaphragm. Its upper course along the superior cavoatrial junction, and adjacent to the right superior pulmonary vein, makes it vulnerable to damage when ablations are carried out for supraventricular arrhythmias. The left phrenic nerve

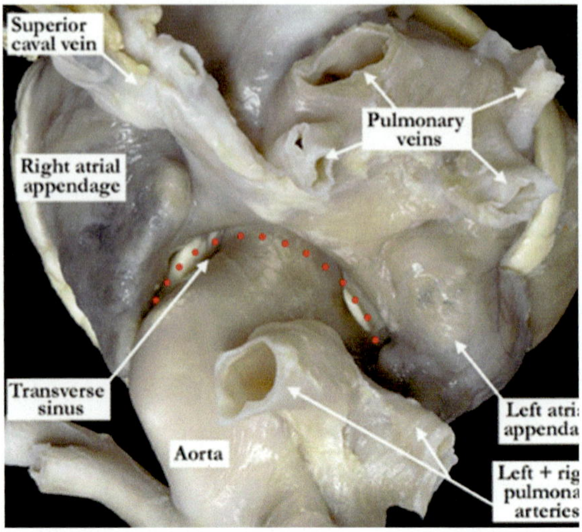

Fig. 14 The heart is photographed from the base with the aorta and pulmonary arteries pulled forward to demonstrate the transverse sinus (red dots). This is the space between the posterior extent of the arterial trunks and the anterior aspect of the atrial chambers

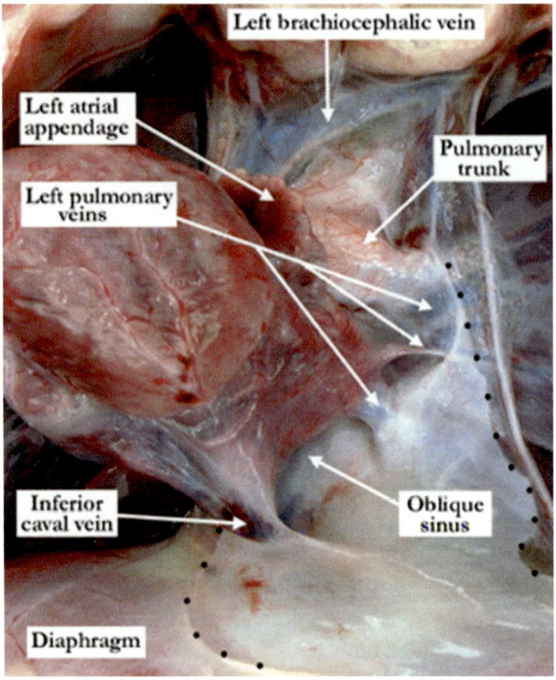

Fig. 15 This in-situ view shows the heart pulled upwards and toward the right, away from the diaphragmatic aspect of the pericardium. The cut edges of the pericardium are marked with black dots. The oblique sinus lies posterior to the left atrium with the left pulmonary veins bordering to the left and the inferior caval vein forming a portion of the right border in this image. The right pulmonary veins are not seen in this image at the right extent of the sinus

passes over the left atrial appendage in its descent. It then takes an anterior course to be related to the great cardiac veins. It becomes at risk during implantation of pacemaker leads into these veins, or when epicardial ablation is attempted in these regions.

Cardiovascular Physiology

Marc Vives

Cardiac Action Potentials

An action potential is a spontaneous depolarisation of the membrane of an excitable cell, usually in response to a stimulus. Two different types of action potential are found in the heart: fast and slow responses. In the myocardium two cell types produce fast-response action potential: contractile myocardial cells and conduction system cells. Slow-response action potential are normally produced by the pacemaker cells in the sinoatrial (SA) node and the atrioventricular (AV) node. These pacemaker cells spontaneously depolarise to produce slow-response action potential, exhibiting a property called automaticity.

Fast-Response Action Potentials

The fast-response action potential of the cardiac muscle cell can be divided into 5 phases (Fig. 1):

- Phase 0—initial rapid depolarisation/upstroke
- Phase 1—early rapid repolarisation
- Phase 2—prolonged plateau phase
- Phase 3—final rapid repolarisation
- Phase 4—resting membrane potential (RMP)

M. Vives (✉)
Hospital Universitari de Girona Doctor Josep Trueta, Avinguda de França, S/N, 17007 Girona, Spain

M. Vives and A. Hernandez (eds.), *Cardiac Anesthesia and Postoperative Care in the 21st Century*, https://doi.org/10.1007/978-3-030-79721-8_2

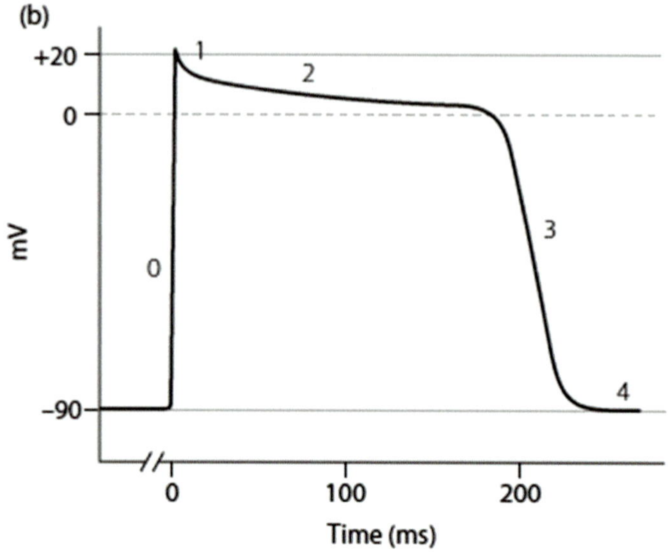

Fig. 1 Myocardial cell fast response action potential

Resting membrane potential

The RMP is the electrical potential across the cell membrane during diastole and is about − 90 mV, the intracellular membrane surface being negative with respect to the extracellular surface (Fig. 2).

RMP is maintained by three mechanisms:

- Retention of many intracellular anions (proteins, phosphates and sulphates) to which the cell membrane is not permeable.
- The resting cell membrane is almost 100 times more permeable to potassium than to sodium, allowing potassium to flow down its concentration gradient out of the cell while keeping sodium extracellular.

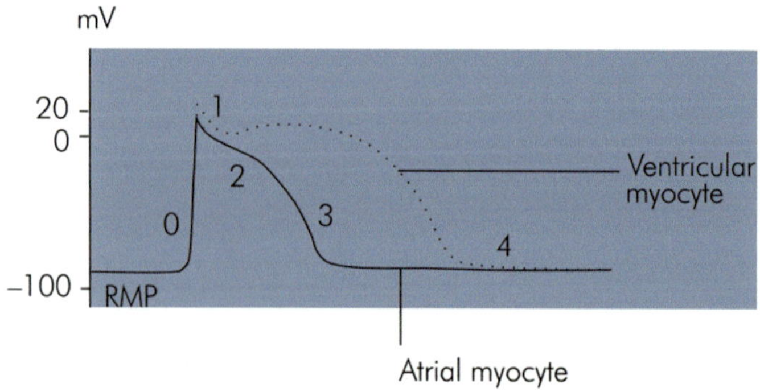

Fig. 2 Atrial and ventricular myocite fast response action potential

- Maintenance of an intracellular–extracellular concentration gradient for potassium ions by a Na + K + ATPase pump. This transports potassium actively into the cell and sodium out of the cell (three Na + ions for every two K + ions) and is dependent on energy supplied by the hydrolysis of ATP.

Slow-Response Action Potentials

The action potential produced when a pacemaker cell depolarises spontaneously is called a slow-response action potential (Fig. 3). The most negative potential reached just before depolarisation is called the 'maximum diastolic potential' (MDP), which is only − 60 mV compared with the resting membrane potential of −90 mV for a myocardial muscle cell. The reason for this is that the pacemaker cell membranes are more permeable to sodium ions in their resting state. Phases can be identified in the slow-response action potential which correspond superficially to some phases of the rapid-response, as detailed below, although the underlying events differ.

Differences Between Pacemaker and Myocardial Cell Action Potential

Pacemaker action potential have the following features which differ from those of the myocardial cells:

- Less negative phase 4 membrane potential
- Less negative Threshold potential
- Spontaneous depolarisation in phase 4
- Less steep slope in phase 0 (dependence on T-type Ca2 + channels)
- Absence of phase 2 (plateau)

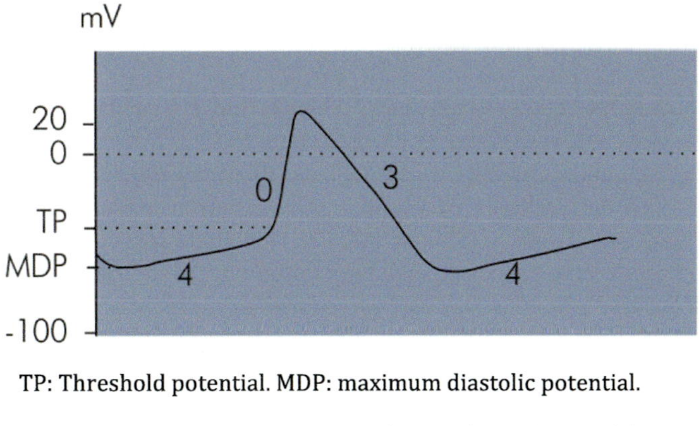

TP: Threshold potential. MDP: maximum diastolic potential.

Fig. 3 Pacemaker cell slow response action potential *TP* Threshold potential. *MDP* maximum diastolic potential

Pacemaker Discharge Rate

Pacemaker discharge rate is controlled primarily by the autonomic system. Control is mediated by changes in action potential characteristics. The following characteristics are associated with variation of the discharge rate:

- Slope of phase 4 in action potential—an increase in the slope of phase 4 reduces the time to reach TP during spontaneous depolarisation, and thus increases pacemaker rate. Similarly, a decrease in the phase 4 slope results in a slower pacemaker rate. Phase 4 slope can be varied by the autonomic nervous system.
- Threshold potential—if this becomes less negative the pacemaker rate will decrease. Drugs such as quinidine and procainamide have this effect.
- Hyperpolarisation potential—if hyperpolarisation is increased, i.e. the membrane potential becomes more negative, spontaneous discharge will take longer to reach threshold potential during phase 4 and the pacemaker rate will decrease. This occurs with increases in acetylcholine levels.

Conduction System

The conduction system of the heart is composed of specialised cardiac tissues that form the following structures:

- Sinoatrial (SA) node
- Atrial conduction pathways
- Atrioventricular (AV) node
- Bundle of His
- Bundle branches
- Purkinje fibres

The SA node is the normal cardiac pacemaker, with a resting rate of between 60 and 100 per minute. It is a group of modified myocardial cells located close to the junction of the superior vena cava with the right atrium. Blood supply is usually from a branch of the right coronary artery. Depolarisation spreads from the SA node through the atria and converges on the AV node.

The two atria are electrically separated from the two ventricles except for three internodal communication pathways, the anterior (Bachmann), middle (Wenckebach) and posterior (Thorel) bundles, which connect the SA node to the AV node. The AV node is located in the right posterior part of the right atrium close to the tricuspid valve and the coronary sinus opening. Anomalous accessory pathways (like the bundle of Kent) can sometimes connect the atria directly to the ventricle or other areas of the conducting system and cause a pre-excitation syndrome with arrhythmias. Blood supply to the AV node is also from a branch of the right coronary artery. The AV node is connected to the bundle of His, which distributes the impulse to the ventricles via the left and right bundle branches in the interventricular septum. There is a slight delay (about 0.13 s) of the impulse before it enters the AV node, inside the AV node and in the bundle of His. This delay permits completion of both atrial electrical activation and conduction before ventricular activation is started. The left bundle branch divides into the anterior and posterior fascicles. These bundles and fascicles run subendocardially down the septum and into the Purkinje system, which spreads the impulse to all parts of the ventricular muscle. Conduction velocity through the bundle branches and the Purkinje system is the most rapid of the conduction system. The AP also begins endocardially and spreads out to the outside of the heart. However, repolarisation occurs from the outside to the inside. Ventricular activation is earliest at the apex and latest at the base of the heart, giving it an apical to basal contraction pattern.

Conduction System Defects

Defects can arise in any part of the conduction system. Some examples of arrhythmias occurring due to lesions in different parts of the conduction system are shown in Fig. 4.

Fig. 4 Arrhythmias due to conduction system defects

Site	Arrhythmia	Features
Sinoatrial node	Sick sinus syndrome	Sinus arrest, sinus bradycardia, tachycardias
Atrial conduction pathways	Wolff–Parkinson–White syndrome	Supraventricular tachycardia
Atrioventricular node	AV junctional rhythm	Bradycardia with abnormal P waves
Bundle of His	Complete (3° block) AV block	Bradycardia with dissociated P waves
Bundle branches	Bundle branch block	abnormal broad QRS complexes (>0.12 s)

Refractory Period

Period during and following the action potential during which the neurone is insensitive to further stimulation.

It is subdivided in:

- Absolute: no excitation, regardless how strong the stimuli is (It includes phase 0, 1, 2 and beginning of 3).
- Relative: excitation may follow if stimuli is stronger than normal.

Cardiac Innervation

Parasympathetic System

It is located mainly in the atrium and conduction system. It acts by acethylcoline through Muscarinic type 2 Receptors to produce negative chronotropism, inotropism and dromotropism.

Acethylcoline increases permeability of potassium in sinus atrial (SA) node and conduction nerves. Consequently, it decreases SA node and conduction nerves excitability.

Sympathetic System

Na permeability in all areas is increased by Noradrenaline. Consequently, the following event occur: (1) conduction velocity in all areas of the heart is increased, (2) contractility in both ventricles and atrium is increased, (3) Heart Rate in SA node is increased and lastly (4) calcium permeability is increased by Noradrenaline. Therefore, contractility is also increased.

Cardiac Cycle

Each cardiac cycle consists of a period of relaxation (diastole) followed by ventricular contraction (systole). During diastole the ventricles are relaxed to allow filling. In systole the right and left ventricles contract, ejecting blood into the pulmonary and systemic circulations respectively.

Ventricles

The left ventricle pumps blood into the systemic circulation via the aorta. The systemic vascular resistance (SVR) is 5–7 times greater than the pulmonary vascular resistance (PVR). This makes it a high-pressure system (compared with the pulmonary vascular system) which requires a greater mechanical power output from the left ventricle (LV). A normal LV can develop intraventricular pressures up to 300 mmHg. Coronary perfusion to the LV occurs mainly in diastole, when the myocardium is relaxed.

The right ventricle receives blood from the vena cava and coronary circulation, and pumps it via the pulmonary vasculature into the LV. Since PVR is a fraction of SVR, pulmonary arterial pressures are relatively low and the wall thickness of the right ventricle (RV) is much less than that of the LV. The RV thus resembles a passive conduit rather than a pump. Coronary perfusion to the RV occurs continuously during systole and diastole because of the low intraventricular and intramural pressures.

In spite of the anatomical differences, the mechanical behaviour of the RV and LV is very similar.

The cardiac cycle can be examined in detail by considering the ECG trace, intracardiac pressure and volume curves, and heart valve function (Fig. 5).

Phase 1: **Atrial Contraction:** It has a 30% contribution of Stroke Volume.

Phase 2: **Isometric Ventricular Contraction**: It goes from the closing of the Tricuspid and Mitral Valve until ventricular pressure exceeds aortic and pulmonary valves.

Phase 3: **Ventricular Ejection:** Most rapid at the start of systole. It lasts until the aortic and pulmonary valves close.

Phase 4: **Isometric Ventricular Relaxation:** It lasts until Tricuspid and Mitral valves open.

Phase 5: **Passive Ventricular Filling:** Most rapid at the start of diastole.

Diastolic Function

Diastole can be broken down into the following stages:

- Isovolumetric ventricular relaxation
- Rapid ventricular filling
- Slow ventricular filling (diastasis)
- Atrial contraction

Although diastole appears to be a passive part of the cardiac cycle, it has some important functions:

- Myocardial relaxation—a metabolically active phase. One essential process is the reuptake of calcium by the sarcoplasmic reticulum. Incomplete reuptake leads to diastolic dysfunction due to decreased end-diastolic compliance. The

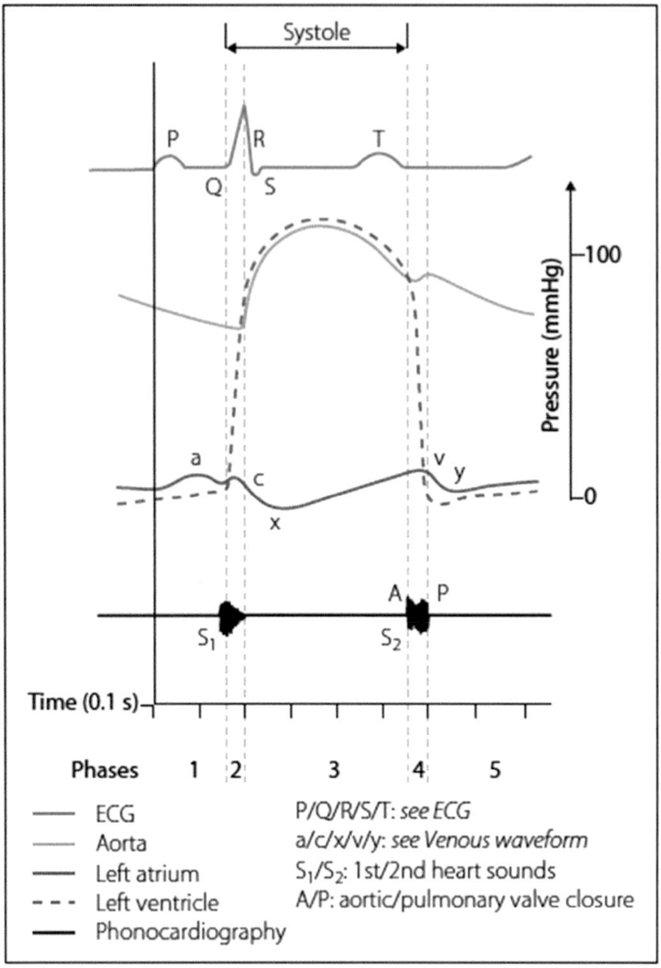

Fig. 5 Cardiac cycle, showing ventricular volume, ventricular pressure, aortic pressure and atrial pressure

negative slope of the ventricular pressure–time curve during isovolumetric relaxation (termed dP/dt (max)) indicates myocardial relaxation. Increased sympathetic tone or circulating catecholamine levels give rise to an increased dP/dt (max). This is known as positive lusitropy.

- Ventricular filling—provides the volume for the cardiac pump. Most of the ventricular filling occurs during early diastole. There is only a small increase in ventricular volume during diastasis. As the heart rate increases diastasis is shortened first. When the heart rate exceeds about 140 bpm, rapid filling in early diastole becomes compromised and the volume of blood ejected during systole (stroke volume, SV) is significantly decreased.

- Atrial contraction—contributes up to 25–30% of total ventricular filling in the normal heart. This atrial contribution can become of greater importance in the presence of myocardial ischaemia or ventricular hypertrophy.
- Coronary artery perfusion—the greater part of left coronary blood flow occurs during diastole.

Central Venous Pressure

Central venous pressure (CVP) is usually monitored in the large veins feeding the superior vena cava, i.e. the internal jugular or subclavian veins. The CVP waveform reflects right atrial pressure, and therefore consists of ‘a’, ‘c’ and ‘v’ waves that correspond to atrial contraction, isovolumetric contraction and opening of the tricuspid valve, as described above. There are also two labelled downward deflections, the ‘x’ and ‘y’ descents, which occur after the ‘c’ and ‘v’ waves respectively (Fig. 6). The ‘x’ descent reflects the fall in right ventricular pressure when the pulmonary valve opens. The ‘y’ descent corresponds to the initial drop in atrial pressure caused by rapid ventricular filling when the AV valves open. Various pathological conditions affect mean CVP or alter the CVP waveform. For example, if the timing of atrial and ventricular contraction become dissociated (as in 3° block) the right atrium contracts against a closed tricuspid valve and produces prominent or ‘cannon’ ‘a’ waves (Fig. 7).

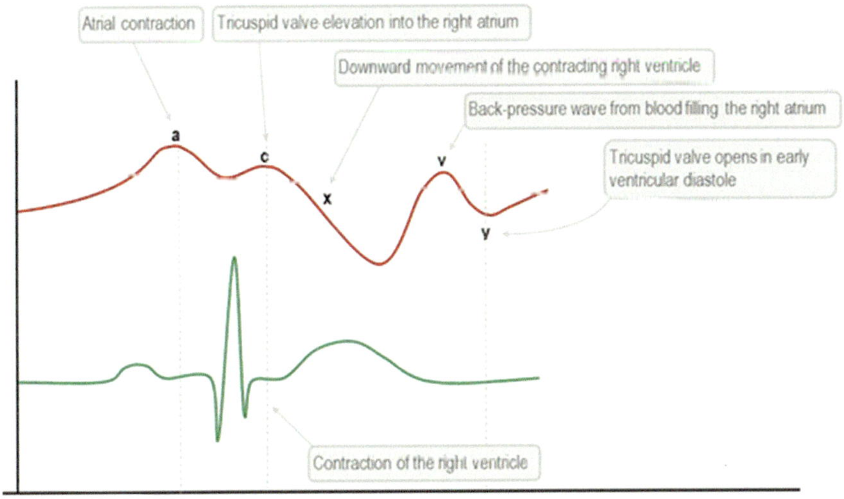

Fig. 6 Central venous pressure waveform

Factor	Change in CVP
Depleted intravascular volume	↓ mean CVP
Excessive intravascular volume ('overloading' with intravascular fluid)	↑ mean CVP
Cardiac failure	↑ mean CVP
Pericardial tamponade	↑ mean CVP
Bradycardia	More distinct 'a', 'c' and 'v' waves
Tachycardia	Fusion of 'a' and 'c' waves
AV junctional rhythm	Regular cannon 'a' waves
3° AV block	Irregular cannon 'a' waves
Tricuspid regurgitation	Loss of 'c' wave and 'x' descent Prominent 'v' waves

Fig. 7 Factors affecting the central venous pressure waveform

Right Atrium Pressure Curve

1. a wave: It is secondary to atrial contraction (late diastole).
2. c wave: It is secondary to the tricuspid valve elevation into de right atrium (isometric ventricular contraction).
3. x wave: Downward movement of the contracting right ventricle (ventricular ejection).
4. v wave: Back-pressure wave form of blood filling the right atrium (isometric ventricular relaxation).
5. y wave: It is secondary to the opening of the tricuspid valve in early ventricular diastole (early diastole).

RV Volume or Pressure Overload

Clinically, CVP is crucial for early diagnose of RV volume or pressure overload. Specifically, for diagnosing **cardiac tamponade** after cardiac surgery in a sedated and ventilated patient. Cardiac tamponade is a clinical diagnosis consisting of tachycardia, hypotension (or increasing dose of vasopressors), high CVP (usually CVP > 14 mmHg) with or without oliguria and signs of organ hypoperfusion. Echocardiography is useful for confirming the clinical suspicion of cardiac tamponade triggered by high CVP, tachycardia and hypotension (Fig. 8). Pericardial effusion collapsing right atrium in systole or right ventricle collapse in diastole

Hypotension (Systolic BP <100mmHg or increasing dose of vasopressors)
Tachycardia (HR >100bpm)
High CVP (>13-14mmHg)
Hyoperfusion parameters (High lactate, oliguria, high delta CO2)
If decreasing bleeding flow from the chest drainage, pericardial effusion should be rule out due to malfunctioning drainage

Fig. 8 Clinical signs of Cardiac Tamponade

along with dilated inferior vena cava (>21 mm) with distensibility less than 50% and mitral inflow variation of more than 25% and tricuspide inflow variation of more than 40%.

The Cardiac Work

Ventricular Pressure–Volume Loop

The mechanical performance of the heart as a pump can be summarised using a ventricular pressure–volume (PV) loop. An example for the left ventricle is shown in Fig. 9.

The cycle starts at the end-diastolic point (EDP). Isovolumetric contraction follows, represented by a vertical ascending segment which ends with the opening of the aortic valve. The ejection phase segment passes across the top of the loop from right to left. Ejection ends at the end-systolic point (ESP) when the aortic valve closes. Isovolumetric relaxation follows next as a vertical descending segment ending when the mitral valve opens. The final lower segment corresponds to ventricular filling and ends when the mitral valve closes at EDP.

The PV loop can be used to derive several parameters reflecting ventricular function including SV, stroke work (SW), end-diastolic volume (EDV) and end-systolic volume (ESV).

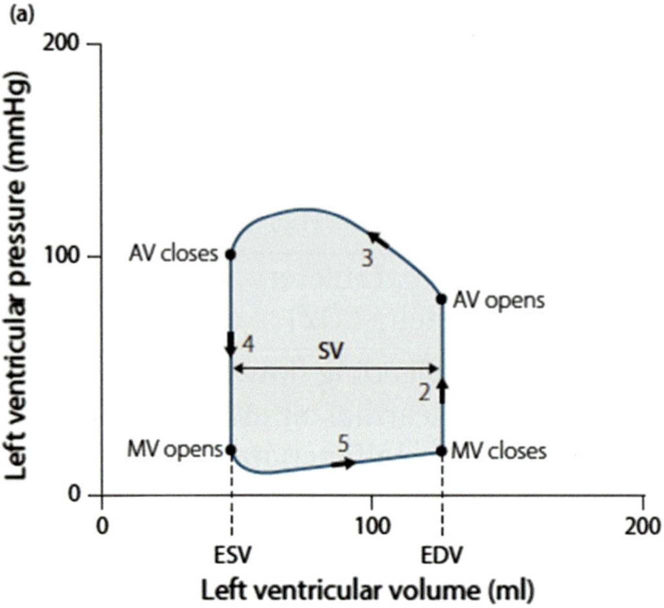

Fig. 9 Pressure–volume loop for left ventricle

- Phase 2: **Isometric Ventricular Contraction:** From the closing of the Mitral Valve until ventricular pressure exceeds the aortic valve.
- Phase 3: **Ventricular Ejection:** Most rapid at the start of systole. It lasts until the aortic valve closes.
- Phase 4: **Isometric Ventricular Relaxation:** It lasts until the Mitral valve opens.
- Phase 5: **Passive ventricular filling + atrial contraction**.
- Stroke Volume: It consists of the difference between End-Diastolic Volume and End-Systolic Volume.
- Stroke Work: Area within the loop.

End-Diastolic Pressure–Volume Relationship

On the ventricular PV loop, the EDP records volume and pressure at the end of diastole. If different PV loops are plotted for a given ventricle, different EDPs are obtained (Fig. 10).

These points form a PV relationship for the ventricle at end-diastole when plotted. This is called the end-diastolic PV relationship (EDPVR). EDPVR is a useful indicator of diastolic function, and in particular ventricular filling performance, since its gradient is equal to the elastance (or compliance $^{-1}$) of the ventricle during filling. The steeper this gradient, the lower the compliance of the ventricle during filling. Over the normal range of ventricular filling volumes the EDPVR gradient is approximately linear and the ventricle is relatively compliant. As EDV

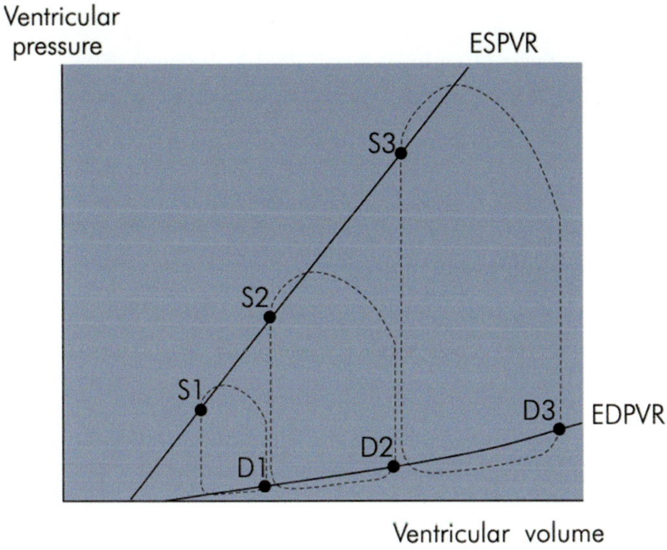

Fig. 10 End-diastolic and end-systolic pressure–volume relationship curves

increases and the ventricle becomes more distended at the end of diastole, the EDPVR gradient becomes steeper, showing a marked decrease in ventricular compliance to filling. Pathological conditions such as ischaemic heart disease and ventricular hypertrophy can shift the EDPVR up and to the left, demonstrating ventricular diastolic dysfunction (Fig. 11).

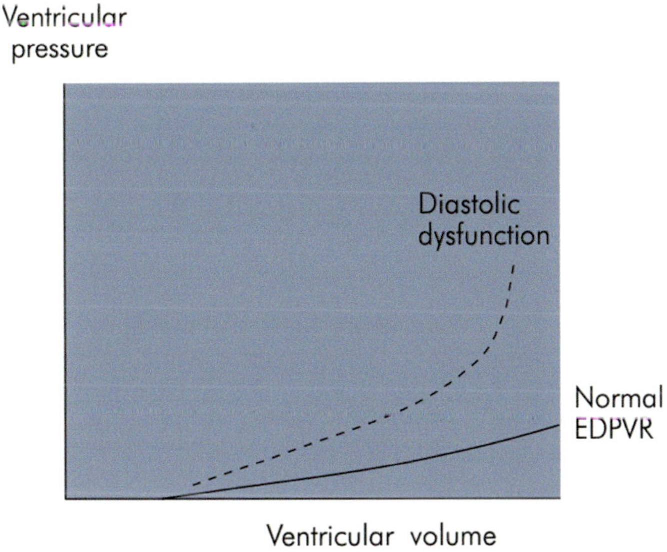

Fig. 11 Effects of diastolic dysfunction on the end-diastolic pressure–volume relationship curve

Increasing Preload or End-diastolic Volume

Secondary to an increase of preload or end-diastolic volume there is, not only, an increase in Stroke Volume, but also, an increase in stroke work (Fig. 12).

Increasing Afterload or End-systolic Pressure

Secondary to an increase of afterload there is a decrease in stroke volume and consequently, there is an increase in end-systolic volume (Fig. 13).

Increasing Cardiac Contractility

Secondary to an increase of cardiac contractility there is an increase in stroke volume ejected, hence, there is a decrease in end-systolic volume and an increase in stroke work (Fig. 14).

Stroke Work

It is defined as stroke volume x mean Ejection pressure-mean filling pressure.

As the mean filling pressure increases, the stroke work decreases (the area within the loop is smaller).

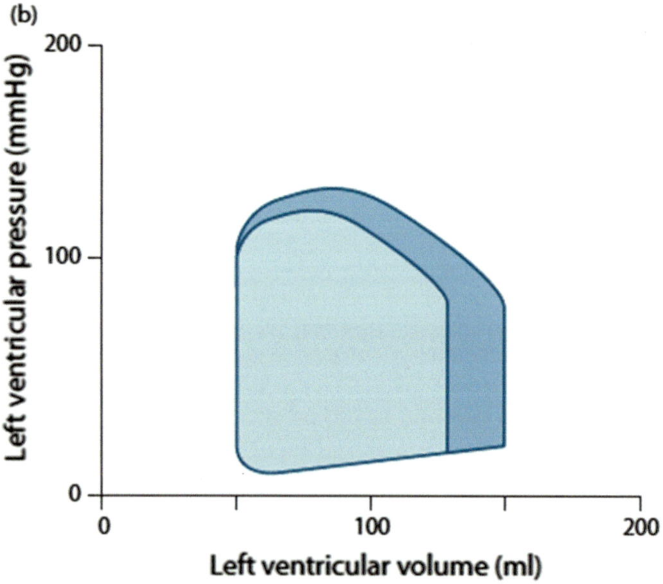

Fig. 12 Effects of pressure–volume relationship curve with increasing preload

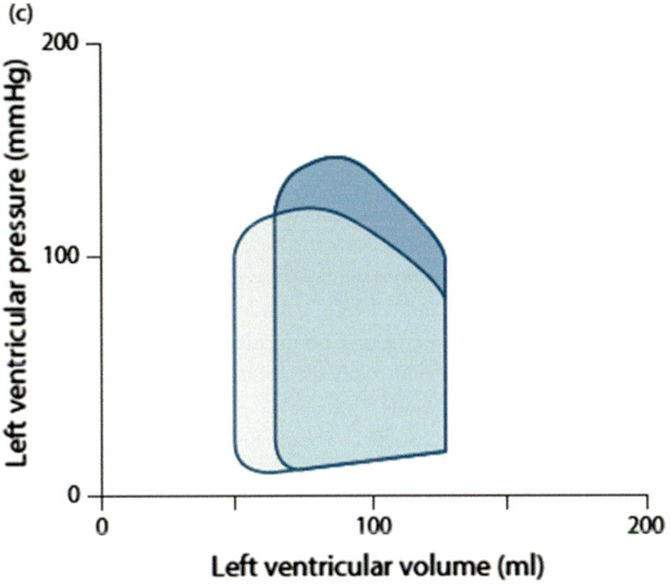

Fig. 13 Effects of pressure–volume relationship curve with increasing afterload

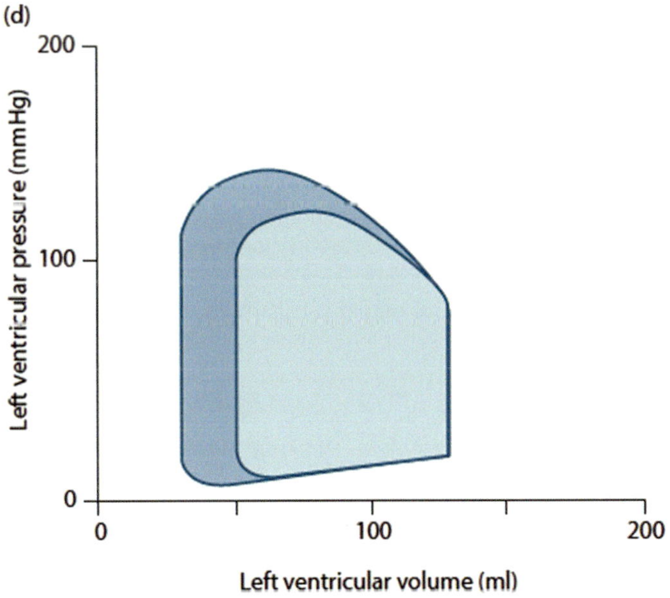

Fig. 14 Effects of pressure–volume relationship curve with increasing contractility

Cardiac Output

Cardiac output gives a measure of the performance of the heart as a pump. It is defined as the volume of blood pumped by the LV (or RV) per minute, and is equal to the product of the SV and heart rate:

$$CO = SV \times HR$$

With a normal HR = 70–80 bpm and SV = 70–80 ml, the average CO of a 70 kg person varies between 5 and 6 l min $^{-1}$ under resting conditions. To compare patients of different body sizes, CO can be divided by the patient's body surface area to give a normalised parameter called the cardiac index (CI):

$$CI = CO / BSA$$

BSA can be estimated from the height (cm) and weight (kg) of an individual and is quoted in m^2. The average 70 kg adult has a BSA = 1.7 m^2 and a CI = 3–3.5 L min^{-1} m^{-2}.

When the oxygen demand of the body increases during exercise, the CO of a young, healthy individual can increase up to five-fold. CO should always be evaluated with reference to the oxygen demand at the time.

There is a clear interventricular dependence between LV/RV.

Cardiac Output Measurement

CO is usually measured by indirect methods. Some current methods of monitoring cardiac output in clinical practice are outlined in Fig. 15.

Indicator Dilution Techniques

Thermodilution is at present the most commonly used method to measure CO at the bedside. A pulmonary artery catheter (PAC) is inserted, cold saline is injected into the RA, and the change in blood temperature is measured by the PAC thermistor in the pulmonary artery. The cardiac output is calculated using the modified Stewart–Hamilton equation:

$$CO = \frac{V(T_B - T_1) \times K_1 \times K_2}{\int_0^\infty T_B(t)\, dt}$$

where.

V = volume of injectate; TB = initial blood temperature (○C); TI = initial injectate temperature (○C); K1 = density constant; K2 = computation constant

$$\int_0^\infty T_B(t)\, dt = \text{integral of blood temperature change}$$

Cardiac output (CO) monitor	Method of CO measurement	Advantages	Disadvantages
Pulmonary artery catheter (Swan–Ganz)	Pulmonary artery thermodilution: cold saline bolus injected into PAC, thermodilution principle, measured by thermistor in PAC tip in the pulmonary artery	Continuous PA pressures PACWP measurement Can be used with intra-aortic balloon pump (IABP) Heat dissipation minimised by short travel from injection to catheter tip 'Gold standard' for comparison with newer methods	Invasive – sheath in large vein, catheter through right heart Risk of injury to heart and pulmonary vessels, catheter migration No evident outcome benefit Not continuous
LiDCO	Transpulmonary lithium dilution. Calibration by lithium chloride bolus into CVP or vein while sampling arterial blood past lithium electrode. Continuous CO by arterial wave form analysis	Avoids heat dissipation errors. Uses routine CVP and arterial lines Provides continuous CO Various displays target CO to aid management	Requires 24-hourly calibration No pulmonary artery pressures Not used in patient with IABP Cannot be used in patients on lithium
PiCCO	Transpulmonary thermodilution: cold saline bolus injected into CVP line. Thermistor in femoral a-line. CO by continuous arterial wave form analysis	Arterial line is also used for blood sampling Continuous CO	Arterial line in femoral artery. Errors due to heat dissipation because of trans-pulmonary passage between injection point and thermistor
Pulse contour CO Vigileo	Analysis of arterial waveform characteristics and calculate CO from patient demographic data	Arterial line transducer supplied by manufacturer No calibration input	Uses extrapolation from patient demographic data Dependent on quality of a-line trace No use in patient with IABP
Doppler	Oesophageal or sternal notch Doppler probe. Calculation of CO using Doppler signals and patient demographic data	Does not require vascular access No calibration needed	Consistency of monitoring depends on Doppler trace quality Cannot be used in patient with IABP

Fig. 15 Current methods of monitoring cardiac output

CO is inversely proportional to the area under the temperature–time curve. This technique is popular because multiple CO estimations can be made at frequent intervals without blood sampling. The accuracy of the technique is influenced by several factors, which include intracardiac shunts, tricuspid regurgitation and positive pressure ventilation.

A modification of this principle is used in the 'continuous' CO monitor. A pulse of electrical current heats up a proximal part of the PAC creating a bolus of warmed blood. The temperature rise is sensed when the warmed blood passes a thermistor in the pulmonary artery. A computer then calculates the 'area under the curve' and, hence, CO.

Dye Dilution

This was the most popular technique prior to thermodilution. Indocyanine green is injected into a central vein, while blood is continuously sampled from an arterial cannula. The change in indicator concentration over time is measured, a computer calculates the area under the dye concentration curve, and CO is computed. Unfortunately recirculation and build-up of the indicator results in a high background concentration, which limits the total number of measurements that can be taken. The dye is non-toxic and rapidly removed from circulation by the liver.

Fick Method

The Fick principle states that the amount of a substance taken up by an organ (or the whole body) per unit time is equal to the arterial concentration of the substance minus the venous concentration (a–v difference), times the blood flow. This can be applied to the oxygen content of blood to determine CO.

First, the steady-state oxygen content of venous (CvO2) and arterial blood (CaO2) are measured. Then oxygen uptake in the lungs is measured over 1 min (VO2).

Finally, the Fick principle is applied to calculate the blood flowing in 1 min:

$$\text{Cardiac output} = \frac{\dot{V}O_2}{(CaO_2 - CvO_2)}$$

Errors in sampling, and the inability to maintain steady- state conditions, limit this technique.

Doppler Techniques

Ultrasonic Doppler transducers have been incorporated into pulmonary artery catheters, endotracheal tubes, suprasternal probes and oesophageal probes. These probes can then be used to measure mean blood flow velocity through the aorta or any valve orifice. Using an estimation for the cross-sectional area of flow, the flow velocity–time integral, heart rate and a constant, CO can be calculated.

Control of Cardiac Output

The product of stroke volume (SV) and heart rate (HR) gives cardiac output (CO). The factors determining CO can thus be divided into those affecting HR and those that determine SV. Overall control of CO is a combination of the mechanisms controlling SV and HR. Factors controlling SV and HR are considered in detail below.

Stroke Volume

Several factors determine SV. The three major determinants of SV are:

- Preload
- Afterload
- Contractility

Overall control of SV is summarised in Fig. 16. The above factors are based on physiological concepts arising from the performance of isolated muscle preparations. They have become useful in clinical practice when applied to the intact heart, but are difficult or impractical to measure directly. Hence more easily monitored parameters are used as practical indices.

Preload

A strict definition for preload can be obtained from the Frank relationship between muscle fibre length and developed tension. Here preload is the initial length of the muscle fibre before contraction. Relation between SV and EDV is based on Frank-Starling Law. With a constant HR, SV is directly related to EDV, until a point which it decreases (Fig. 17). In the intact ventricle the preload would, therefore, be equivalent to the end-diastolic volume, since the presystolic length of the myocardial fibres will be directly related to EDV (Fig. 18).

Determinants of preload or EDV

- Venous Return
- Left ventricle filling
  - Atrial contraction
  - Heart Rate
  - LV compliance (diastolic function)

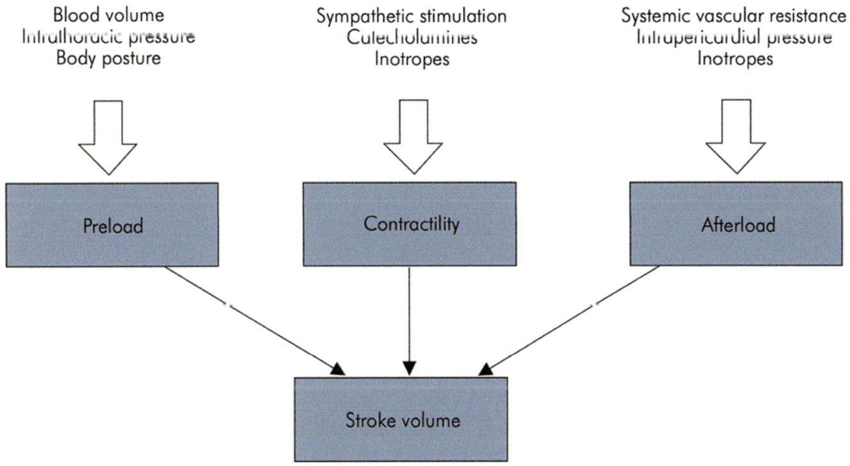

Fig. 16 Determinants of stroke volume

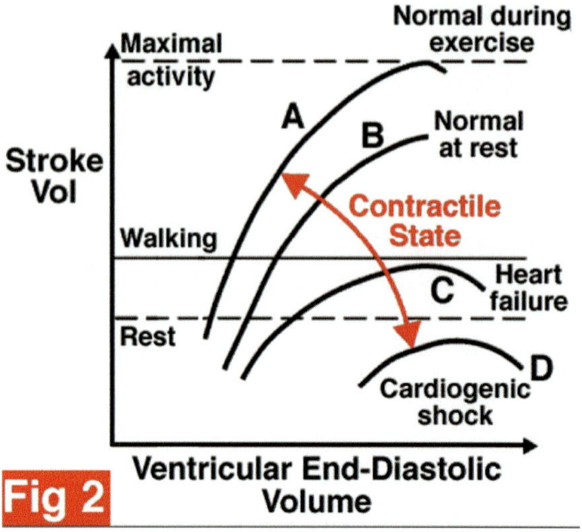

Fig. 17 Frank-Starling law

Fig. 18 Preload

- Physiological definition – Pre-systolic length of cardiac muscle fibres
- Physiological index – End-diastolic volume
- Practical concept – Filling pressure of ventricles
- Practical index – CVP or PCWP

Various factors affecting EDV include:
Total blood volume
Body position
Intrathoracic and intrapericardial pressures
Venous tone and compliance
Pumping action of skeletal muscles
Synchronous atrial contribution to ventricular filling
Ventricular end-diastolic compliance

Venous Return

- Depends mainly on venous tone
- 64% of SV is in venous territory
- If O2 metabolic rate increases, venous return increases by increasing venous tone

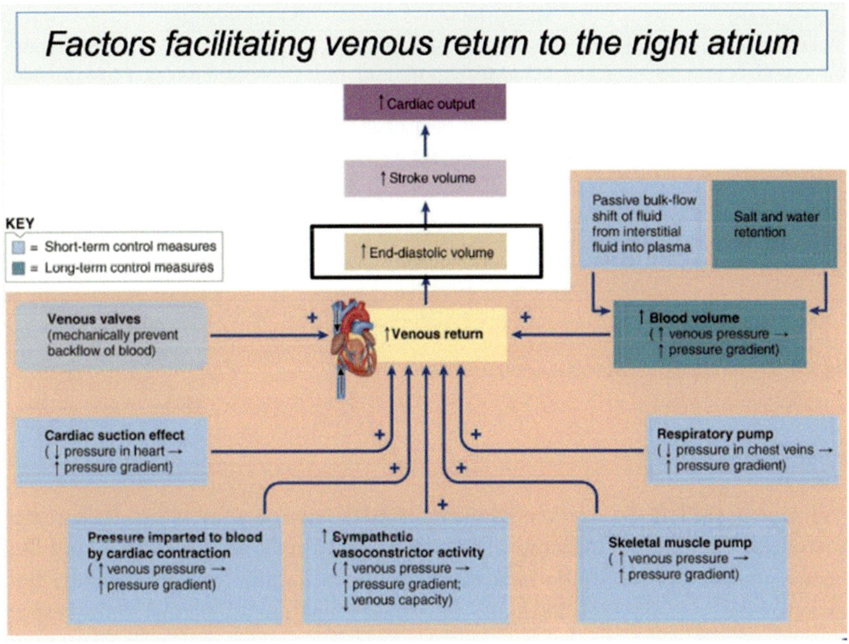

Fig. 19 Factors facilitating venous return to the right atrium

- Depends on pressure gradient between venous pressure and Right Atrium (Fig. 19).

Measurement of Preload

There are no convenient or practical methods of measuring EDV directly. EDP is related to EDV by the ventricular end-diastolic PV curve and is sometimes referred to as the 'filling pressure' of the ventricle. EDPVR is approximately linear at normal filling pressures, but the gradient (ventricular elastance = compliance^{-1}) gradually increases as filling pressure increases. EDP is, therefore, only a reasonable index of preload under normal conditions.

In practice, EDP can be estimated on the left side of the heart, by measuring left atrial pressure (LAP), pulmonary capillary wedge pressure (PCWP) or pulmonary artery diastolic pressure (PADP). On the right side, preload is reflected by right atrial pressure (RAP) or central venous pressure. These measurements can be made using a pulmonary artery catheter, but the most common measurements used are CVP and PCWP as indices of right and left preload respectively.

Parameters	Measured by	Comments
Increase SV >12% by PLRT	Either measured by Echocardiography or pulse contour analysis	Useful in spontaneous ventilation or arrhythmias. Best discrimination.
Increase SV >10% by mini-fluid challenge	Either measured by Echocardiography or pulse contour analysis	Useful in spontaneous ventilation or arrhythmias.
SVC distensibility >36%	TEE	Not influence by IAP
SVV >12%	Either measured by Echocardiography or pulse contour analysis	Note criteria of reliability
IVC distensibility >18%	Echocardiography	Note criteria of reliability

Fig. 20 Dynamic fluid responsiveness parameters

Fluid Responsiveness

With a constant HR, SV is directly related to EDV, until a point which it decreases. As a result, it is crucial to know whether the patient may benefit from giving fluid therapy (increasing his EDV) increasing his stroke volume or not. Dynamic fluid responsiveness parameters have the best discrimination to predict fluid responsiveness (Fig. 20).

Dynamic fluid responsiveness parameters

1. Increase of Stroke Volume by 12% secondary a passive leg raising test, measured either by echocardiography or pulse contour analysis.
2. Increase of Stroke Volume by 10% secondary a mini-fluid challenge of 100 ml en 1 min, measured either by echocardiography or pulse contour analysis.
3. Superior Vena Cava (SVC) distensibility (Diameter max—Diameter min/ Diameter min) during mechanical ventilation > 36% measured by trans-esophageal echocardiography (TEE).
4. Stroke volume variation (SV max—SV min / SV mean) with positive pressure ventilation > 12% measured by either echocardiography or pulse contour analysis. Reliable only if: sinus rhythm with no premature ventricular or atrial contraction, mechanical ventilation with tidal volume >8 ml/kg with no inspiratory efforts or assisted ventilation, normal RV systolic function, intra-abdominal pressure (IAP) < 12 mmHg, a compliance of >30 ml/cm H20 and lastly a closure chest is required.
5. Inferior Vena Cava (IVC) distensibility (Diameter max – Diameter min/ Diameter min) during mechanical ventilation >18% measured by echocardiography.

   Not reliable if: Tidal volume <8 ml/kg or PEEP >5, assisted or spontaneous ventilation, severe tricuspide regurgitation or RV systolic dysfunction, cardiac tamponade, intra-abdominal hypertension or mechanical compression of the IVC.

Abbreviations: IVC: Inferior vena cava; IAP: intra-abdominal pressure; PLRT: passive leg raising test; SV: stroke volume. SVC: superior vena cava; SVV: stroke volume variation. TEE: transesophageal echocardiography.

Afterload

In an isolated muscle fibre preparation, afterload is defined as the tension developed during contraction. Thus, afterload is related to the mechanical resistance to shortening of the muscle fibre. In the intact heart, afterload becomes the tension per unit cross section (T), developed in the ventricular wall during systole. This can be related to the intra- ventricular pressure during systole, by applying Laplace's law for pressure in an elastic sphere as follows:

$$\text{Intraventricular pressure} = \frac{2hT}{r}$$

where.

h = ventricular wall thickness.

r = radius of the ventricular cavity.

Afterload is thus a measure of how forcefully the ventricle contracts during systole to eject blood (Fig. 18).

The normal ventricle has an intrinsic ability to increase its performance in response to increases in afterload, to maintain SV. If the afterload increases suddenly, it causes an initial fall in SV. The ventricle then increases its EDV in response to the change, which in turn restores the SV. This is called the Anrep effect.

Measurement of Afterload

Systematic vascular resistance (SVR), SVR index and elastance may be used to give an estimate of afterload.

- Arterial pressure or ventricular pressures during systole normally follow each other and are indirect indices of ventricular wall tension. Arterial systolic pressure is often the available measurement, but its accuracy is limited if there is a significant gradient between aorta and ventricle, e.g. as in aortic stenosis.
- Systemic vascular resistance is the most commonly used index of afterload in clinical practice, and can be calculated from mean arterial pressure (MAP), central venous pressure and CO, as follows:

$$SVR = \frac{MAP - CVP}{CO} \times 80\,\text{dyne.s cm}^{-5}$$

The normal value for SVR ranges from 900 to 1400 dynes. s cm $^{-5}$. SVR is not a good estimate of afterload, as it is only one component determining afterload, and does not provide any index of intraventricular pressures generated during systole (i.e. how hard the ventricle is contracting). Clearly, if the ventricle only generates low intraventricular pressures by contracting softly, the afterload is low irrespective of SVR.

In a similar manner the pulmonary vascular resistance (PVR) may be calculated as an index of RV afterload, using mean pulmonary arterial pressure (MPAP), pulmonary capillary wedge pressure and CO:

$$PVR = \frac{MPAP - PCWP}{CO} \times 80\,\text{dyne.s}\,\text{cm}^{-5}$$

The normal PVR ranges from 90 to 150 dynes.s cm $^{-5}$.
PAP and PCWP have to be obtained with a PAC to calculate SVR and PVR.

- Systemic vascular impedance is the mechanical property of the vascular system opposing the ejection and flow of blood into it. This is composed of two components. One is the resistive or steady-flow component, which is the SVR (see above). This component is mainly due to the frictional opposition to flow in the vessels. The other component is the reactive or frequency-dependent component, which is due to the compliance of the vessel walls and inertia of the ejected blood. This component is dependent on the pulsatile nature of the flow and rapidity of ejection. A major part of this reactive component is formed by the arterial elastance (Ea).
- Arterial elastance is the inverse of arterial compliance and is a measure of the elastic forces in the arterial system that tend to oppose the ejection of blood into it. Determination of Ea involves plotting a PV curve for the arterial system using different SV and recording end-systolic pressures. The slope of the curve then gives the effective elastance (compliance^{-1}) of the arterial system.

Circulation—Ohm and Poiseuille Law

The equation to calculate SVR and PVR is derived from Ohm's law.

Ohm's Law

Ohm's law states that flow is related to pressure gradient and inversely related to resistance.

$$\text{Flow} = \text{P1} - \text{P2(Perfusion Pressure)}/\ \text{Resistance}$$

Therefore, the equation for systemic flow (or cardiac output) is the following:

$$CO = MAP - CVP\ /\ SVR$$

Abbreviations: CO: cardiac output; MAP: mean arterial pressure; CVP: central venous pressure; SVR: systemic vascular resistance.

Therefore,

$$SVR = MAP - CVP / CO$$
$$MAP - CVP = SVR \text{ x } CO$$
$$MAP = CO \times SVR (\text{assuming CVP is 0 or 1})$$

Poiseuille's Law

Resistance is related to length and viscosity and inversely related to radius.

$$\text{Resistance} = L \cdot v \cdot 8/r4 \cdot k$$

where,
L: length; v: viscosity; r: radius.

Recommended Reading

1. Guyton AC, Hall JE. Textbook of medical physiology, 13th ed. Philadelphia: Elsevier Saunders; 2016.

Cardiovascular Pharmacology

Geoff Lockwood

Introduction

In this chapter we will approach cardiovascular pharmacology from the perspective of four common clinical situations.

I. Drugs to use when the systemic arterial pressure is too low.
II. Drugs to use when the systemic arterial pressure is too high.
III. Drugs to control rate and rhythm
IV. Drugs to use for the failing right heart

I. Drugs to use when the systemic arterial pressure is too low.

Why is the blood pressure low? General points on clinical decision-making. Before starting drug therapy in this situation it is essential to decide whether the hypotension is due to a reduced cardiac output or a reduced systemic vascular resistance. This is usually easy to determine on physical examination of the patient but nowadays invasive and non-invasive equipment is available to guide the clinical decision.

If the cardiac output is inadequate, it may be more appropriate to give fluids than drugs. Devices are available that estimate cardiac filling from arterial pulse contour analysis, but observing blood pressure variation with respiration and a leg-raising manoeuvre may be enough to form a clinical decision.

G. Lockwood (✉)
Department of Anaesthesia, Hammersmith Hospital, London W12 0HS, UK
e-mail: g.lockwood@imperial.ac.uk

M. Vives and A. Hernandez (eds.), *Cardiac Anesthesia and Postoperative Care in the 21st Century*, https://doi.org/10.1007/978-3-030-79721-8_3

It is essential that cardiac output is adequate when vasoconstrictors are used. The physiological situation is dynamic after cardiac surgery and so the state of the circulation must be re-assessed frequently. Vasoconstriction may be appropriate at first assessment but focussing attention thereafter exclusively on arterial blood pressure and treating it with vasoconstrictors without making any estimate of cardiac output can lead to impaired perfusion and ischaemic injury.

Catecholamines.

The most common agents used to increase cardiac output after cardiac surgery are β-adrenergic agonists. Although the simple physiological teaching is that β_1 receptors are the cardiac adrenoceptors and β_2 receptors are located in the lungs and peripherally, this is a gross simplification even in the healthy subject. Typically 20% of ventricular β-adrenoceptors are β_2, but in chronic heart failure this may reach 50% as a result of depopulation of all adrenoceptors – but particularly β_1-adrenoceptors—in response to chronically increased concentrations of circulating catecholamines.

It might appear from Box 1 that isoprenaline would be the ideal agent in this situation. However, although it will indeed increase cardiac output, the other effects of β_2-agonism on the peripheral vasculature are likely to result in a further reduction in arterial pressure! Adrenaline may be preferred because the α-adrenoceptor stimulation will more than counter the β_2-induced vasodilation, but its use is associated with an increased serum lactate concentration. Although this is a physiological consequence of increased peripheral lactate production, many intensivists prefer to avoid its use if possible because, in other situations, increased serum lactate is associated with adverse outcomes. They turn instead to noradrenaline as a first-line treatment. Noradrenaline has less effect on the cardiac output than adrenaline because its inotropic activity has little β_2 component and the increased afterload from relatively unopposed α-adrenoceptor stimulation works against the inotropic drive. Although catecholamines improve the immediate situation there is no evidence that they reduce mortality.

Potencies of drugs at adrenoceptors, based on the EC50 (the concentration required to produce 50% of maximal response). +++++ indicates an EC50 of a few nM; ++++ indicates an EC50 a few tens of nM and so on in orders of magnitude. The relative potency at the different receptors is more important than the absolute value because it is always possible to give a larger dose. The effect of stimulating different receptors is also important: although α1 and β2 receptors are equally sensitive to noradrenaline, the effect on the systemic vascular resistance is dominated by α1-mediated vasoconstriction, far outweighing β2 vasodilation.

Drug	α_1	β_1	β_2
Adrenaline	+ + + + +	+ + + +	+ + + +
Noradrenaline	+ + + + +	+ + + +	+ + +
Isoprenaline	-	+ + + + +	+ + + + +
Dopamine	+ + +	+ + + +	+ +
Dobutamine	+	+ + + + +	+ + +
Dopexamine	-	+	+ +

Phosphodiesterase Inhibitors

β-adrenoceptor stimulation causes a G-protein second messenger system to activate adenyl cyclase and increase production of intracellular cyclic adenosine monophosphate (cAMP) to produce the intracellular β-adrenergic effect. Acute hyperstimulation of β-receptors, such as occurs during cardiac surgery, impairs the coupling between the receptor and its G-protein messenger so that less cAMP is produced and the effect of receptor stimulation is reduced. Phosphodiesterases (PDEs) convert cAMP to inactive AMP. The isoform relevant to tissues with β-receptors is PDE III, so its inhibition counters the acute decoupling found after cardiac surgery and consequently many anaesthetists administer a PDE III inhibitor routinely. These drugs restore and enhance the function of β-receptors and are often referred to as inodilators. Their use as sole agents is limited by hypotension (β_2-adrenoceptor effect) so they are most commonly used with noradrenaline.

PDE inhibitors

Drug	**Action**	$t_{1/2}$	**Notes**
Aminophylline	Non-specific PDE inhibition, adenosine antagonism	8 h	Dose up to 6 mg kg^{-1} for PDE inhibition. The anti-inflammatory effect of PDE IV inhibition may also be useful. More potent as an adenosine antagonist then PDE inhibitor
Enoximone	Imidazole PDE III inhibitor	6 h	Elimination prolonged in heart failure and renal impairment
Milrinone	PDE III inhibitor, enhances calcium flux on sarcoplasmic reticulum to improve lusitropy	2 h	A derivative of inamrinone but lacking the latter's association with thrombocytopenia. Elimination prolonged in

(continued)

(continued)

Drug	Action	$t_{½}$	Notes
			heart failure and renal impairment
Levosimendan	PDE III inhibitor, sensitises troponin to improve myocardial contractility	1 h	Active metabolites have an elimination half-time of 80 h

Aminophylline is the archetypal PDE inhibitor (and also an adenosine antagonist) but it is non-selective for PDE III and so enoximone is usually preferred in the cardiac patient. Other PDE III inhibitors have additional effects on calcium metabolism within the cardiac myocyte. Milrinone and inamrinone (previously amrinone) enhance calcium flux on the sarcoplasmic reticulum, improving lusitropy and giving them greater clinical effect than enoximone. Levosimendan has a very specific action that is dependent on the intracellular calcium concentration: it enhances myocardial contraction by binding to troponin C when the cytosol calcium concentration is increased during systole but, when the cytosol calcium concentration reduces during diastole, levosimendan dissociates and so does not inhibit diastolic relaxation. A single dose has an effect for several days, partly because its main metabolite has similar pharmacological properties. Its use is limited by its high cost, its slow onset of action—rapid infusion is associated with marked vasodilatation and hypotension – and a lack of convincing evidence of improved patient outcome. In fact there is no evidence that inodilators reduce mortality and there has been concern over their safety following the PROMISE trial (in which long term oral milrinone was associated with up to a 50% increase in mortality in heart failure patients). However, their short term use can provide an immediate improvement in haemodynamics and does not seem to be associated with increased mortality.

Vasoconstrictors

The vasoconstrictive pathways that can be controlled clinically are α-adrenoceptors and V_1 vasopressin receptors; angiotensin and endothelin agonists are not available although they are also very potent systems. In extreme states of pathological vasodilation (vasoplegia) when the circulation is unresponsive to α and V_1 agonists, drugs that inhibit vasodilation have a role.

Calcium Hypocalcaemia is common after cardiopulmonary bypass and many clinicians routinely correct it. Calcium administration increases blood pressure, predominantly through vasoconstriction - the inotropic effect is modest and does not increase cardiac output. All vascular beds are sensitive to calcium, including all conduits used for coronary grafts, and graft flow is reduced after calcium administration in spite of the increased arterial pressure and so it should be used with caution.

The first line in cardiac intensive care is usually noradrenaline. This is safer than a pure α-agonist such as phenylephrine because its β_1 stimulation supports the cardiac output. The internal mammary artery and saphenous veins are not densely populated with α-adrenoceptors but the radial artery is very sensitive to α-agonism and care must be taken when the radial is used as a conduit. Vasopressin is usually used as a second line constrictor for when the dose of noradrenaline is becoming a matter of concern or arrhythmias are significant. Opinions vary as to the relative benefits of the two drugs: the ideal agent will constrict the vascular beds where flow is excessive while preserving flow to vital organs, but this is probably determined by both the patient phenotype and the aetiology of the vasodilation, two unknowns for the clinician. Most patients can be managed with modest doses of one or both of these drugs.

When the patient is more resistant, small doses of hydrocortisone (50 mg qds) may improve the efficacy of both α and V_1 agonists. Vasoplegia is a term used to describe the situation when there traditional vasoconstrictors have negligible effect, and it is thought to be a result of pathologically increased production of nitric oxide. The vasoplegic patient may benefit from methylthioninium chloride or hydroxycobalamin, or both. Methylthioninium, also known as methylene blue, is an irreversible antagonist of inducible nitric oxide synthase. It is usually well tolerated but may cause serotonin syndrome by inhibition of monoamine oxidase in patients taking selective serotonin reuptake inhibitors, and may also induce methaemoglobinaemia. There has been less clinical experience with hydroxycobalamin in this situation but, in the very large doses used to treat cyanide poisoning (5 g), it also inhibits nitric oxide synthase and has few adverse effects. The immediate beneficial effects of these drugs is established but they have not been shown to improve outcome: in septic vasoplegia, the competitive nitric oxide synthase antagonist l-NMMA also increased mean arterial pressure but reduced cardiac output and increased mortality.

II. Drugs to use when the systemic arterial pressure is too high.

General points on the management of acute hypertension In the context of cardiac surgery, arterial pressure needs to be controlled primarily to minimise aortic dissection or protect anastomoses in the proximal aorta. If hypertension is treated simply with vasodilators, homeostatic mechanisms, working through the sympathetic system, will increase inotropy and may place increased stress on the proximal aorta. Best management will therefore both suppress cardiac drive and reduce the systemic vascular resistance.

There is no perfect way to achieve this aim. In a sedated patient on mechanical ventilation, it may be enough to simply increase the sedation, but often a specific therapy is more desirable.

In the intensive care environment, the choice of drug is often determined by the desired timescale of its action, and vasodilators are no exception. There is no point turning to oral medication in an emergency situation, and a long-acting drug will be undesirable if surgery is imminent or very tight control is required. In an emergency, choice is dominated by availability. An immediate reduction in afterload can usually be achieved with an intravenous α-adrenoceptor antagonist such as phentolamine, or hydralazine can be used for a slightly less brief and less dramatic effect. Such drugs are often followed by an intravenous infusion of a short-acting vasodilator such as glyceryl trinitrate or sodium nitroprusside, allowing tight control and rapid termination of effect when required. These fast acting drugs are both associated with rebound hypertension so the infusions should not be stopped abruptly.

Vasodilators for acute control of hypertension. Note that all will produce the adverse effects of vasodilatation: reflex tachycardia, increased intracranial pressure, headache and flushing.

Drug	Action	$t_{½}$	Notes
Phentolamine	α-adrenoceptor antagonist	20 min	Start with a small dose! 0.5 mg usually has a noticeable effect
Hydralazine	Unknown but may involve the epoprostenol PGI_2 receptor	2 h	Adverse effects, such as a lupus-like syndrome, are associated with long term use only
Glyceryl trinitrate (GTN)	Degraded by mitochondrial aldehyde dehydrogenase to release nitric oxide	3 min	Particularly affects the venous capacitance vessels
Sodium nitroprusside	Reacts with oxyhaemoglobin to release nitric oxide (and cyanide)	2 min	Degrades in light. Cyanide ions are sequestered in erythrocytes but consider toxicity after a large dose if there is metabolic acidosis and treat with hydroxycobalamin and sodium thiosulphate

In calmer situations there is a wide choice of oral preparations: α_1-selective adrenoceptor antagonists such as prazosin and doxazosin, an angiotensin converting enzyme (ACE) inhibitor such as ramipril or calcium channel antagonists such as nifedipine or amlodipine. An ACE inhibitor or angiotensin receptor antagonist is particularly indicated in patients with reduced left ventricular function, provided renal function is adequate. Starting 48 h after surgery and continuing in the long term, they reduce adverse effects: the addition of an aldosterone antagonist increases this benefit.

It is important to prevent reflex tachycardia and inotropy when vasodilators are used, and β-blockers are the obvious choice. Metoprolol is commonly available as an intravenous preparation, and labetalol is popular with some physicians because of its dual action at both α- and β-adrenoceptors. There are many β-blockers available for oral administration with differing pharmacological properties, but none shown to be associated with better outcomes than others in this situation. β-blockade may reduce mortality after cardiac surgery, especially in patients with impaired left ventricular function.

All of the drugs mentioned so far suffer from the common disadvantage that a surge in endogenous catecholamines will break through and increase blood pressure. Ganglion blocking drugs overcame this issue by also blocking adrenal activation, but they are no longer available. Perhaps the closest alternative is an α_2 adrenoceptor agonist such as clonidine or dexmedetomidine, which reduce sympathetic outflow through a central action and allow smoother control of haemodynamics.

III. **Drugs to control rate and rhythm**

Perioperative dysrhythmias are common in cardiac surgery and may not require treatment, such as brief disturbances associated with surgical manipulation of the heart. Everyone is happier to see their patients in a stable sinus rhythm, but it is worth checking plasma electrolyte concentrations (particularly potassium and magnesium) and excluding physical causes a central venous catheter that is too long and irritates the atrium or a pacing box that has not been set up properly— before starting drug treatment.

Bradycardia is a problem when it reduces cardiac output. In the presence of regurgitant valves, even a normal heart rate may be insufficient to maintain the circulation. After cardiac surgery, epicardial pacing wires are often available to allow immediate pacing, but pharmacological treatment has advantages when only ventricular pacing wires are present. An anticholinergic drug is usually first line, but the central action of atropine may cause confusion in susceptible patients. Glycopyrronium, on the other hand, is slower in onset and inappropriate in urgent situations. Anticholinergics are very effective against clonidine-induced bradycardia but less effective when the bradycardia is secondary to β-blocker therapy.

If the bradycardia is due to ischaemia of the sinus or atrio-ventricular nodes, adenosine may be inhibiting conduction and aminophylline is a useful antagonist in modest doses (the K_m for adenosine antagonism is about one tenth the K_m for phosphodiesterase inhibition). If neither of these approaches work, then a sympathomimetic such as isoprenaline might be used. Bear in mind that β-adrenergic infusions are probably a step up in risk and ventricular pacing would often be preferred. Finally, if the bradycardia is the result of β-blocker overdose, glucagon (50 μg kg^{-1}) can be used: it stimulates the β-agonist pathway but acts downstream of the β-receptor itself.

Sinus tachycardia may embarrass cardiac output, especially in patients with stenotic valves, and will increase myocardial oxygen consumption. It may be a response to hypovolaemia, in which case fluids rather than specific drug therapy would be appropriate. The first choice of drug is likely to be a β-blocker, administered intravenously or orally according to the urgency of the situation.

New onset atrial fibrillation (AF) occurs after one third of cardiac operations. Prophylaxis with β-blockers reduces this risk to about 20% and is especially important in patients taking β-blockers pre-operatively. Amiodarone is the most effective pharmacotherapy for preventing and treating AF but has a greater risk of adverse effects compared to a β-blocker. If the ventricular rate is compromising the circulation and DC cardioversion is not appropriate, amiodarone should be given intravenously, using central venous access if available because thrombophlebitis occurs in 10% of patients when a peripheral vein is used. Oral amiodarone is no less effective in reverting AF to a regular rhythm but is likely to take several hours longer. In spite of a number of small trials showing a useful prophylactic effect of magnesium, larger trials do not support its use and opinion remains divided. AF may be provoked by the inflammatory response to cardiac surgery and anti-inflammatory strategies (e.g. pre-bypass steroids, post-operative colchicine) have been tried, but none have has found widespread favour. It may not be possible to convert AF to sinus rhythm, in which case a β-blocker or digoxin (if hypotension precludes β-blockade) may be preferred to amiodarone for control of the ventricular response rate, and the question of anticoagulation must then be addressed.

Drugs are never first-line treatment for ventricular fibrillation (VF), but adrenaline may be used to coarsen fine VF and improve the likelihood of cardioversion. Drugs do have an important place in suppressing VF; they may increase the chance of successful cardioversion and they certainly reduce the chance of a repeat episode of VF. Lidocaine is a first line therapy, being easily obtainable and safe with a rapid onset of effect. It binds transiently to open sodium channels, prolonging their refractory period (Class I action). Amiodarone has a slower onset of effect. β-blockers also reduce the risk of a relapse into VF by obtunding the pro-dysrhythmic effect of catecholamines. In addition, sotalol has an action on phase 3 that is similar to, though less efficacious than, that of amiodarone.

Ectopic beats are usually of little concern in themselves, although increasingly frequent or multi-focal ectopics may be a harbinger of a more malignant dysrhythmia. They may disappear if the underlying rate is increased, but β-blocker therapy is more commonly used to suppress them. Alternatively a lidocaine infusion or amiodarone may be justified if there is particular concern that the ectopic beats may degenerate into fibrillation.

Amiodarone is the most effective antidysrhythmic for use after cardiac surgery but it has the worst adverse effect profile. It is a Class III drug, acting on potassium channels to prolong the cardiac action potential, but it also affects sodium and calcium channels to inhibit AV conduction. It is used to convert AF to sinus rhythm and controls the rate even when sinus rhythm is not restored, it suppresses ventricular ectopics and is part of the European Resuscitation Council protocol for managing ventricular fibrillation resistant to DC cardioversion, and for pulseless ventricular tachycardia. The risk of side effects (thyroid dysfunction, corneal deposits, optic nerve damage, hepatitis, skin lesions, pneumonitis) increases with duration of treatment and active surveillance is essential. Toxic effects in the acute situation are rarer but more serious. Lung and liver injury have been reported within a few hours of starting treatment and are associated with a high mortality; if they are suspected then amiodarone should be discontinued and steroids given, possibly with acetylcysteine in cases of acute hepatitis. If amiodarone converts AF the underlying rhythm may be very slow, especially if beta-blockers or calcium channel antagonists are being used, and complete heart block may develop. A prolonged loading regime is required to overcome the large volume of distribution (>100 L kg−1) and the elimination half time varies from a few hours for a single dose to weeks for a patient on long term therapy. Its major metabolite, desmethylamiodarone, is also pharmacologically active. Dosages of digoxin, warfarin and calcium channel antagonists may need to be reduced.

IV. Drugs to use for the failing right heart

The differences between the management strategies for right and left heart failure are little to do with differences between the right and left ventricles but rather the differences between the pulmonary and the systemic circulations. Cardiac drugs have similar effects on both sides of the heart, but the right heart copes less well with increases in afterload than the left, and so particular efforts must be made to reduce pulmonary vascular resistance (PVR). If a systemic vasoconstrictor is required, vasopressin is a good choice because V_1 receptors are not expressed in pulmonary vasculature, whereas α-adrenoceptor agonists will increase PVR. Although there are drugs specifically licenced for pulmonary hypertension (endothelin antagonists such as bosentan, phosphodiesterase 5 inhibitors such as sildenafil) these are mostly oral medications, unsuited to the intensive care situation. Recently intravenous sildenafil has become available but clinical experience is very limited. Milrinone is a popular inotrope in this situation - PDE inhibitors generally reduce pulmonary arterial pressure.

The pulmonary circulation can be selectively treated by delivering drugs via the inhalational route. Several drugs have been tried in this way but the gas nitric oxide and the thromboxane A2 receptor antagonist epoprostenol (prostacyclin) are licensed for this route. These vasodilators are delivered to the better ventilated areas of lung and improve ventilation-perfusion matching, but may have little effect on total PVR. Epoprostenol has a half-life of about 40 s and, when it is delivered intravenously, the pulmonary circulation receives the full vasodilatory effect but effect is diminished by the time the circulation has carried the drug systemically. Because the drug caused indiscriminate pulmonary vasodilation, it may reduce arterial oxygen saturation by allowing blood to flow through underventilated alveoli but, by helping right heart function and thereby improving cardiac output, oxygen delivery to the tissues may be increased. Neither drug has been shown to improve survival in acute illness, but continuous intravenous epoprostenol has been shown to reduce mortality in pulmonary arterial hypertension, possibly through other effects of nitric oxide such as suppression of smooth muscle proliferation or platelet inhibition.

Recommended Readings

1. Schumann J, Henrich EC, Strobi H et al. Inotropic agents and vasodilator strategies for the treatment of cardiogenic shock or low cardiac output syndrome. Cochrane Database Syst Rev 2018.
2. Arsenault KA, Yusuf AM, Crystal E et al. Interventions for preventing post-operative atrial fibrillation in patients undergoing cardiac surgery. Cochrane Database of Syst Rev 2013.
3. Sousa-Uva M, Head SJ, Milojevic M et al. 2017 EACTS Guidelines on perioperative medication in adult cardiac surgery. European J Cardio-thoracic Surg 2018: 53:5–33.

Preoperative Assessment and Decision-Making

Anna Jarosz and Marcin Wąsowicz

Introduction

Anesthesia preoperative assessment for cardiac surgical patient is in essence not very different to one for any other general anesthesia. All cardiac surgical patients are having extensive cardiac workup and this needs to be reviewed thoroughly in context of perioperative planning and possible intraoperative and postoperative complications. On the other hand, several aspects of assessment are unique to this population and require additional expertise and knowledge, which is an essential part of training of cardiothoracic anesthesiologist. The size of this chapter does not allow for comprehensive discussion of all facets of preoperative assessment and optimization, therefore, we will focus only on some important topics, which recently became a challenge and task for cardiac anesthesiologist.

Frailty

Due to complexity of cardiac interventions, in particular those requiring use of CPB and their impact on normal body physiology, more attention is being paid to these patient characteristics that may influence the perioperative outcome. Among all comorbidities and conditions, frailty seems to have been out of focus of researches for many years. However, as the patient's population is aging and demands from

A. Jarosz
Department of Anesthesia and Intensive Care, University Hospital in Wroclaw, Wroclaw, Poland

M. Wąsowicz (✉)
Department of Anesthesia and Pain Medicine, University Health Network, Toronto General Hospital, Toronto, ON, Canada
e-mail: marcin.wasowicz@uhn.ca

M. Vives and A. Hernandez (eds.), *Cardiac Anesthesia and Postoperative Care in the 21st Century*, https://doi.org/10.1007/978-3-030-79721-8_4

society increasing, it becomes one of the most important factors, which impact on recovery and outcome cannot be overrated. Frailty focuses not only on age, but rather all these characteristics that might be age related, yet in a non-linear manner like malnutrition, wasting, weakness, slowness, inactivity and dependence. Unlike any specific medical condition, frailty is believed to express patients' vulnerability and influences health and recovery even from minor insults in a disproportional manner. Since none of the features regarded as frailty is easy to be quantified, there are numerous scales that try to grade and describe frailty, some better validated than others. Out of all, Clinical Frailty Scale (CFS) (Table 1) is worth mentioning, as it is a simple 9-point scale that assesses patient clinically, often on a basis of first impression. It is being mentioned as a screening tool in a systematic review focused on the impact of frailty on outcomes after cardiac surgery, where this characteristic is identified as a risk factor increasing mortality by fivefold. It also increases morbidity, functional decline and incidence of major adverse cardiac and cerebrovascular events. It is essential to recognize these vulnerable patients before planning surgery and post-operative care, providing information to patients and their families, particularly in context of protracted ICU stay. Cardiac rehabilitation programs, especially these run before surgery improve patients outcomes (prehabilitation), partially by improving their nutritional status, activity level, muscle mass so by addressing some of the components of frailty syndrome. Therefore it is advocated that all elective patients presenting with frailty should be considered to be enrolled in prehabilitation programs that need to be continued after surgery.

Anemia

One of the very few chronic conditions that can and should be optimized before elective cardiac surgery is anemia. It is a disease, which can be easily diagnosed and rising of hemoglobin (Hb) (treating anemia) level requires only 14 days prior to surgery. It is defined as a Hb concentration < 12 g/dL for women or < 13 g/dL for men. It is proven, that there is an independent association of anemia with transfusion rates (odds ratio (95% confidence interval) 2.75 (2.55–2.95), $p < 0.001$), mortality (1.42 (1.18–1.71), $p < 0.001$) and length of hospital stay (geometric mean ratio (95% confidence interval) 1.15 (1.13–1.17), $p < 0.001$). Its prevalence in cardiac surgical population is 20–30% and is a result of either impaired erythropoiesis (iron deficiency, vitamin B6 or B12 deficiency, malabsorption, chronic kidney failure, bone marrow disorders) or chronic blood loss. All sorts of chronic occult bleeding sources must be investigated, as they pose risk of severe, unexpected bleeding once full anticoagulation is instituted. More often, however, it is the impaired erythropoiesis due to iron deficiency that leads to anemia, hence preoperative substitutive therapy is proven to be beneficial in cardiac surgical population. There is evidence that preoperative supplementation with intravenous iron and erythropoietin improves perioperative outcomes. In case of documented vitamin B12/B6 deficiency they should be substituted as well (Fig. 1). Even ultra-short anemia treatment with

Table 1 Clinical frailty scale

Level	Description
1. Very fit	People who are robust, active, energetic and motivated. These people commonly exercise regularly They are among the fittest for their age
2. Well	People who have no active disease symptoms but are less fit than category 1. Often, they exercise or are very active occasionally, e.g.'. seasonally
3. Managing well	People whose medical problems are well controlled, but are not regularly active beyond routine walking
4. Vulnerable	While not dependent on others for daily help, often symptoms limit activities. A common complaint is being "slowed up", and/or being tired during the day
5. Mildly frail	These people often have more evident slowing, and need help in high order activities of daily living (finances, transportation, heavy housework, medications). Typically, mild frailty progressively impairs shopping and walking outside alone, meal preparation and housework
6. Moderately frail	People need help with all outside activities and with keeping house. Inside, they often have problems with stairs and need help with bathing and might need minimal assistance (cuing, standby) with dressing
7. Severely frail	Completely dependent for personal care, from whatever cause (physical or cognitive). Even so, they seem stable and not at high risk of dying (within - 6 months)
8. Very severely frail	Completely dependent, approaching the end of life. Typically, they could not recover even from a minor illness
9. Terminally ill	Approaching the end of life. This category applies to people with a life expectancy of < 6 months, who are not otherwise evidently frail

single dose of iron/erythropoietin/Vit B12/Folic acid right before surgery reduces perioperative transfusion rates, yet there is no data supporting any difference in perioperative mortality. Therefore the problem of pre-operative anemia needs to be addressed as part of the routine preoperative assessment and preferably supplemented in a timely, elective manner prior to surgery.

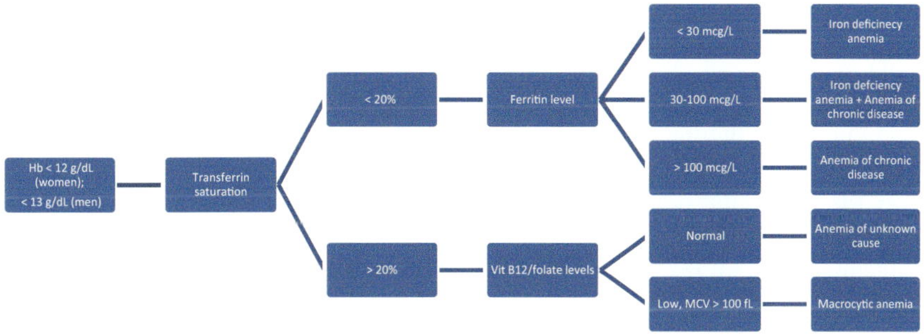

Fig. 1 Diagnostic algorithm of perioperative anemia. Algorithm modified from Muñoz et al. [2]

Heart Team

There are three main approaches to the management of heart conditions. The first one is medical treatment and optimization of symptoms that is usually reserved for patients who are presenting too early or too late for invasive intervention. The second and third are percutaneous or surgical interventions, respectively. Our initial understanding of risk–benefit balance for surgical revascularization vs percutaneous intervention (PCI) for coronary artery disease comes from SYNTAX trial. Rates of major adverse cardiac or cerebrovascular events (primary end point: death from any cause, stroke, myocardial infarction, or repeat revascularization) at 12 months were significantly higher in the PCI group than in surgical (17.8, vs. 12.4% for CABG; $P = 0.002$), in large part because of an increased rate of repeat revascularization (13.5% vs. 5.9%, $P < 0.001$). Despite the fact that stroke was significantly more likely to occur with CABG (2.2%, vs. 0.6% with PCI; $P = 0.003$), SYNTAX trial proved that cardiopulmonary bypass grafting (CABG) is superior to PCI in patients with left main stenosis or multivessel disease. This prompted publication of guidelines on cardiopulmonary revascularization in 2010, later revised in 2019. In this document the authors introduced the concept of Heart Team as a multidisciplinary decision making team that proposes treatment based on evidence-based guidelines. The core of the team comprises of cardiologist, interventional cardiologist and cardiac surgeon but it is expected that additional input may be needed from general practitioners, anesthetists, geriatricians and intensivists. Revised 2019 version of guidelines not only stresses the importance of Heart Team in proper patient management, but also gives positive feedback on this intervention by minimizing specialty bias (cardiologists as "gate keepers") and optimizing patient care. Successful introduction of Heart Team concept into perioperative management of patients suffering from coronary artery disease led to incorporation this form of decision making in qualification for valvular procedures, and surgical treatment of patients with end stage congestive heart failure. It is being mentioned in 2012 update of Guidelines on the Management of Valvular Heart Disease (VHD), where the authors emphasize "the importance of collaborative approach between cardiologists and cardiac surgeons in the management of patients with VHD—in particular when they are at increased perioperative risk". This approach was feasible with the advancement in diagnostic as well as minimal invasive surgical and percutaneous interventional techniques. More recent guidelines (2017) define a Heart Team as a group of specialists with particular expertise in VHD comprising cardiologists, cardiac surgeons, imaging specialists, anesthetists and, if needed, general practitioners, geriatricians and heart failure, electrophysiology or intensive care specialists, who are all involved in decision-making regarding valvular intervention. Over the years, the concept of Heart Team has proven to be a part of routine evaluation tool for all cardiac patients that guarantees adequate management compatible with up-to-date evidence-based standards.

Scores

One of the tools used for decision making are scores predicting perioperative morbidity and mortality. Numerous scores have been developed and further validated but unfortunately the complexity of the intervention itself, along with heterogeneity of patients and their comorbidities make such multifactorial analysis very difficult. Yet, scores are being designed in order to balance risk–benefit. They are important for decision-making process and for explaining the potential risk to patient and his family, finally comparing center outcomes with expected morbidity and mortality. Choosing a score that is tailored for given patient is very difficult, and one needs to keep in mind, that some older scores might not reflect up-to-date protocols, that there might be some intercontinental differences in prevalence of some conditions or interventional approaches and last but not least, that despite very little predicted risk, unpredictable could take place that might completely change the outcome of the particular patient.

STS Short Term Risk Calculator

STS (The Society of Thoracic Surgeons) risk calculator is a tool design to assess the impact of patient risk factors on perioperative mortality and morbidity. The latest update, released in 2018 acknowledges recent changes in both patient population's characteristics and surgical and perioperative management. In essence this online calculator predicts the risk for operative mortality, stroke, renal failure, prolonged ventilation, reoperation, composite major morbidity or mortality, deep sternal wound infection/mediastinitis and prolonged (> 14 days) or short (< 6 days) postoperative length of stay for patients undergoing isolated coronary artery bypass grafting surgery (CABG), isolated aortic or mitral valve surgery and combined valve plus CABG procedures. Predicted risk models are validated against patients' outcomes database, and are subject to elicit statistical analysis hence their accuracy is expected to reflect true patient's risk. Older versions of STS calculator were believed to overestimate the risk in low risk patients, as well as older patients and combined surgeries and the latest revision is yet to be further validated in terms of observed-to-expected ratio of adverse effects.

Euroscore

The most recent revision of The European System for Cardiac Operative Risk Evaluation called EuroSCORE II was published in 2012, replacing older versions dating back in late 90's. Similarly to other scores it focuses on patients characteristics (age, gender), comorbidities (creatinine clearance, presence of extracardiac arteriopathy, chronic lung disease, severe muscular/neurologic condition, insulin dependent diabetes, infective endocardiatis), critical preoperative state (ventricular tachycardia or fibrillation or aborted sudden death, cardiac massage, ventilation before arrival in the operating room, use of inotropes, intra-aortic balloon counterpulsation or ventricular-assist device before arrival in the anaesthetic room, acute renal failure (anuria or oliguria <10 ml/h)), cardiac function and symptoms (LV function, history of recent MI, NYHA class, CCS class, presence of pulmonary hypertension) and urgency and complexity of surgery (first time vs redo surgery, isolated procedure vs revascularization and valve procedure, involvement of thoracic aorta) in predicting risk of in-hospital mortality. Its accuracy was subject of a meta-analysis and proved to significantly overestimate risk in isolated coronary artery bypass grafting (observed/expected ratio of 0.829) and slightly underestimate the predictions in high-risk patients (observed/expected ratio 1.253). However, the overall performance of the EuroSCORE II in terms of discrimination and accuracy of model predictions for operative mortality is believed to be good. Therefore, it is routinely used in most of European countries.

Summary

Current review briefly summarized the most important aspects of preoperative assessment and cardiac surgical patients. Authors focus on these aspects which relates to risk assessment and multidisciplinary approach towards qualification. Additionally, we briefly discussed essential principles of perioperative blood management. This single intervention is one of the easiest to implement in every department and has potentially huge influence on outcome. Concluding this chapter, we would like to emphasize once again that all other aspects or preoperative anesthesia assessment applies to every cardiac surgical patient.

Recommended Readings

1. Muñoz M, Gómez-Ramírez S, Besser M, Pavía J, Gomollón F, Liumbruno GM, Bhandari S, Cladellas M, Shander A, Auerbach M. Current misconceptions in diagnosis and management of iron deficiency. Blood Transfus. 2017;15(5):422–437. https://doi.org/10.2450/2017.0113-17.
2. Muñoz M et al., Perioperative anemia management in colorectal cancer patients: a pragmatic approach. World J Gastroenterol. 2014;20(8):1972–85.
3. McCann et al., Cardiac prehabilitation. J Cardiothorac Vasc Anesth. 2019;33(8):2255–65.
4. Meybohm P et al., Perioperative anemia management as part of PBM in cardiac surgery—a narrative updated review. J Cardiothorac Vasc Anesth. 2019.

Monitoring for Cardiac Surgery

Ricard Navarro-Ripoll and Albert Carramiñana Domínguez

Abbreviations

CPB	Cardiopulmonary bypass
CO	Cardiac output
ECG	Electrocardiography
IBP	Invasive blood pressure
DHCA	Deep hypothermic circulatory arrest
BIS	Bispectral index
CPP	Cerebral perfusion pressure
MAP	Mean arterial pressure
CVP	Central venous pressure
ICP	Intracranial pressure
NIRS	Near-infrared spectroscopy
PAC	Pulmonary artery catheter
ECMO	Extra-corporeal membrane oxygenation
VAD	Ventricular assist device
PEEP	Positive End Expiratory Pressure
$ScvO_2$	Central venous saturation
TCD	Transcranial Doppler

R. Navarro-Ripoll (✉) · A. C. Domínguez
Anaesthesia and Intensive Care Department, Hospital Clinic Barcelona, Barcelona, Spain
e-mail: rnavarr1@clinic.cat

A. C. Domínguez
e-mail: carraminana@clinic.cat

M. Vives and A. Hernandez (eds.), *Cardiac Anesthesia and Postoperative Care in the 21st Century*, https://doi.org/10.1007/978-3-030-79721-8_5

Hemodynamic Monitoring

Hemodynamic parameters are essential during cardiac surgery because of sudden changes in cardiovascular stability may happen during and after general anaesthesia in patients with important comorbidities, primary advanced cardiac disease and before, during and after cardiopulmonary bypass (CPB). The main purpose is to maintain the balance between oxygen demand and supply. There are some standard parameters and some other more controversial and that are in constant evolution with new monitors. According to the authors, these are the most important hemodynamic parameters in cardiac surgery..

A. *Electrocardiography (ECG)*
   Main objectives in monitoring ECG during general anaesthesia are detection of ischemia and dysrhythmias, as well as electrolyte disorders.
   It is crucial to monitor for all cardiac patients a 5 electrode surface ECG that displays 6 frontal limbs plus one precordial limb, registering two leads at the same time. Evidence suggests that II and V_5 leads are the most accurate to diagnose around 90% episodes of myocardial ischemia. The electrodes should be protected with waterproof tape to avoid loss of signal, and placed in the back of the patient when possible.
B. *Invasive Blood Pressure (IBP)*
   Invasive arterial pressure monitoring is mandatory in patients undergoing cardiac procedures because of the likelihood of hemodynamic instability, use of vasopressors/inotropic support and abrupt blood volume or arterial tone changes. For radial artery cannulation, Seldinger technique has better success rate than direct insertion of peripheral intravenous cannula.
   More frequent sites for cannulation:

   – Radial artery: easier, cleaner and good correlation with aortic pressure. Special attention should be paid in coronary artery bypass surgery as radial artery may be used as free graft.
   – Femoral artery: especially useful in patients undergoing deep hypothermic circulatory arrest (DHCA), such as aortic dissection or pulmonary endarterectomy. Be aware of patients with previous vascular groin surgery or with groin skin infections.
   – Humeral artery: used as an alternative to femoral artery when both radial arteries are unavailable. Has a good correlation with aortic pressure but there is a potential risk of limb ischemia.
   – Aortic root: punctually used through the aortic root surgical cannula, to compare measurements between radial or femoral artery when concerns regarding reliability arise. Extreme attention to avoid air emboli is crucial.

C. *Central Venous Pressure (CVP)*
   Defined as the right atrium pressure, its normal values range between 0 and 7 mmHg. Very useful to assess systemic drainage and right ventricle function, but poorly correlated with fluid responsiveness. Central venous catheter tip should be located between the junction of the superior vena cava and the right atrium.

Main accesses for central venous catheterisation:

- Internal jugular vein (IJV): Most common access route.
- Subclavian vein: is an acceptable alternative.
- Femoral vein: more often in pediatric cardiac surgery.
- Arm veins: not recommended for cardiac surgery.

Depending on the insertion site, placement of central catheters may present significant complications: accidental artery puncture, nerve damage, air embolism, pneumothorax, infection, thrombosis, etc. The use of ultrasound decreases the rate of complications and should always be considered.

D. *Cardiac Output (CO)*

One of the most interesting and controversial monitoring parameters. There are various modalities for CO monitoring during the perioperative period. In the following lines some of the most important will be exposed.

- Pulmonary Artery Catheter (PAC, Swan-Ganz): considered the gold standard since the 70s. CO is measured after a cold saline bolus is injected into the proximal port and a thermodilution curve is generated. The use of PAC is controversial because of the morbidity and mortality reported, nevertheless some authors do not agree with those findings. Probably not a routine but a proper patient selection is the key to advocate for this monitor (see Table 1).
- Minimally invasive methods: Based on the pulse power analysis and pulse contour analysis, there are multiple monitors and each have is main advantages and disadvantages (see Table 2).

E. *Central venous saturation ($ScvO_2$)*

Indicator of the balance between oxygen consumption and delivery and the adequacy of CO (normal $ScvO_2$ is >70%). A low value may indicate tissue hypoxia due to low blood concentration of haemoglobin, hypoxemia or to insufficient cardiac output. On the other side, a high value may suggest hypervolemia, anatomic shunt or inability to extract oxygen in the peripheral tissue, the latter with an extremely poor prognosis.

Table 1 Main PAC indications

Main indications for PAC colocation
Impaired left ventricular systolic function (EF <30%)
Impaired right ventricular systolic function
Severe left ventricular diastolic dysfunction
Acute ventricular septal defect
Left ventricular assist device
Complex valve surgery
Heart transplantation
Emergency aortic surgery

Table 2 Main semi-invasive CO monitors

Device	Advantage	Disadvantage
PiCCO	– Continuous CO measurement – Quantifies pulmonary oedema and fluid responsiveness	– Requires calibration – Low accuracy during hemodynamic instability/ OPCAB
Transesophageal echocardiography	– Useful for GDT – Judge adequacy of valve or congenital disease repair	– Operator dependency – No continuous monitoring
LiDCO	– Continuous measures CO and SVV	– Requires regular calibration – Poor reliability in cardiac surgery
FloTrac/Vigileo	– Only arterial line – No external calibration – Operator independent	– Low liability in severe vasoconstriction (arterial waveform) – Low accuracy in arrhythmias, IABP, morbid obesity
PRAM	– No external calibration	– Still not validated

Respiratory Monitoring

General anaesthesia induces many changes in respiratory system, as well as formation of atelectasis and decrease in functional residual capacity, etc. Respiratory monitoring is basic to detect and treat appropriately any event and to adjust properly protective ventilation parameters.

A. *Pulse oximetry* (SpO_2)
   Simple and non-invasive method useful to monitor oxygen saturation (SpO_2), peripheral perfusion and cardiac rate based on the amount of oxyhaemoglobin and deoxygenated haemoglobin in arterial blood (Fig. 1). Finger probe is normally used as first option, being the earlobe probe a good alternative when distal perfusion is compromised.
B. *Capnography* ($EtCO_2$)
   Non-invasive monitor that assesses end-expiratory CO_2, an indirect measurement of $PaCO_2$ (Fig. 2). It reflects alterations in alveolar ventilation, cardiac output, pulmonary perfusion or accidental ventilator disconnection.

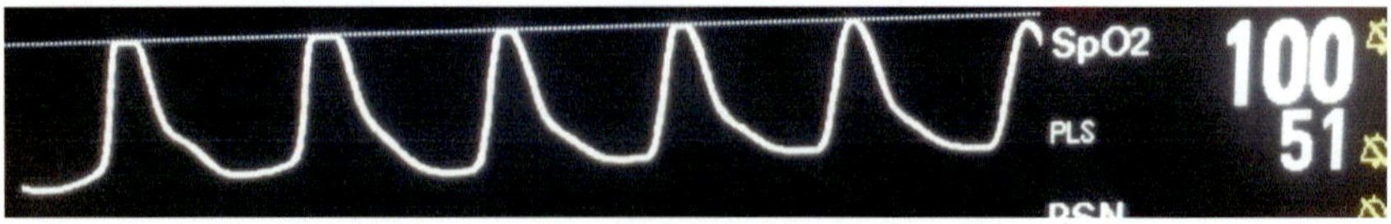

Fig. 1 Pulse oximetry curve

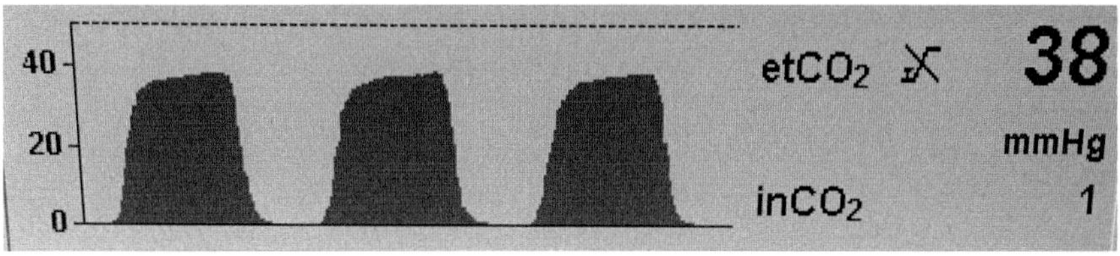

Fig. 2 Capnography curve with end-expiratory CO_2

C. *Respiratory Mechanics*
Measurement of airway pressure (Peak, Plateau, and Driving Pressure) and compliance is helpful to optimize ventilator parameters as well as to adjust individualized PEEP and perform recruitment manoeuvres if needed (Fig. 3). General anaesthesia and CPB facilitate the formation of atelectasis as well as hypoxemia and ARDS.

Temperature Monitoring

Temperature is a paramount parameter during cardiac surgery where wide changes may happen during CPB. Choosing an appropriate site of monitoring has relevant consequences as hypothermia may be needed in order to properly protect organs during CPB or DHCA. Cooling and rewarming at a certain temperature and temperature rate change imply deep physiologic changes and reliable monitoring is mandatory to ensure optimal management. It is well known that hyperthermia during CPB may cause neurologic injury and that excessive fast rewarming after cooling may result in rebound hypothermia after resuming spontaneous circulation. Although temperature management and monitoring site is not uniform between centres, monitoring should include at least two locations. Main advantages and disadvantages of different monitoring sites are showed in Table 3.

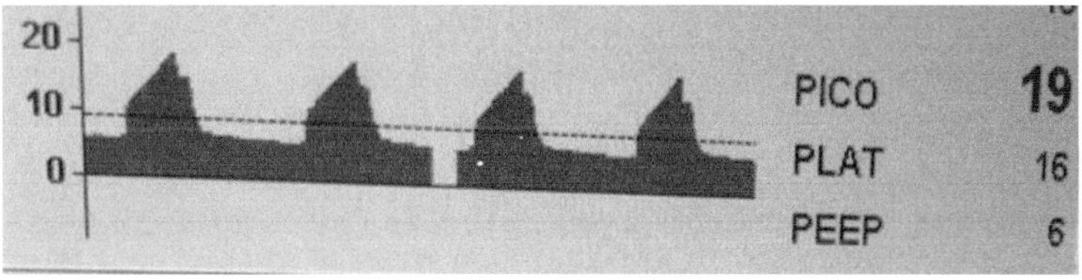

Fig. 3 Respiratory mechanics and airway pressure values (Peak and plateau, PEEP)

Table 3 Main sites of temperature monitoring during cardiac surgery

Temperature monitoring site	Advantage	Disadvantage
Intravascular	Gold standard	Not useful when the heart is not ejecting
Nasopharyngeal	Reliability and availability	Risk of epistaxis
Urinary bladder	Easy to place, availability, no added risk	Delay in rapid core temperature changes, reliability depends on urinary output
Oesophageal	Ease of placement, minimal risk	Incorrect positioning can alter its reading, transoesophageal echocardiography
Tympanic membrane	Estimation of brain temperature	Risk of tympanic damage
Rectal	Ease of placement, minimal risk	Artefacts, lower reliability

Monitoring sites:

- *Intravascular*: devices that monitor intravascular temperature are the gold standard of core temperature measurement. They directly monitor the blood temperature through a thermistor located at the tip of the catheter and are normally used to measure cardiac out through thermodilution. The pulmonary catheter is the most frequently used in the cardiac surgery environment, but it has strong limitation as it can only be used when there is pulmonary flow but not during CPB.
- *Nasopharyngeal*: probably one of the most commonly used sites thanks to its reliability. When correctly positioned in the upper pharynx, it is surrounded by highly irrigated mucosa and it reflects the brain and core temperature. Its main drawback is the risk of epistaxis that may be significant in patients who receive systemic heparinisation.
- *Bladder*: after nasopharyngeal, the most common site used. The temperature is measured through a thermistor attached to a Foley catheter. It is may have a delay of up to 3 °C compared to nasopharyngeal temperature in rapid cooling or rewarming. Its accuracy decreases when there is low urinary output.
- *Oesophageal*: it correctly reflects the heart and core temperature. The temperature probe should be placed in the distal oesophagus; about 45 cm form the nose. Positioning is important because false measurements may be obtained if placed proximal to the trachea. Its main limitations consist in false measurements due to pericardial cold solutions applied during myocardial protection, pericardial saline irrigation and probe displacement during transoesophageal echocardiography assessment during the surgery.

- *Tympanic membrane*: mostly used as a surrogate of brain temperature, very useful during DHCA. The tympanic membrane lies next to the hypothalamus and is irrigated by the carotid artery. There is a risk of tympanic membrane damage.
- *Rectal*: it can be used to estimate the core temperature but some artefacts such as splanchnic vasoconstriction, the presence of stool and heat generated by bacteria limit its reliability. Rectal temperature usually exceeds core temperature. Frequently used for general cases but less commonly for active cooling and rewarming due to its drawbacks.

Neurologic Monitoring

Neurologic monitoring has a potential to facilitate anaesthetic titration, improve cerebral perfusion and decrease postoperative neurologic dysfunction. Different devices are available to estimate neuronal transmission and brain perfusion. However, there is still no non-invasive monitor that can reliably assess global cerebral perfusion. The integration of different data including clinical parameters and specific monitoring such as the bispectral index, near-infrared spectrometry or transcranial doppler is probably the best available information when trying to optimize neurologic outcomes.

Clinical parameters:

Basic clinical neurologic monitoring includes hemodynamic parameters and temperature. Although there is a lack of consistent evidence, ensuring appropriate cerebral perfusion during cardiac surgery seems a promising strategy to decrease neurological injury. The cerebral blood flow (CBF) will depend on the cerebral perfusion pressure (CPP), calculated as:

$$\text{CPP} = \text{MAP} - (\text{CVP} + \text{ICP})$$

where MAP = mean arterial pressure, CVP = central venous pressure, ICP = intracranial pressure.

Maintaining an optimal CPP during all the procedure will depend on maintaining an adequate MAP and avoiding significant increase in CVP and ICP. Cerebral hypo-perfusion and hypotension should be avoided as they may be related to an increase in postoperative neurological dysfunction, in particular in those with previous neurologic conditions and in the elderly. The main problem arises when trying to define an "adequate" MAP for every patient. Cerebral auto-regulation curve may be shifted rightwards in hypertensive and in the elderly and higher values of MAP may be necessary. Moreover, there are some specific situations in cardiac surgery that may impair cerebral venous drainage, due to inadequate positioning of drainage cannula, superior vena constriction or surgical manoeuvres.

Temperature affects cerebral metabolic rate and hypothermia has been used to minimize cerebral metabolism during DHCA. There is little evidence regarding the effect of mild to moderate hypothermia but there is consistent evidence regarding the deleterious effect of hyperthermia. In fact, cerebral hyperthermia associated to actively rewarming during CPB is related to worse neurologic outcome. Monitoring the temperature to avoid hyperthermia (>37 °C) and limiting the arterial line temperature to 37 °C might be useful to avoid cerebral hyperthermia.

Bispectral index:

The bispectral index (BIS) is one of the most common neurophysiologic monitors used in cardiac surgery. One of the most important reasons why it gained such popularity is that cardiac surgery has been deemed at high risk for intraoperative awareness, especially when low dose of hypnotics and high dose of opioids to avoid hemodynamic instability were used. Modern anaesthetics techniques and drugs suppose a different scenario but the bispectral index has continued to gain more acceptation. Different reasons may explain why. Anaesthetic dose titration may be facilitated using BIS and therefore it can help to limit hemodynamic side effects of anaesthetic drugs. Moreover, excessive anaesthetic depth and over-suppression (prolonged BIS of <40) has been related to worse neurologic outcomes and increased mortality. BIS can also help when aiming for isoelectrical cerebral activity during DHCA and avoiding excessive neuronal activity in the periods of rewarming. Despite these potential benefits, the main limitation is that there is a lack of evidence that BIS may contribute to better outcomes in cardiac surgery. Another limitation is artefacts due to signal contamination and sensor mobilization.

Other neurophysiologic monitoring:

Some other methods have been assessed but they are rarely used. Electroencephalogram and somatosensory evoked potentials could be helpful but to the moment there is scarce evidence in general cardiac population. They are more complex and difficult to interpret and are sensitive to many artefacts that make them less attractive for clinical practice.

Cerebral oximetry:

Near-infrared spectroscopy (NIRS) technology is used to assess haemoglobin oxygen saturation in the brain. In a different manner than pulse-oximetry does, NIRS measures the haemoglobin oxygen saturation of not only of the pulsatile blood but also venous blood and tissue. When placed in the forehead, it theoretically measures regional saturation of the frontal lobe, a zone irrigated by both mean and anterior cerebral arteries with transitional zones susceptible to ischemia. Cerebral oximetry has the potential to assess the mismatch of oxygen supply and demand in the brain and it can help to assess cerebral auto-regulation during cardiac surgery.

One of the main limitations of NIRS is the lack of normal values. 75% of saturation has been used as a desired target and desaturation below 50% or more than 20% below the baseline (obtained in the non-sedated awake patient breathing

Table 4 Main benefits and pitfalls of NIRS

Benefits	Pitfalls
Non-invasive	Not well-defined baseline value
Easy to interpret	Only anterior perfusion is assessed
Continuous monitoring	Extra-cranial signal contamination
Bilateral assessment	Cost-efficiency
Interventional algorithms created	Lack of evidence

room air) seem to be related to worse outcomes. Recent studies suggest that desaturation episodes can successfully be treated in 95 97% of the patients and that may have an impact in a reduction of postoperative complications. Main advantages and disadvantages of NIRS are showed in Table 4.

Despite its limitations, NIRS is a useful tool when used combined to clinical parameters in many situations. As said before, cerebral auto-regulation curve is different between patients and NIRS can help to elucidate the desired MAP during CPB and to assess tolerance to hypotension. It can also help to assess correct cannulation and perfusion during arch surgery and antegrade cerebral perfusion, tolerance to circulatory arrest during DHCA (Fig. 4) and can help in the decision making on when to transfuse. Use of cerebral oximetry differs widely between

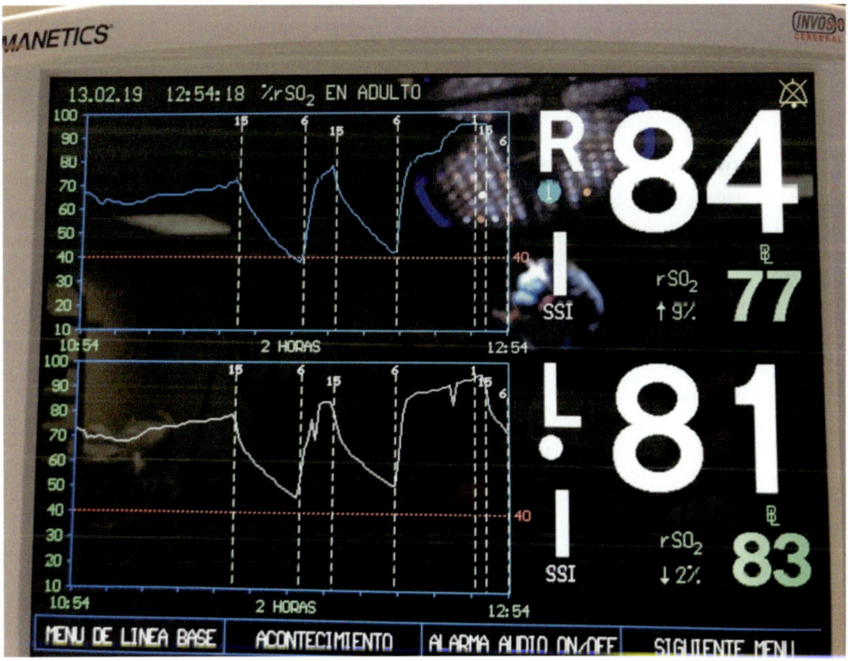

Fig. 4 Desaturation observed in the NIRS monitor during DHCA in a pulmonary endarterectomy

Table 5 Suggested indications of NIRS in cardiac surgery

Suggested indications of NIRS
Aortic arch surgery/aortic dissection
Increased risk of postoperative neurological dysfunction (frailty, age, anaemia, previous cerebrovascular disease)
Risk of cerebral blood flow impairment (significant carotid stenosis)
DHCA
Advanced heart failure and mechanical support (ECMO/VAD)

institutions and no clear indications have been established, being part of the standard monitoring in some centres whereas in some others it is only used in selected patients (see Table 5).

Transcranial Doppler:

Transcranial doppler (TCD) has been used in cardiac surgery to assess cerebral blood flow during both pulsatile spontaneous flow and during CPB. The doppler beam interrogates the mean cerebral artery and reduction of systolic velocity or absence of diastolic velocity suggests cerebral hypo-perfusion. TCD can also be helpful to detect embolic phenomena and to assess correct flow during selective cerebral perfusion. However, some drawbacks limit its use due to the time consuming learning curve, presence of artefacts, difficult probe positioning and position maintenance during all the surgery. These limitations have made other perfusion monitoring such as cerebral oximetry much more popular.

Recommended Readings

1. Saad H, Aladawy M. Temperature management in cardiac surgery. Glob Cardiol Sci Pract. 2013;2013(1):44–62. https://doi.org/10.5339/gcsp.2013.7.
2. Kowalczyk AK, Bachar BJ, Liu H. Neuromonitoring during adult cardiac surgery. J Biomed Res. 2016;30(3):171–3. https://doi.org/10.7555/JBR.30.20150159.
3. Green DW, Kunst G. Cerebral oximetry and its role in adult cardiac, non-cardiac surgery and resuscitation from cardiac arrest. Anaesthesia. 2017;72(Suppl 1):48–57. https://doi.org/10.1111/anae.13740.
4. Kobe J, et al. Cardiac output monitoring: technology and choice. Ann Card Anaesth. 2019;22(1):6–17. https://doi.org/10.4103/aca.ACA_41_18.
5. Arora D, Mehta Y. Recent trends on hemodynamic monitoring in cardiac surgery. Ann Card Anaesth. 2016;19(4):580–3. https://doi.org/10.4103/0971-9784.191557.

Coronary Angiography

Daniel Rivero Cerda and David Viñas Fernández

Introduction

In recent decades there has been an enormous advance in cardiac catheterization technique in both diagnostic and therapeutic procedures. In this chapter we will focus in Coronary Angiography as a technique for the study of coronary anatomy.

Main indications for cardiac catheterization include assessing coronary anatomy (including by-pass grafts in case of previous surgical revascularization), ventricular function (ventriculography), aortic anatomy (aortography can be performed during the procedure), endocavitary pressures and the evaluation of heart valves can be studied through a diagnostic cardiac catheterization (Table 1). It is also possible to perform therapeutic procedures both at the coronary level and in different cardiac structures. However, a correct indication and clinical evaluation of the patient is required to perform this procedure safely since despite presenting a low percentage of complications some of them may be major.

Performing a coronary angiography requires a specialized team consisting of a interventional cardiologist and specialized nurses. It is also necessary a room equipped with X-rays, continuous hemodynamic monitoring, iodinated contrast, some specific drugs (Table 2), specific material to treat possible complications and advanced CPR equipment. All of this equipment is the so-called catheterization laboratory (*cath lab*).

Supplementary Information The online version contains supplementary material available at https://doi.org/10.1007/978-3-030-79721-8_6.

D. Rivero Cerda (✉)
Department of Interventional Cardiology, Hospital Universitari Dr J Trueta, Girona, Spain
e-mail: driveroc.girona.ics@gencat.cat

D. Viñas Fernández
Department of Cardiology, Hospital Universitari Dr J Trueta, Girona, Spain

M. Vives and A. Hernandez (eds.), *Cardiac Anesthesia and Postoperative Care in the 21st Century*, https://doi.org/10.1007/978-3-030-79721-8_6

Table 1 Main indications of diagnostic coronary angiography (Based on the latest ESC guidelines and recommendations)

Acute coronary syndrome	Unstable angina, non ST-segment elevation myocardial infarction (NSTEMI) and ST-segment elevation myocardial infarction (STEMI)
Stable coronary artery disease	Especially in symptomatic patients with prior revascularization (percutaneous or surgical), suspicion of ongoing ischemia, worsening of left ventricular function or arrhythmias
Patients with angina and suspected coronary artery disease	In patients with high clinical likelihood of coronary artery disease. In cases of inconclusive non-invasive testing. Exceptionally in patients from particular professions due to regulatory issues
Heart Failure	In some cases of left ventricular dysfunction (rule out coronary artery disease)
Cardiogenic shock	Especially if there is suspicion of underlying ischemic cause
Valvular heart disease	Coronary angiography prior to valve surgery
Ventricular arrhythmias of unknown origin	In case of moderate probability of coronary heart disease or if non-invasive studies cannot rule out arrythmogenic substrate
Hypertrophic cardiomyopathy	Before surgery or in chest pain despite treatment
Heart transplant/Ventricular assist devices	Before surgery. Some cases of follow-up
Survivors to cardiac arrest of unknown cause	Particularly in haemodynamically unstable patients
Congenital heart disease	As part of the anatomical and functional study

Table 2 Main drugs used during a diagnostic coronary angiography

Indication	Drug
Anxiety	e.g. Diazepam. Mainly administered routinely before the procedure
Anticoagulation	Unfractioned Heparin or Low-molecular weight heparin
In case of access through the radial artery different drugs are used to vasodilate the vessel	Verapamil, nitroglycerin
Assess the real diameter of the coronary vessels	nitroglycerin
Fractional Flow Reserve (FFR) in a pressure wire study	Adenosine
Pain	Morphine, fentanyl, benzodiazepines

Contraindications to Diagnostic Coronary Angiography

There are no absolute contraindications to perform coronary angiography. However, in certain situations, the procedure may be delayed until patient stabilization or appropriate management of specific situations (Table 3).

Steps to Perform a Coronary Angiography

1. Patient must be informed in advance of the indication as well as the potential benefit and risks of the procedure. As long as the clinical situation permits it, written informed consent must be read and signed by the patient or the legal tutor.
2. Assess the possible personal risks of the patient. Some clinical scenarios (Table 3) will require special preparation, for instance cases of allergy to iodinated contrast, chronic anticoagulation, history of peripheral artery disease, previous cardiac surgery, ventricular systolic dysfunction, chronic kidney disease, diabetes mellitus, hemodynamic instability or patients requiring sedation and invasive ventilation.

Table 3 Special concerns and clinical situations to consider and manage before a coronary angiography. (DOAC = direct oral anticoagulants, LMWH = Low-molecular weight heparin, VKA = vitamin-K antagonists). (Based on recommendations from International Guidelines)

Active infection	Delay the test as far as possible until stable and afebrile
Chronic kidney disease or acute kidney injury	Apply specific renal protection protocols through prior and subsequent hydration
Active bleeding, coagulopathy, severe thrombocytopenia	Delay the test as far as possible until the underlying cause or condition is resolved. Correct using vitamin K, prothromplex, coagulation factors or platelets if required
Severe hydroelectrolytic disturbance	Delay the test or correct
Iodine contrast allergy	Apply specific protocols based on pre and post treatment with intravenous corticoids, oral antihistaminic and hydration
Drugs	VKA: safely if INR <1.8 in femoral access or INR <2.2 in radial access DOAC: stop 24 h before the procedure if radial access (more if femoral access or renal function impairment) LMWH: hold medication 12 h before the procedure Metformin: recommended holding 48 h before the procedure although lack of robust evidence Antiplatelet drugs: do not discontinue

3. In outpatient setting, performing the procedure in the best possible conditions is the best way to reduce the risk of complications. A low dose of oral benzodiazepine is usually given before entering the cath lab so patient patient will be relaxed.
4. Peripheral venous access is necessary to administer drugs during the procedure.
5. Asses the best vascular access. The radial artery is the preferred one since a clinical benefit has been demonstrated in trained operators (Fig. 1b); other options would be the common femoral artery (Fig. 1c) and the brachial artery.
6. The arterial puncture is performed with Seldinger's technique. In case the common femoral artery is chosen, puncture can be performed by anatomy and palpation of the femoral pulse, however to reduce complications it can be guided by angiography or ultrasound.

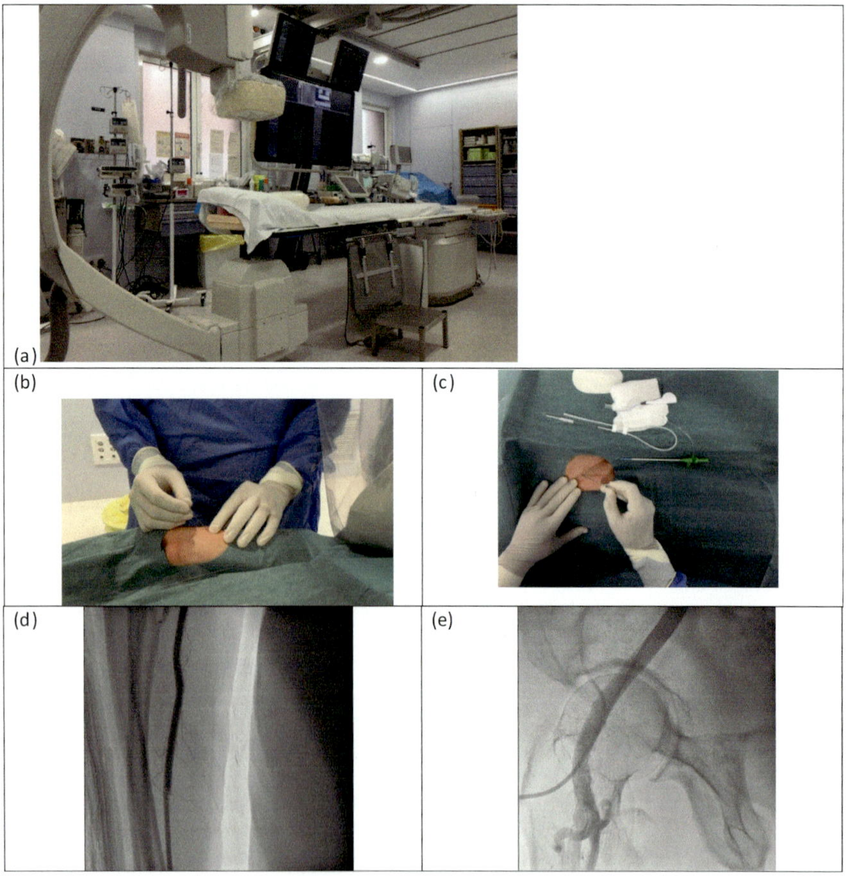

Fig. 1 **a** Catheterization laboratory and monitors. **b** Radial access. **c** Femoral access. **d** Radial access angiography (video 1). **e** Femoral access angiography (video 2)

7. After performing the puncture, using Seldinger's technique a valved introducer is used to enter the necessary catheters to carry out the study. In diagnostic angiography the introducer is usually 5 French (Fr), but it could also be 4 or 6 Fr.
8. Diagnostic catheters for coronary angiography are specific for each coronary and there are different curves due to anatomical variability. A Pig-Tail catheter is usually used to perform aortography and ventriculography (Fig. 2).
9. With the use of iodinated contrast injections and X-ray cinemas the coronary anatomy is assessed looking for anatomical abnormalities or coronary stenosis.
10. To end the procedure effective haemostasis on the vascular access is performed with manual compression. In case the puncture is through the femoral artery, haemostasis can also be performed with a percutaneous closure mechanism. Puncture areas should be assessed in the follow-up to rule out vascular and hemorrhagic complications.
11. Complications should be ruled-out in the follow-up according to the procedure performed (Table 6).

Coronary Anatomy

The coronary arteries are three main or epicardial with their secondary branches. Here we will describe the normal anatomy with some different anatomical variations and anomalies.

The left main (LM) is originated from the left Valsalva sinus and usually divides into the left anterior descending (LAD) and the circumflex (LCx). The third epicardial coronary is the right coronary artery (RCA) originated in the right coronary sinus. The artery from which the posterior descending artery (PDA) is originated is called the dominant coronary. Approximately 85% of the population has right coronary dominance; however, the percentage of dominance varies in different series. The rest of patients would have left dominance by having the origin of the PDA from the LCx. In a smaller percentage there may be another epicardial artery called intermediate artery which is originated from the LM between the origin of the LAD and the LCx. These main arteries have a proximal, middle and distal segment, except for the CX which in most anatomical maps is considered with only a proximal and middle segment.

The LAD runs through the anterior interventricular groove as it rises its secondary branches: the septal arteries (S) and the diagonal arteries (D). Through the septal arteries gives flow to the anteroseptal segments and, through the diagonals, the anterior and part of the anterolateral segments of the left ventricle.

In turn, the LCx runs through the left atrioventricular groove and through the marginal obtuse arteries (OM) gives flow to the anterolateral and part of the posterolateral segments of the left ventricle.

Left Anterior Descending (RAO 10º/CRAN 40º)	
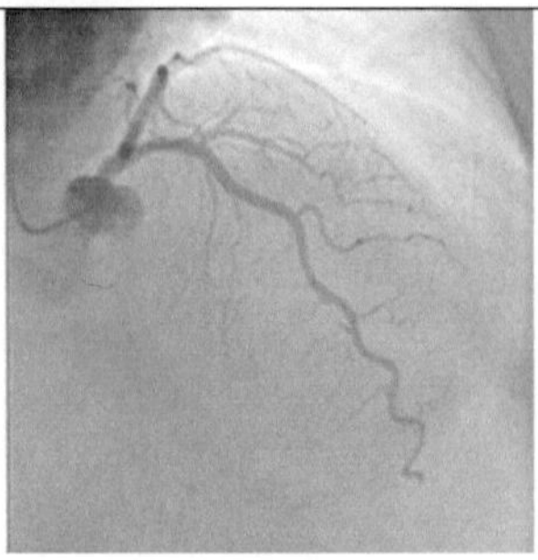	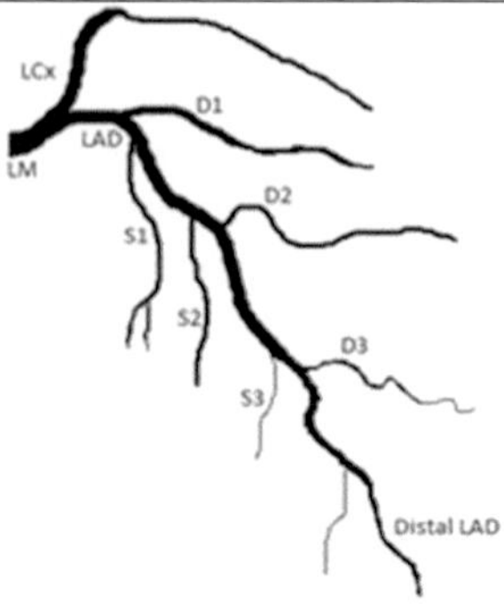
Left Circunflex (RAO 30º / CAU 25º)	
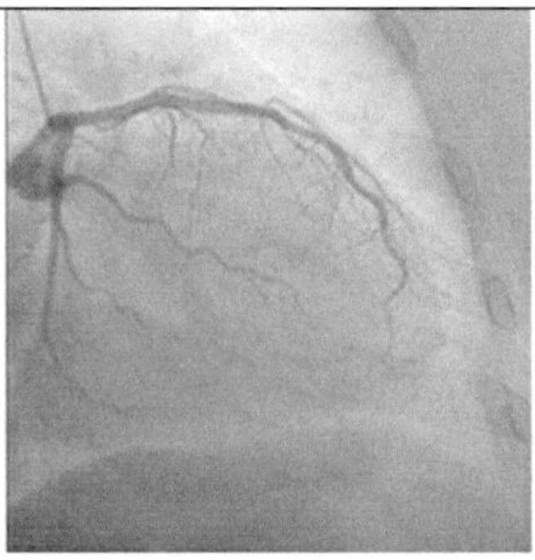	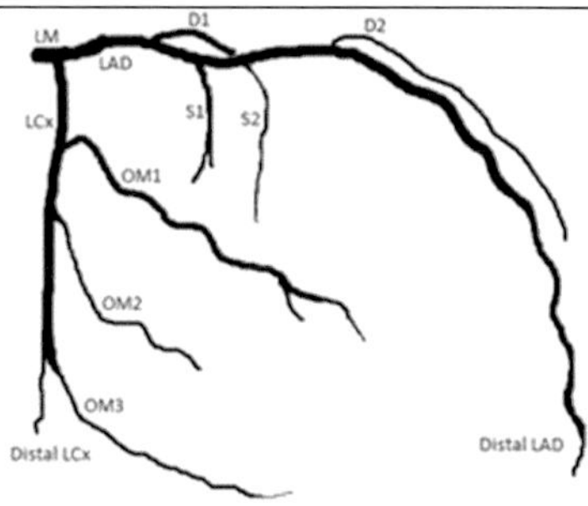
Right Coronary artery (CRAN 30º)	
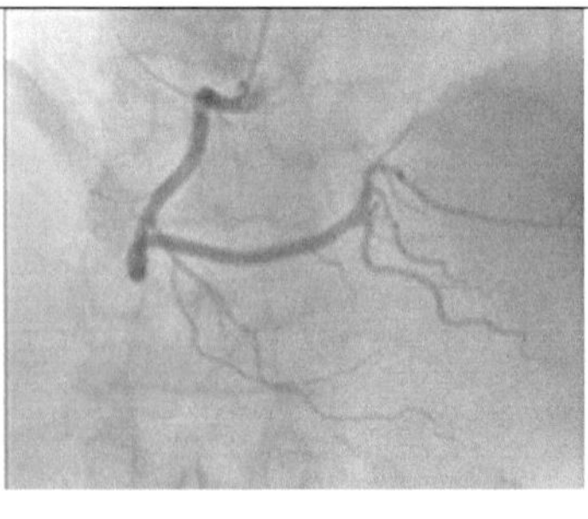	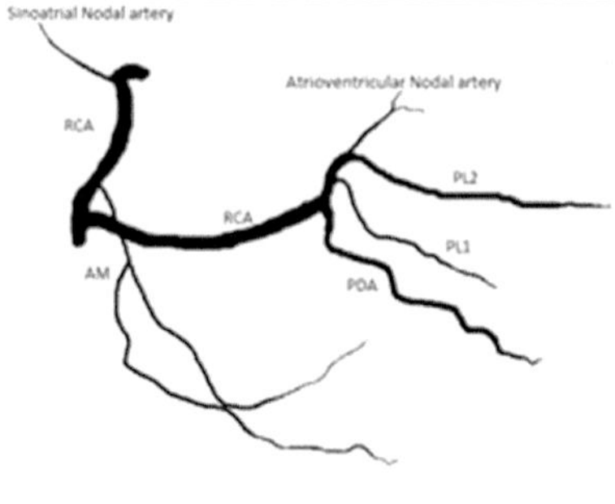
By-pass grafts	

Fig. 2 Main basic projections in diagnostic coronary angiography as well as examples of other anatomical structures (LM = Left Main, LAD = left anterior descending, LCx = Left Circunflex, OM = Obtuse Marginal, RCA = Right Coronary Artery, PDA = Posterior Descending Artery, PL = Posterolateral, S = Septal, D = Diagonals, RAO = Right Anterior Oblique angulation, LAO = Left Anterior Oblique angulation, CRAN = Cranial angulation, CAU = Caudal angulation)

Left internal mammary artery – Video 3	Distal anastomosis of the left internal mammary artery to the LAD and native mid and distal segments of the LAD.
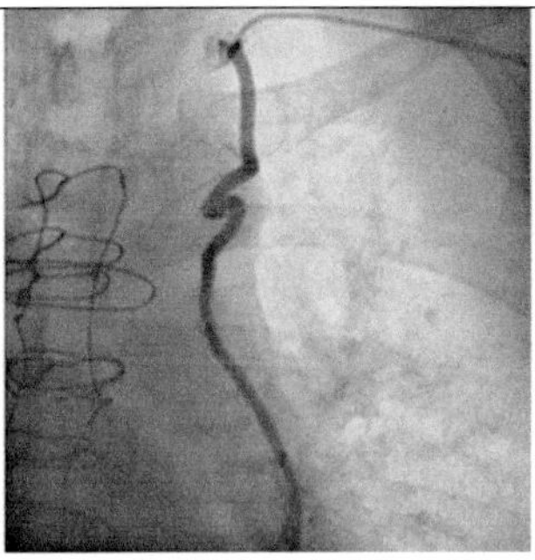	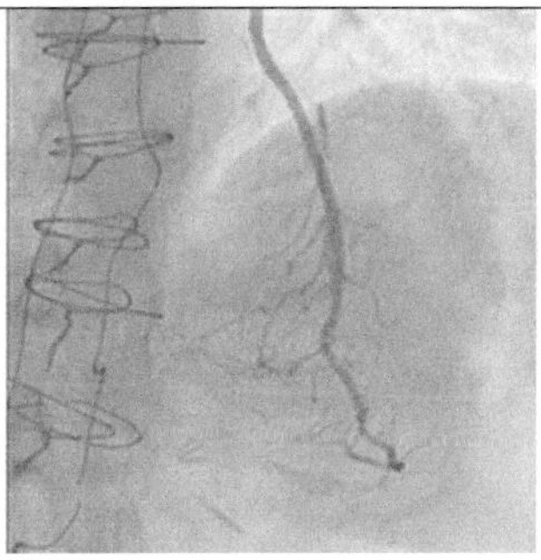
Sequential saphenous vein coronary graft to Obtuse Marginals – Video 4	Saphenous vein coronary graft to PDA – Video 5
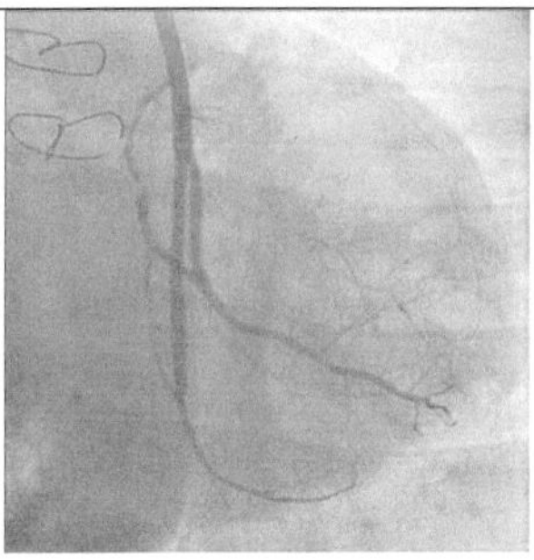	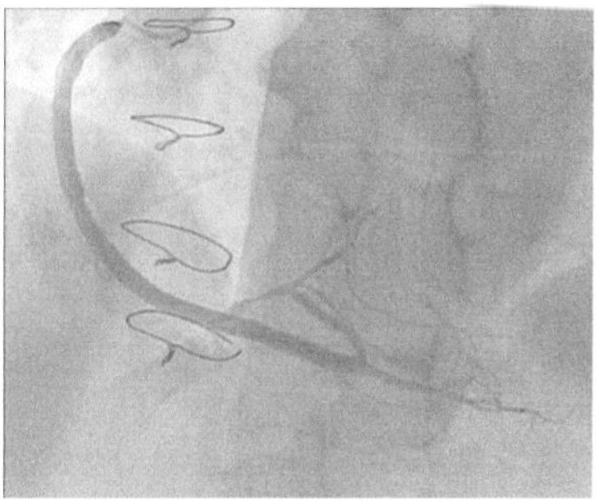
Aortography (LAO 45º / CAU 5º)	
Normal aorta – Video 6	Dilated aorta – Video 7
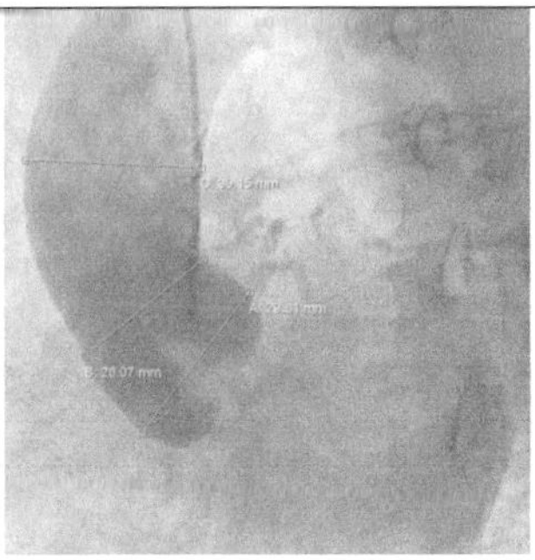	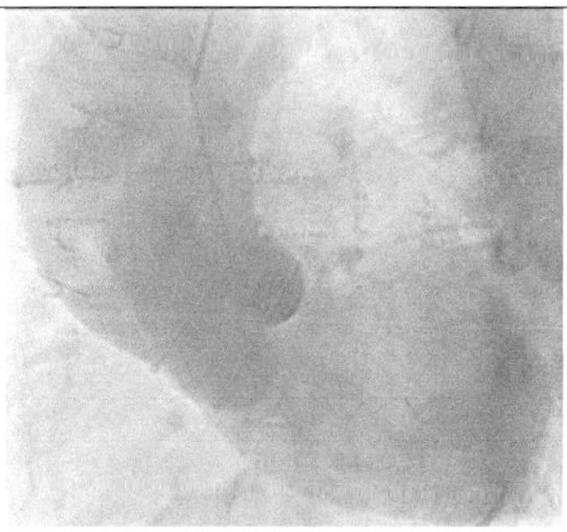

Fig. 2 (continued)

Ventriculography – Video 8	
Normal telediastole	Normal telesistole
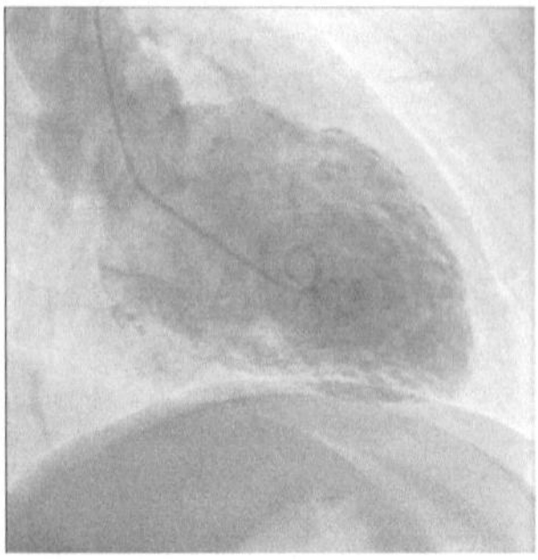	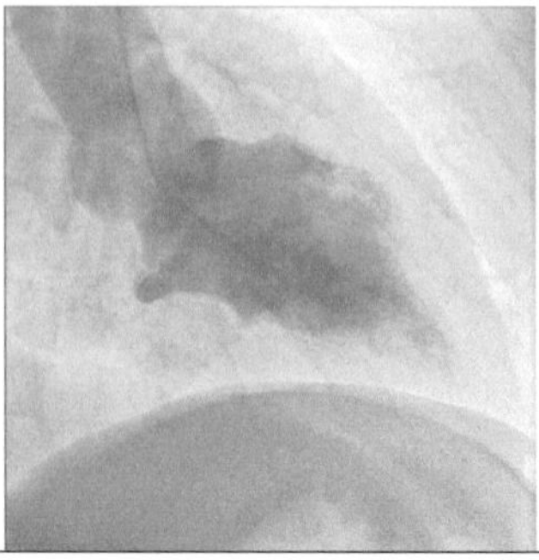

Fig. 2 (continued)

The RCA runs through the right atrioventricular groove and gives flow to the right ventricle through the acute marginals (AM). In case of right dominance, RCA through the PDA gives flow to the inferior and inferoseptal segments of the left ventricle. Through the posterolateral arteries (PL) it can give flow to the infero-lateral segments. There are two important branches of the RCA although not very big: the sinoatrial nodal artery and the atrioventricular nodal artery.

At the catheterization laboratory the study of the coronary arteries and other anatomical structures is carried out by means of the x-ray tube that has the capacity to rotate in two axes of space. This provides the ability to capture images from different positions, also called projections. To locate the projections, the angular deviation from the Antero-Posterior or neutral projection (0°/0°) is called in two axes: cranio-caudal and right-left. Figure 2 shows the main basic projections in diagnostic coronary angiography as well as examples of other anatomical structures.

Coronary Evaluation by Angiography

Coronary angiography allows seeing the luminogram of the coronaries in different projections and as previously said to see the coronary anatomy. Assessing coronary arteries for stenosis or obstructions (coronary artery disease) is the main indication for a coronary angiography (see example in Fig. 3). Usually visual estimation is the parameter to assess the severity of the lesions as the percentage of stenosis of the arterial diameter, comparing the reference segment before and after the area of greater stenosis with the smaller luminal diameter. A stenosis of 50% or greater can produce significant ischemia, being 100% a total occlusion.

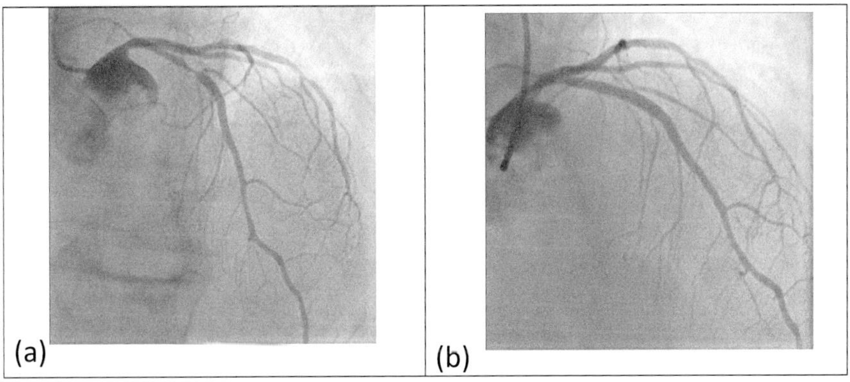

Fig. 3 Patient with a proximal LAD severe stenosis (**a**) treated effectively via PCI (percutaneous coronary intervention) with a drug-eluting stent (**b**)

Table 4 Invasive intracoronary diagnostic techniques

Classification	Intracoronary diagnostic technique	Information provided
Imaging	Ultrasound based (IVUS) Optical coherence tomography (OCT) Angioscopy	Tissue and stenosis characterization. Measurement of the luminal diameter and length of a lesion. Mainly used are IVUS and OCT
Physiological	Pressure wire study with Fractional Flow Reserve (FFR) Pressure wire study with instantaneous wave-free ratio (iFR) Intracoronary Doppler Infrared Thermography	Functional assessment of coronary stenosis (significant ischemia). Mainly used the pressure wire studies (FFR and iFR)

Invasive Intracoronary Diagnostic Techniques

Sometimes additional information may be necessary to assess whether a stenosis is significant or not. In this direction intracoronary diagnostic procedures have been developed. They can be classified in imaging techniques and physiological techniques (Table 4).

Table 5 Correlation between coronary severity stenosis assessed by visual estimation and FFR pressure wire study [2, 7]

Angiographic visual estimation of stenosis (%)	Positive pressure wire study (FFR $\leq$ 0.80) (%)
50–70	35
71–90	80
> 90	96

Intravascular Ultrasound (IVUS)

It is the most experienced intracoronary diagnostic technique providing characterization of coronary anatomy and coronary plaques. The transducers can be 30–40 MHz achieving a resolution of 150 μm and a penetration of 5 mm [3]. There are also ultrasounds with higher frequency (60–80 Mz) with a higher resolution [3, 4]. The lastest ESC 2018 revascularization guide recommends using IVUS to assess the severity of unprotect left main lesions with an IIa B recommendation [2].

Optical Coherence Tomography (OCT)

Generates an intracoronary image based on reflected light. It has a resolution of 15 μm which is higher than the IVUS but with less penetration. OCT is optimal for characterization of atheromatose plaques, for instance for the detection of fine capsule related to vulnerable plaques [5].

Pressure Wire Study of Coronary Stenosis and Fractional Flow Reserve (FFR)

With this technique, intermediate coronary lesions are assessed individually (Table 5). Fractional flow reserve (FFR) is a pressure-wire–based index that is used during coronary angiography to assess the potential of a coronary stenosis to induce myocardial ischemia. The quotient between the coronary pressure distal to the lesion and the aortic pressure is calculated, requiring maximum hyperemia that is achieved with the perfusion of drugs such as Adenosine. If the quotient value is less than or equal to 0.80 it is a functionally significant lesion (the lesion causes significant ischaemia) and revascularization may be justified. While if the FFR is greater than 0.80 the clinical evolution without revascularization is excellent [6].

In patients that have already been studied with non-invasive techniques sometimes significant ischemia and its location has already been identified. In this setting, pressure-wire study may only be indicated if ischemia has not been previously demonstrated or to assess, in multivessel disease, the significance of each individual lesion. In this both scenarios, the latest ESC 2018 revascularization guide mentions that when evidence of ischemia is not available, FFR or iFR (instantaneous wave-free ratio) are recommended to assess the intermediate-grade lesions with a I A recommendation and that FFR-guided PCI in multivessel disease undergoing PCI with a IIa B recomendation.

Coronary Angiography Complications

As any invasive procedure, coronary angiography has risk of complications. Nevertheless, the overall risk of major complications of the diagnostic procedure is around 1.5–2%, which is considered low. The risk of major complications in the case of intervention increases with respect to the diagnostic angiography. Higher incidence of complications has been described in the presence of: advanced age, diabetes mellitus, acute renal failure, shock and left ventricular dysfunction. More frequently major complications in diagnostic coronary angiography are detailed in Table 6.

Table 6 Major complications in diagnostic coronary angiography

Major complication	Incidence (%)	Comment
Death	0.1	Increased risk in clinical instability and urgent procedures (acute myocardial infarction, shock, etc.)
Acute myocardial infarction	0.05	Rare cases of coronary dissection because of contrast injection or catheter lesion
Stroke	0.07	Manly embolic aetiology. Some cases of haemorrhagic events due to necessary heparinization during angiography, especially in patients with uncontrolled hypertension during the procedure
Arrythmia	0.38	Atrial fibrilation or Atrial Flutter that usually disappear in the 2–3 h after angiography. Ventricular Tachicardia or Fibrilation very rare in the setting of diagnostica procedure
Iodinated contrast reactions	0.37	Allergy or contrast induced nephropathy
Hemodynamical instability	0.26	Most frequent vagal induced hypotension. Other situations may include volume overload or shock
Cardiac perforation	0.03	It could be resolved with intracoronary balloon prolonged inflation, implantation of a coated stent or with coils. It may require heparin reversal with protamine and urgent pericardiocentesis. First treatment option is percutaneous but surgical repair may be indicated
Other major complications	0.28	Highlighting the cholesterol crystals systemic embolization (0.15% of coronary angiography)

References

1. Grossman's cardiac catheterization, angiography and intervention. Seventh edition. 2005.
2. Neumann F-J, et al. 2018 ESC/EACTS Guidelines on myocardial revascularization. Eur Heart J. 2019;40(2):87–165.
3. Alfonso F, Botas J (editors). Intracoronary dianostic techniques. Madrid. McGraw-Hill Interamericana; 2003.
4. Li X et al. Intravascular photoacoustic imaging at 35 and 80 MHz. J Bioned Opt 2012;17 (10):106005.
5. Prati F et al. Expert's OCT Review Document. Expert review document part 2: methodology, terminology and clinical applications of optical coherence tomography for the assessment of international procedures, Eur Heart J 2012;33(20): 2513–20.
6. De Bruyne B et al. FAME 2 Trial Investigators. Fractional flow reserved-guided PCI versus medical therapy in stable coronary disease. N Engl J Med 2012;367(11):991–1001.
7. Tonino PAL et al. FAME trial investigators. Fractional flow reserve versus angiography for guiding percutaneous coronary intervention. N Engl J Med 2009;360:213–24.
8. Johnson, LW, Lozner EC, Johnson S, et al. Coronary arteriography 1984–1987: a report of registry of Society for Cardiac Angiography and Interventions. I. Results and complications. Cathet Cardiovasc Diagn 1989;17:5–10
9. Tommaso CL. Contrast-induced nephrotoxicity in patients undergoing cardiac catheterization. Cathet Cardiovasc Diagn. 1994;31:316–21.

Transesophageal Echocardiography

Massimiliano Meineri and Asad Mashari

Introduction

From its introduction into clinical practice in the early seventies using monoplane probes to the development of real three-dimensional (3D) imaging technology, transesophageal echocardiography (TEE) (Fig. 1) has gain a key role in the perioperative and acute care settings. The decreased in cost of TEE probes, the availability of single used ones and the increased availability of portable more affordable Ultrasound (US) systems has contributed to the spread of this imaging modality outside Cardiology and Cardiac Anesthesia. Nevertheless, the availability of image storage systems and expertise among anesthesiology and critical care physicians still constitutes the main burden for further spread of this imaging modality.

TEE (Figs. 2 and 3) has become standard of care in the intraoperative management of patients undergoing cardiac surgical procedures. In the hand of cardiac anesthesiologists, it is used to confirm indication, to guide surgical and catheter-based intervention, to assess results and to monitor hemodynamics [1, 2]. This requires advanced TEE competences, typically acquired through a Cardiac anesthesia fellowship and subsequent Board Certification and imply performing a comprehensive intraoperative examination. A simplified TEE examination has also

M. Meineri (✉) · A. Mashari
Professor of Anesthesiology, University of Toronto, Toronto, ON, Canada
e-mail: Massimiliano.Meineri@medizin.uni-liepzig.de

A. Mashari
e-mail: Azad.Mashari@uhn.ca

M. Meineri
Co-Chair Department of Anesthesia, Herzzentrum Leipzig, Struempell Strasse 39, 04289 Leipzig, Germany

A. Mashari
Director API, Staff Anesthesiologist Toronto General Hospital, 200 Elizabeth Street EN3, Toronto, ON M5G 2C4, Canada

M. Vives and A. Hernandez (eds.), *Cardiac Anesthesia and Postoperative Care in the 21st Century*, https://doi.org/10.1007/978-3-030-79721-8_7

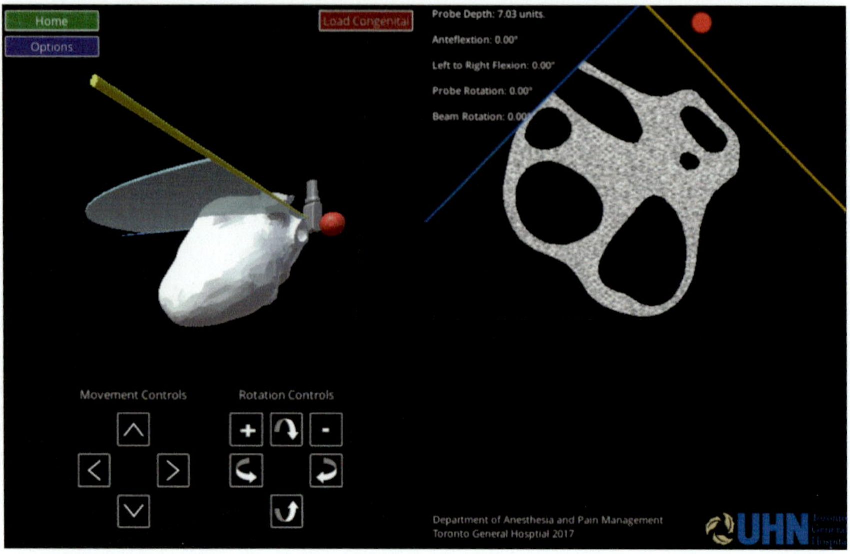

Fig. 1 On-line TEE simulator displaying (on the left) a 3D rendering of the TEE probe head, the ultrasound scanning plane and the heart. On the right is a simulation of the ultrasound imaging. (https://apil.ca/echocardiography-simulator/)

been defined to be used outside of cardiac surgery as a "basic" TEE examination [3] (Fig. 1) to define gross structural and functional cardiac abnormalities and provide hemodynamic monitoring. Furthermore, Focused TEE, including only five views, has been successfully introduced in emergency medicine as an effective tool to answer dichotomous questions and guide treatment in hemodynamically unstable patients [4]. Each application of TEE in the intraoperative or acute care setting mandate clear definition of scope of practice that include indication, imaging protocol, training pathway and quality assurance. In this chapter we will provide a practical overview of intraoperative Advanced and Basic TEE for novices.

Probe Manipulation and Standard Views

The TEE probe has been developed by integrating a single line of piezoelectric crystals on the tip of a gastroscope. The TEE probe head is a phased array that generated a single 2D pie-shaped US scanning plane, similarly to transthoracic echocardiography (Fig. 2). Different TEE scanning planes were obtained by rotating the probe right and left, withdrawing and advancing the probe in the esophagus. The probe's tip can be anteflexed, retroflexed, bent right and left bending, through the knobs of a gastroscope. TEE probes also allow to rotate the scanning plane clockwise (if facing the probe) by increments of one degree from 0

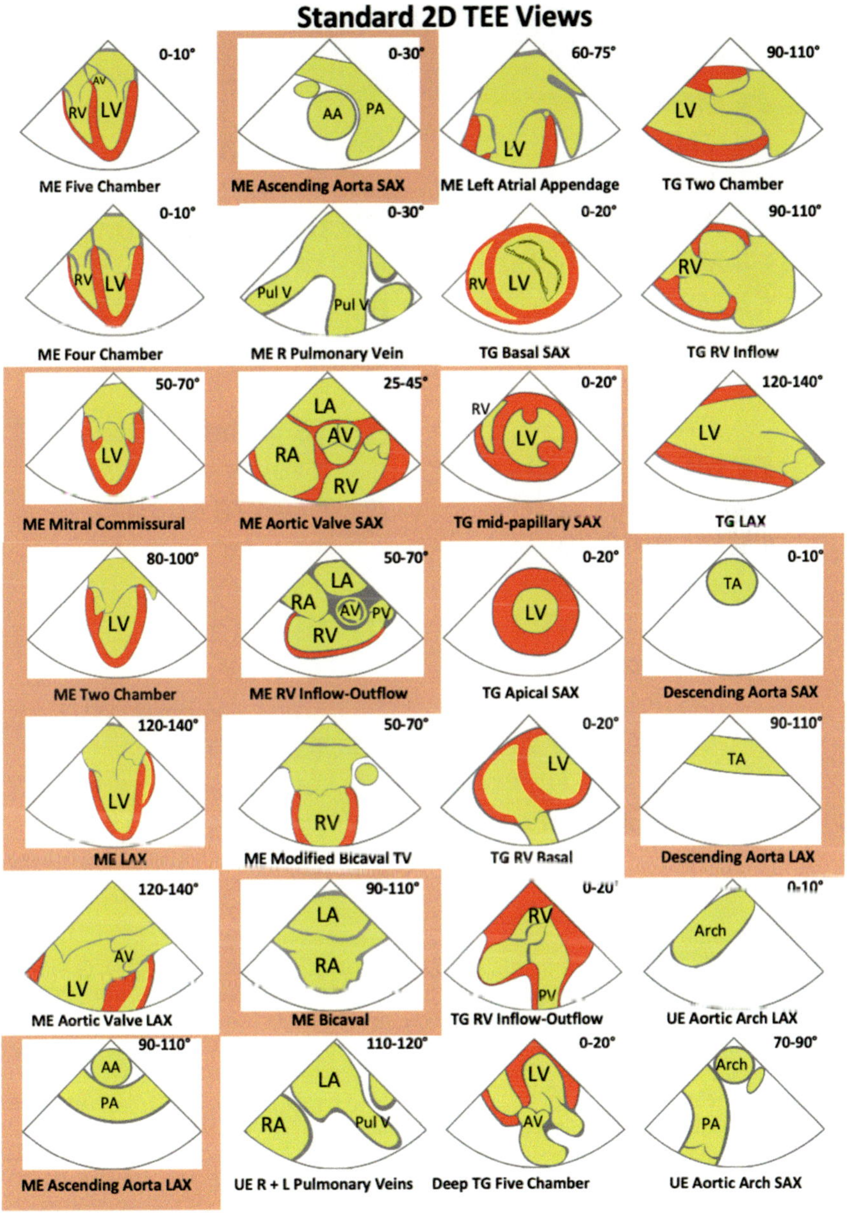

Fig. 2 28 Standard TEE View. The 11 Basic views are highlighted. ME: Mid Esophageal; UE: Upper esophageal; TG: Trans gastric; SAX: Short Axis; LAX: long Axis; LV: Left Ventricle; RV: Right Ventricle; AV: Aortic Valve; AA: Ascending Aorta; PA: Pulmonary Artery; Pul V: Pulmonary vein; LA: Left Atrium; RA: Right Atrium; PV: Pulmonic Valve; TA: Thoracic Aorta; TV: Tricuspid Valve; Arch: Aortic Arch

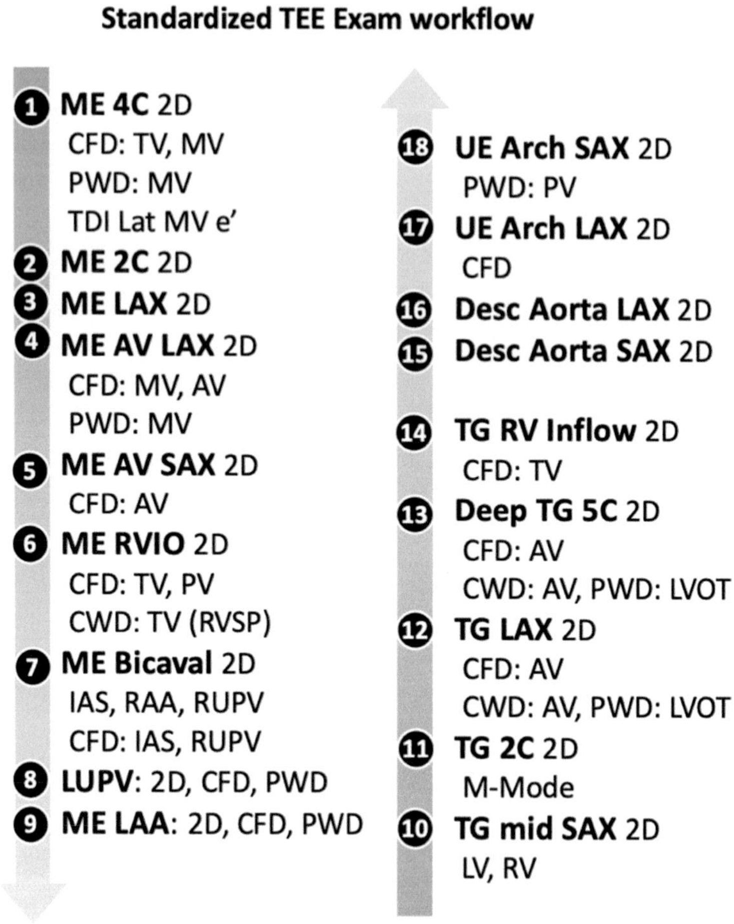

Fig. 3 TEE examination workflow. ME: Mid Esophageal; 4C: Four chambers; CFD: Color Flow Doppler; PWD: Pulsed Wave Doppler; TDI: Tissue Doppler; Lat: Lateral; E′: E′wave; 2C: Two Chambers; RVIO: Right Ventricle Inflow-outflow; RVSP: Right Ventricular Systolic pressure; CWD: Continuous Wave Doppler; IAS: Interatrial Septum; RAA: Right Atrial Appendage; RUPV: Right Upper Pulmonary Vein; LUPV: Left Upper Pulmonary Vein; LAA: Left Atrial Appendage; Arch: Aortic Arch; Desc: Descending; 5C: Five Chambers; LVOT: Left Ventricular Outflow Tract; UE: Upper esophageal; TG: Trans gastric; SAX: Short Axis; LAX: long Axis; LV: Left Ventricle; RV: Right Ventricle; AV: Aortic Valve; AA: Ascending Aorta; PA: Pulmonary Artery; LA: Left Atrium; RA: Right Atrium; PV: Pulmonic Valve; Aorta; MV: Mitral Valve; TV: Tricuspid Valve

to 180°, where 180° would be a mirror image of 0. A single line of 64–128 Ultrasound crystals is rotated by an eclectically powered motor. Modern TEE probes utilize Matrix arrays where the piezoelectric crystals are organized in a checkerboard of 50 by 50 micro elements in less than a centimeter square. Matrix arrays can generate a single or simultaneous two-dimensional US scanning planes.

The scanning planes are rotated electronically by activating different lines of crystals without any mechanically moving parts. These probes also generate real-time 3D images.

The TEE probe is introduced into the esophagus and advanced to the stomach. Through this path the probe's tip can be moved from the aortic arch to the apex of the left ventricle (LV).

Images of the heart are obtained at four levels: upper-esophageal (above the aortic valve), mid-esophageal (at the level of the left atrium), trans-gastric (in the stomach), deep trans-gastric (at the level of the LV apex). At any given level right and left rotation, as well as change in the scanning plane angle allows to obtain infinite cuts of the heart. Three basic movements (insert/withdraw, turn right/left and angle change) with anteflexion when the probe is advanced into the stomach allow navigation through all of the standard views (Fig. 4). In order to set a standardization and comparison between studies a number of standard cutting planes have been defined for a complete TEE exam [2]. A comprehensive exam includes 28 scanning planes, a basic 11 [3] and a focused 5 (Fig. 1).

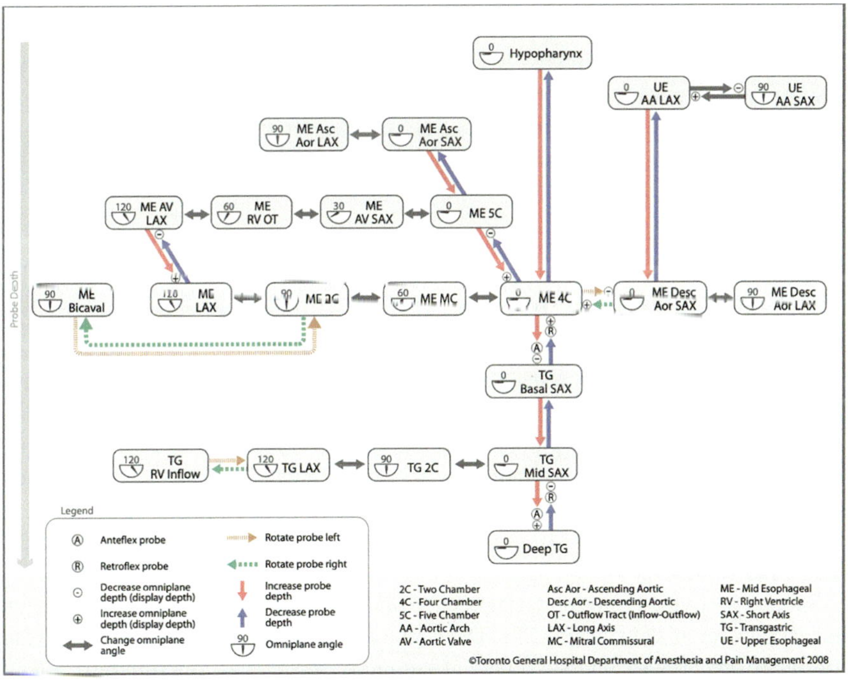

Fig. 4 Navigation between view (www.pie.med.utoronto.ca)

Safety and Indications

Although routinely performed, intraoperative TEE is relatively invasive and carries a risk of overall complication of 0.2%. The majorities of reported complications are mechanical and are related to the introduction and the manipulation of the probe. The most feared one is an esophageal perforation, that occurs between 0 and 0.3% of cases and carries a very high morbidity and mortality. Other complications include: dental damage, oral bleeding, endotracheal tube displacement, postoperative dysphagia and dysphonia. Absolute contraindications for TEE are: perforated viscus, esophageal strictures/perforation/tumor/diverticulum and active esophageal bleed. Hiatus hernia, esophageal/gastric surgery, esophagitis, coagulopathy are considered only relative contraindications [2].

The indication for an intraoperative TEE exam [2] varies depending on the type of exam. According to the American guidelines, a comprehensive intraoperative TEE exam is indicated in all types of open-heart surgeries, in some coronary artery bypass surgeries and in non-cardiac surgery when the patient is known to have cardiac pathology. TEE is also indicated when TTE to guide transcatheter cardiac interventional procedures such as interatrial septal and left atrial appendage closures, valve implantation and clipping. Basic TEE exam is indicated on a case-to-case base to qualitatively assess left ventricular function, wall motion abnormalities, right ventricular function, pulmonary embolism, pericardial effusion, thoracic trauma, gross valvular abnormalities and air in course of neurosurgical procedures [3]. TEE is finally indicated outside the operating room whenever transthoracic echocardiography provided suboptimal images.

Left Ventricular Function

Assessment of LV function remains one of the most common indications for the use of TEE in and outside the operating room. Assessment of LV includes assessment of LV morphology, size, global and regional systolic and diastolic function. Assessment of diastolic dysfunction by TEE is complex and has at the moment minimal impact in clinical decision making in the operating room therefore will be omitted in this chapter. The LV has a grossly oval shape that can be simplified to the geometrical shape of an ellipsoid. It has four walls: anterior, inferior, septal and lateral and is divided into three segments from the base to the apex (basal, mid and apical) plus an apical cap (Fig. 5). The septal and lateral segments at the basal and mid-level are further divided into antero/infero septal and antero/infero lateral. These altogether with the apical cap constitute the 17 segments. For a full assessment of wall motion abnormality all 17 segments must be evaluated. This requires a minimum of three TEE views: mid esophageal four chamber (ME4C), mid esophageal two chamber (ME2C) and mid esophageal long axis (MELAX) [5].

Left Ventricle Anatomy and Views

- ❑ **LV Function**
  - o Systolic: Global, Regional
- ❑ **LV Dimensions**
  - o EDD, ESD
  - o Wall thickness
- ❑ **Associated**
  - o MV annulus size
  - o MR
  - o LA size
  - o AV/LVOT cardiac output

LV Systolic Function	Abnormal
Ejection Fraction	< 55%
Mild	40-49%
Moderate	30-39%
Severe	<30%
S' velocity MV annulus	< 5cm/s
GL strain	< -20%
No longer recommended: Fractional Shortening (<25%) Fractional Area Change (<40%)	

LV Anatomy Normal

- Geometric shape ellipse
- Inlet, apex, outlet
- 17 segment model
- TG and ME views
- TG views measure size
- Examine wall motion and thickening

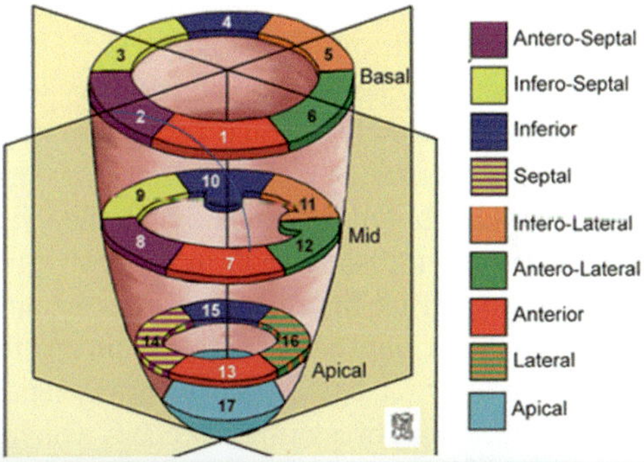

LV Views

- ME 4C
- ME 2C
- ME LAX
- TG Basal SAX
- TG Mid SAX
- TG Apical SAX
- TG 2C
- TG LAX
- TG deep 5C

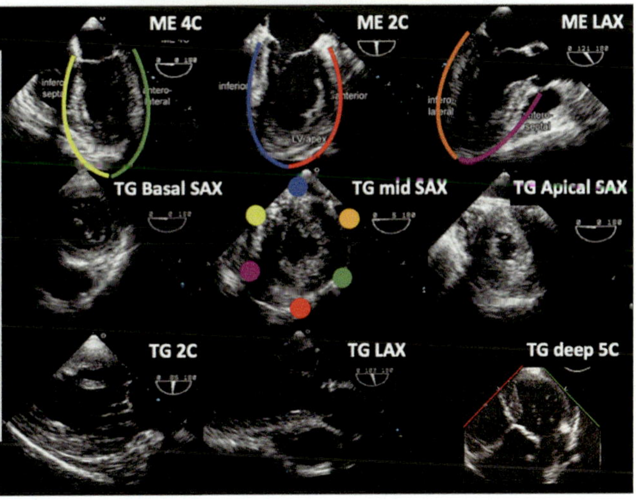

Fig. 5 Left Ventricular Anatomy and Views. LV: Left Ventricle; EDD: End Diastolic Diameter; ESD: End Systolic Diameter; MV: Mitral Valve; MR: Mitral Regurgitation; LA: Left Atrium; AV: Aortic Valve; LVOT: Left Ventricular Outflow Tract; S': S' Doppler Wave; GL: Global Longitudinal; ME: Mid-Esophageal; TG: Trans Gastric; 4C: Four Chambers; 2C: Two Chambers; SAX: Short Axis; LAX: Long Axis; 5C: Five Chambers

It is important to optimize each of these views to make the endocardium and the epicardium visible to assess myocardial contractility and cut through the true apex of the heart to avoid LV foreshortening. The LV contraction results in the displacement of the mitral valve (MV) and the base towards the apex therefore the latter remain relatively still. Movement of the apex means that the view is cutting through the lateral wall and not the real apex therefore resulting in foreshortening of the LV chamber. For each segment we need to assess systolic thickening of the myocardium resulting in displacement of the endocardium towards the center of the ventricle. Reduced thickening in comparison to adjacent segment is defined as hypokinesis, lack of movement as akinesia and outward movement as dyskinesia. New onset of hypo/akinesia typically represent coronary ischemia. Each of the mid-esophageal views only allow assessment of two coronary territories at each time. The trans-gastric midpapillary short axis view (TG mid SAX) displays all three coronary territories at the mid papillary level at the same time. For this reason, this view is the view of choice for monitoring myocardial ischemia. Automatic endocardial detection and speckle tracking strain further enhance the ability to assess wall motion abnormalities by simple eyeballing.

LV diameter is measured in the trans-gastric long axis view (TG LAX) at the level of the papillary muscle tips. Normal values are approximately <5 cm. LV thickness is measured in the TG mid SAX at the septum and the inferolateral walls, normal values are approximately <1 cm. LV chamber dilatation and hypertrophy (thickness > 1) are always the result of a chronic process which etiology should be identified.

Quantification of LV function (Fig. 6) relies on measurement of ejection fraction (EF). EF is the ratio of LV stroke volume (SV) and LV end diastolic volume (EDV). In order to estimate volumes from 2D LV cuts we use two perpendicular views (ME 4C and ME 2C) and assume the LV is a stack of disks constituting an ellipsoid. Modern echocardiographic system simply require manual tracing of the endocardium in systole and diastole in these two views and the LV volume is automatically calculated. Speckle tracking technology further simplifies this process by automatically identifying the blood-tissue interface. As previously mentioned, the LV systolic contraction results in the displacement of the MV towards the apex of the heart. The velocity of systolic displacement of the MV annulus is directly related to the strength of LV contraction. Tissue doppler is a technology that uses the Doppler signal to quantify the movement of the cardiac tissues. In the ME 4C the velocity of displacement of the lateral MV annulus can be measured and provides a reliable estimation of global LV function.

Finally, speckle tracking strain is a semi-automated technology that allows following the grey speckles within the myocardium to quantify their movement in respect to each-others. When we follow the movement of two speckles at the proximal and at the distal end of each LV segment in any mid-esophageal view, we can detect the shortening of the longitudinal myocardial fibers. In systole the base of the heart moves towards the apex and the longitudinal fibers shorten resulting in a negative strain value that can also be expressed as an absolute percentage. Different strain values for adjacent LV segments would detect wall motion abnormalities while the average longitudinal strain (global longitudinal strain) correlates with LVEF.

Left Ventricle Size and Systolic Function

LV Size	Female				Male			
Diameter Index (diameter/BSA)	Refer. range	Mild	Moderate	Severe	Refer. range	Mild	Mod	Severe
Diastole, cm	3.8-5.2	5.3-5.6	5.7-6.1	**> 6.2**	4.2-5.8	5.9-6.3	6.4-6.8	**> 6.8**
Diastole index, cm/m²	2.2-3.1	3.2-3.4	3.5-3.7	**> 3.7**	2.2-3.0	3.1-3.3	3.4-3.6	**> 3.6**
Systole, cm	2.2-3.5	3.6-3.8	3.9-4.1	**> 4.1**	2.5-4.0	4.1-4.3	4.4-4.5	**> 4.5**
Systole index, cm/m²	1.3-2.1	2.2-2.3	2.4-2.6	**> 2.6**	1.3-2.1	2.2-2.3	2.4-2.5	**> 2.5**
LV volume								
Diastolic, mL	46-106	107-120	121-130	**> 130**	62-150	151-174	175-200	**> 200**
Diastolic index, mL/m²	29-61	62-70	71-80	**> 80**	34-74	75-89	90-100	**> 100**
Systolic, mL	14-42	43-55	56-67	**> 67**	21-61	62-73	74-85	**> 85**
Systolic index, mL/m²	8-24	25-32	33-40	**> 40**	11-31	32-38	39-45	**> 45**

Simpson's (EF)
- o Acquire 2D ME 4C + 2C
  - Increase gain to highlight endocardial border
- o Use software to trace endocardial border in S and D
  - Identify LV apex
  - Exclude papillary muscles
- o Obtain EDV, ESV, stroke volume, EF

Speckle Tracking (EF)
- o Acquire 2D ME 4C + 2C, FR > 50Hz, similar HR
  - Increase gain to highlight endocardial border
- o Use software (2DQ)
  - Identify MV annular and LV apex points
- o Software automatically tracks, edit if needed
- o Obtain EDV, ESV, stroke volume, EF

S' velocity MV lateral annulus
- o ME 4C use TDI pre-set
- o Narrow sector, TDI color to identify myocardium
- o PW Doppler on myocardium below annulus
- o Obtain spectral trace and measure S' velocity

Global Longitudinal Strain (GLS)
- o Acquire 2D ME views (4C, 2C, LAX)
- o Open CMQ software
- o Position points at mitral annulus + LV apex
- o Software automatically tracks, edit if needed
- o Display bull's eye for regional and GLS

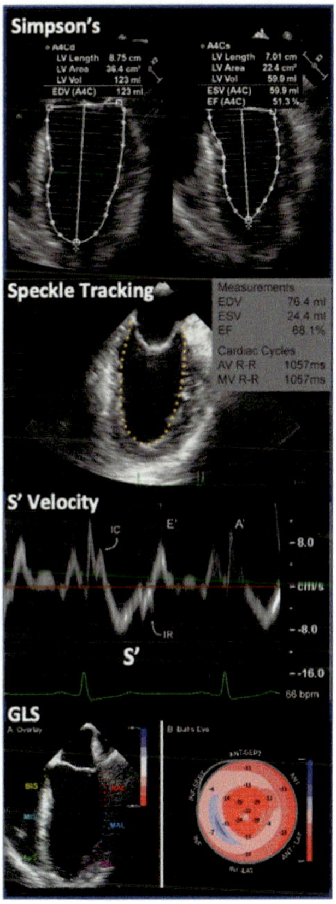

Fig. 6 Left Ventricular Size and Sunction. BSA: Body Surface Area; LV: Left Ventricle; EF: Ejection Fraction; ME: Mid-Esophageal; 4C: Four Chambers; 2C: Two Chambers; LAX: Long Axis; MV: Mitral Valve; EDV: End Distolic Volume; ESV: End Systolic Volume; GLS: Global Longitudinal Strain

Right Ventricular Function

The right ventricle (RV) (Fig. 7) wraps anteriorly around the conical LV. Its shape is irregular: triangular in the coronal plane (ME 4C) and a crescent in the transverse plane (TG mid SAX). Typical anatomical features of the RV are: the attachment of the septal leaflet of the tricuspid valve (TV), presence of a muscle bundle across the apex (moderator band) outflow into the pulmonary artery (PA).

It comprises three portions: the inflow under the tricuspid valve (TV), the apex and the outflow under the pulmonic valve (PV). In the ME 4C the RV appears smaller than the LV and the cardiac apex belongs to the LV. In case of moderate dilatation the RV is as big as the LV and bigger then the LV in case of severe dilatation. The RV diameter is measured at mid ventricle in the ME 4C view. The RV is the only chamber of the heart that can dilate as a result of an acute process. To distinguish between acute and chronic dilatation we need to evaluate right ventricular wall thickness and right atrial (RA) size. RV hypertrophy (thickness in ME 4C, one cm below the TV > 5 mm) and RA dilatation (RA bigger than left atrium) indicate a chronic process. RV dilatation can also be observed in the TG mid SAX where dilatation of the RV would result into flattening of the interventricular septum. Flattening of the septum can occur only in one phase of the cardiac cycle. Systolic flattening would indicate pressure overload (e.g. pulmonary hypertension, PV stenosis or pulmonary embolism), diastolic flattening volume overload (PV insufficiency).

RV contraction results in a displacement of the TV annulus towards the apex, inward movement of the RV free wall and contraction of the outflow. While RV EF can only be measured using 3D TEE, RV function is typically quantified on partial measures such as the displacement of the TV annulus or the percentage change of the coronal plane (Fig. 8) [5].

Tricuspid annular plane systolic excursion (TAPSE) measures the displacement of the lateral TV annul towards the apex in systole. It is measured in the ME 4C using anatomical M Mode (not available on all echo systems) and positioning the M Mode cursor along the RV free wall through the RV apex. Normal values are >1.7 mm. RV fractional area change (FAC) is also measured in the ME 4C by tracing the RV endocardium in end systole and end diastole. Speckle tracking technology allow to trach the myocardial speckles in the free wall of the RV and determine the percentage of shortening of the Myocardial fibers along the RV free wall. Similar to the LV, we observe a shortening of the myocardial fibers in Systole that result in a negative strain value. RV free wall strain seems to allow a more sensitive quantification of RV function. All the above measures of RV function only provide a qualitative assessment that allow classification into normal and abnormal.

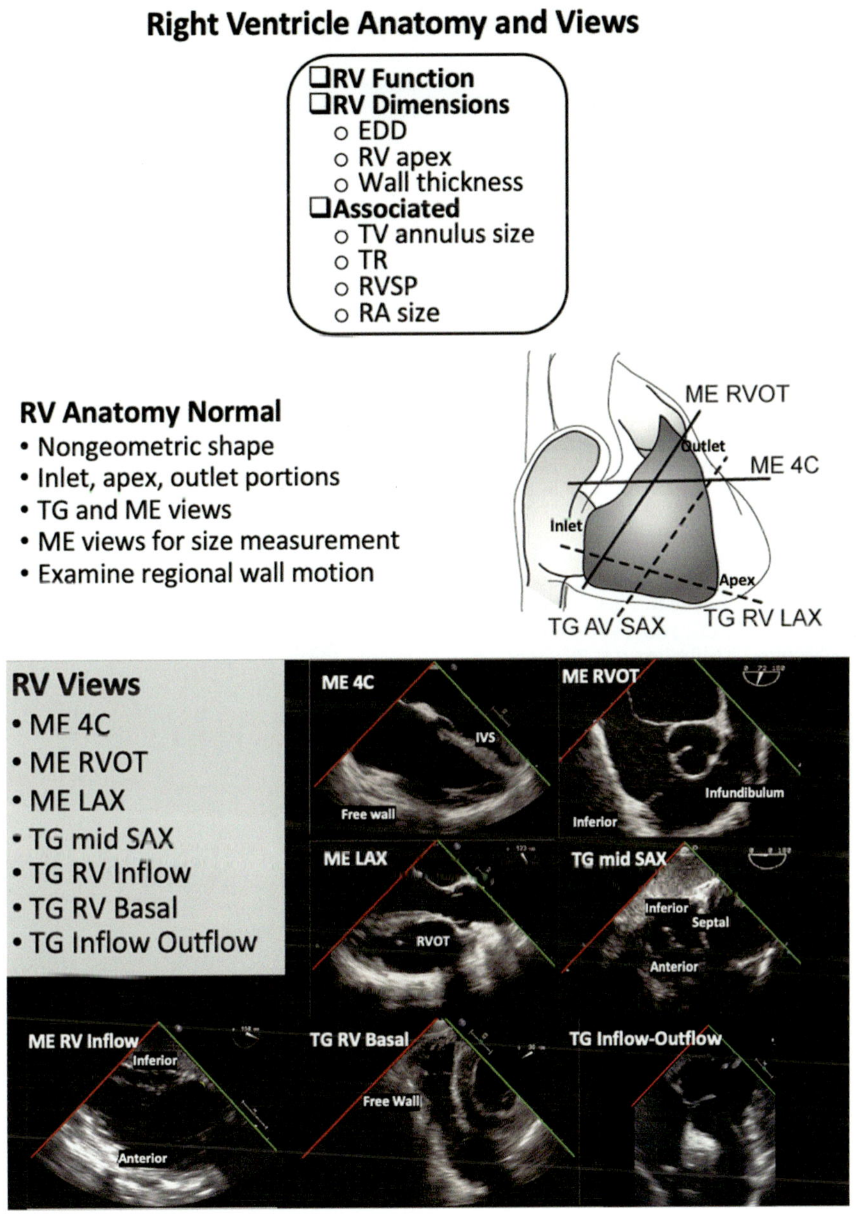

Fig. 7 Right Ventricular Anatomy and Views. RV: Right Ventricle; EDD: End Diastolic Diameter; TV: Tricuspid Valve; TR: Tricuspid Regurgitation; RVSP: Right Ventricular Systolic Pressure; RA: Right Atrium; ME: Mid Esophageal; TG: Trans Gastric; 4C: Four Chambers; RVOT: Right Ventricle Inflow outflow; LAX; Long Axis, SAX: Short Axis; AV: Aortic Valve

Right Ventricle Function and Size

Parameter [Ref 2]	Abnormal
FAC	< 35%
TAPSE	< 17 mm
S' Velocity TV annulus	< 9.5 cm/s
GLS Free Wall	< -20

Measures (mm)	Abnormal
EDD Basal (ME 4C)	> 42
EDD Mid (ME 4C)	> 35
Wall Thickness (TG)	> 5

Fractional Area Change (FAC)

- Acquire 2D ME 4C rotate to show RV
  - Increase gain (endocardium)
  - Retroflex (RV apex)
- Trace endocardial border to TV annulus in S + D
  - Exclude papillary muscles
  - Obtain ED and ES areas
- Calculate **FAC = EDA – ESA / EDA**

Speckle Tracking FAC

- Acquire 2D ME 4C view of RV as above
- Use software (2DQ)
  - Change to area from volume measurement
  - Mark points TV annulus + RV apex
- Software tracks RV area, display FAC
  - Edit if needed to track endocardium

Tricuspid Annular Plane Systolic Excursion (TAPSE)

- Acquire 2D ME 4C view of RV
  - Narrow sector size to TV lateral annulus
- Activate m-mode sample line
  - Align parallel to annular movement
  - Use anatomic m-mode (if available)
- Measure TAPSE
  - Identify similar lower + upper portions

Global Longitudinal Strain (GLS) Free Wall

- Acquire ME 4C 2D view of RV
- Activate CMQ pre-set
  - Mark points TV annulus + RV apex
- Software automatically tracks, edit if needed
  - Obtain GLS that includes IVS
  - Edit to eliminate the IVS for GLS free wall

S' Velocity TV lateral annulus

- TG RV LAX as difficult alignment in ME 4C
- Activate TDI
  - Use TDI color to identify myocardium
- PW Doppler
  - Sample volume on myocardium parallel to motion
- Obtain spectral trace
- Measure S' velocity

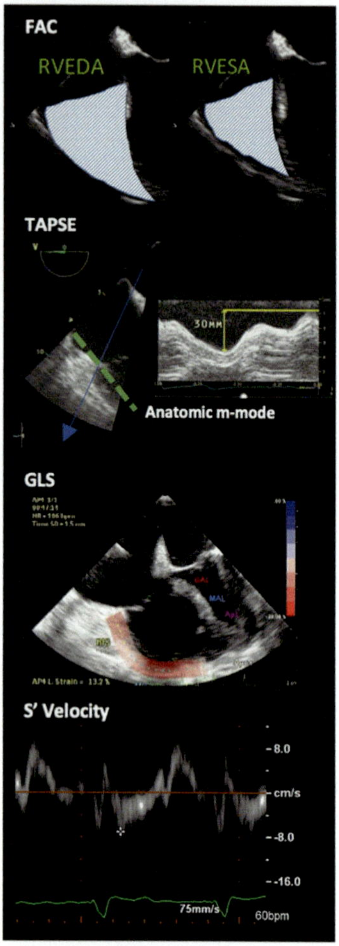

Fig. 8 Right Ventricular Function and Size. RV: Right Ventricle; FAC: Fractional Area Change; TAPSE: Tricuspid Valve Annular Plane Systolic Excursion; S': S' Doppler wave; TV: Tricuspid Valve; GLS: Global Lungitudinal Strain; ME: Mid Esophageal; 4C: Four Chambers; EDA: End Diastolic Area; ESA: End Systolic Area; TG: Trans Gastric; LAX: long Axis; TDI: Tissue Doppler

Aortic Valve

The aortic valve (AV) (Fig. 9) comprises three cusps that correspond to the three sinuses: left, right and non-coronary. The most anterior cusp is the right which explains the risk of right coronary air embolism in a supine patient. The non-coronary cusp is adjacent to the interatrial septum and the left in between. The AV annulus is in close proximity to the posterior MV and to the anterior PV annulus. The PV annulus is rotated 90 degrees in respect to the AV therefore when one is displayed in its short axis the other is in the long axis and vice versa. The only exception is transposition of the great arteries when these valves are on the same plan. The AV functions within a complex of structures that includes: the left ventricular outflow tract, the AV annulus, the AV cusps, the aortic sinuses and the sino-tubular junction (STJ). Alteration of any of these structures would result in AV pathology. Assessment of the AV involves measurement of AV size, leaflet morphology, leaflet function and flow across the valve. The mid-esophageal AV long axis view (ME AV LAX) is the best view to assess leaflet morphology and for measurements. The LVOT and AV annulus should be measured in mid Systole while the aortic sinuses and STJ at end diastole. In the ME AV LAX the more distal, lower cusp is invariably the right while the upper cusp can be the non or the left. In order to obtain the widest AV annular diameter slight movement right and left would allow to cut in the commissure between the non and the left cusps that can be identified by poor definition of the upper cusp. Aortic cusp calcification is typical of degenerative aortic stenosis (AS) it appears as hyperechoic bright cusps that cast a dark shadow and have limited movement. By subtracting 90 degree to the scanning plane of ME AV LAX we can obtain a short axis view of the AV in the mid-esophageal AV short axis view (ME AV SAX) which displays all three cusps and allows tracing the AV opening in systole to estimate aortic valve area. This measure is though not very precise due to the geometry of the AV opening therefore does not constitute the gold standard.

The AV flow cannot be measured in the middle-esophageal views because it is perpendicular to the ultrasound (US) beam therefore, we can only use qualitative color flow Doppler (CFD) assessment. In order to position the Doppler beam though the LVOT and the AV we need to advance the probe in the stomach [6]. CFD is used to quantify the degree of aortic insufficiency (AI) [7] by measuring the width of the regurgitant jet right below the AV (Vena Contracta) which is also further compared to the LVOT diameter. The deep trans-gastric 5 chamber view (DTG) is obtain by advancing the probe deep in the stomach and apply anteflexion. Alternatively, the trans gastric log axis view can be used. It typically allows the best alignment of the doppler beam with the blood flow through the AV. Continuous wave Doppler (CW) is used to assess the flow through the AV and pulse wave Doppler to assess the flow though the LVOT. Based on the principle of conservation of mass the same SV flows through each portion of the heart therefore the SV in the LVOT be the same as through the AV. The SV is the cylinder of blood which base is the LVOT cross-sectional area and the height is the velocity time

Aortic Valve

- **ME AV LAX** 2D
  - Valve morphology
  - CFD AV + LVOT
  - Root Measurements
- **ME AV SAX** 2D
  - Valve morphology
  - CFD
- **Deep TG 5C/TG LAX** 2D
  - CFD
  - PWD LVOT
  - CWD AV
- **Aorta Desc/Asc** 2D
  - CFD
  - PWD

Aortic Measurements

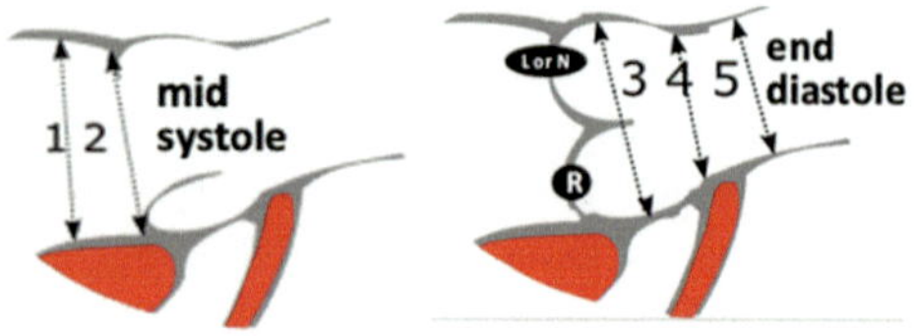

1. LVOT 2. AV Annulus 3. SOV 4. STJ 5. Ascending aorta	**ME AV LAX view** For accurate measure of AV annulus turn probe so upper cusp is not seen, for Asc Ao withdraw probe + decrease angle 110°

Aortic Stenosis

- ❑ **Mechanism** (2D SAX/LAX)
  - Sub/valve/supra: 2D, CFD
- ❑ **Severity**
  - Velocity peak, PG mean
  - AVA: $VTI_{lvot} \times 0.785 D_{lvot}^2 / VTI_{AV}$
  - VR: $Vmax_{lvot} / Vmax_{AV}$
  - DI: VTI_{lvot} / VTI_{AV}
  - Low flow/low gradient AS
  - Planimetry: 2D
- ❑ **Associated**
  - LV: LVH, function, SAM
  - MV pathology, MR
  - Aorta path (aneurysm, coarct)
  - Diastolic dysfunction
  - PHTN, TR

AS Severity	Mild	Mod	Severe
Velocity peak (m/s)	2.6-2.9	3.0-4.0	>4.0
PG mean (mmHg)	<20	20-40	>40
AVA (cm^2)	1.5-2.0	1.0-1.5	<1.0*
VR or DI	>0.50	0.25-0.50	<0.25

VR, velocity ratio; DI, dimensionless index
* AVA indexed < 0.6cm^2/m^2
- Low flow AS (low EF) or low gradient AS (normal EF): AVA ≤1cm^2, Vel peak <4m/s, PG mean <40mmHg
  - If low EF → Dobutamine echo
  - If normal EF → Stroke volume index (SVI) <35cc/m^2

Aortic Insufficiency

- ❑ **Mechanism** (2D SAX/LAX)
  - Valve
  - Aorta
  - Jet direction
- ❑ **Severity**
  - PHT CWD
  - Vena Contracta: 2D,
  - Jet width/LVOT
  - Desc Ao flow reversal
  - Reg Volume, Reg Fraction
  - EROA: 2D
- ❑ **Associated**
  - LV: size, function
  - MV flutter, closure

AI Severity	Mild	Mod	Severe
Jet Width (%LVOT)	<25	25-65	>65
Vena Contracta (mm)	3	3-6	>6
PHT (ms)	>500	200-500	<200
Reg Volume (cc/beat)	30	30-60	>60
Reg Fraction (%)	<30	30-50	>50
EROA (cm^2)	<0.10	0.10-0.30	>0.30

Reg Volume = LV SV – MV SV = $(CSA_{LVOT} \times VTI_{LVOT}) - (CSA_{MV} \times VTI_{MV})$
Reg Fraction = Reg Volume/MV SV
EROA: PISA = $\frac{2\pi r^2 \times \alpha\ angle/180 \times Valias}{V\ peak\ AI}$ or = $\frac{Reg\ Volume}{VTI\ AI}$

Fig. 9 Assessment of the Aortic Valve. ME: Mid Esophageal; AV: Aortic Valve; SAX: Short axis, LAX: Long Axis; CFD: Color Flow Doppler; LVOT: Left Ventricular Outflow Tract; SAX: Short Axis; TG: Transgastric; 5C: Five Chambers; PWD: Pulsed Wave Doppler, CWD: Continuous Wave Doppler; Desc: Descending; Asc: Ascending; AVA: Aortic Valve Area; VR: Velocity Ratio; VTI: Velocity Time Integral; LV: Left Ventricle; LVH: Left Ventricular Hypentrophy; MV: Mitral Valve; MR: Mitral Regurgitation; SAM: Systolic Anterior Motion; PHTH: Pulmonary Hypertension; TR: Tricuspid Regurgitation; PHT: Pressure Half Time; EROA: Effective Regurgitant Orifice Area; DI: Dimensionless Index; AS: Aortic Stenosis; AI: Aortic Insufficiency; Reg: Regurgitation; V: Velocity; PISA: Proximal Isovelocity Surface Area

integral (VTI), which is automatically calculated in cm by tracing the PW doppler trace at the LVOT level. If we obtain the AV VTI by tracing the CW AV velocity envelope, we can derive the AV area (AVA). We define this as the continuity equation, and it is suggested to be used to estimate AVA. Subtracting the SV measured through the MV to that measure in the LVOT allows computation of the AI regurgitant volume and fraction. In case of AI, CW would display the regurgitant diastolic flow. The steep of the AI regurgitant flow velocity in diastole is directly relates to the degree of AI and it is quantified using the Pressure half time. The most precise measurement of AI remains though the measurement of AV effective regurgitant orifice area (EROA). This can be calculated using proximal iso velocity surface area (PISA). This requires the CFD in the DTG and adjusting the lower velocity to approximately 30 cm/s. This will create a blue hemisphere above the AV. The radius of the hemisphere and the upper CFD velocity allows in central jets to precisely estimate the AV EROA.

Mitral Valve

The MV (Fig. 10) is located between the left atrium (LA) and the LV. It comprises two leaflets (anterior and posterior) and a saddle shaped annulus. According the Carpentier's nomenclature the leaflets are further divided into three scallops (P/A 1–3) where P1 is lateral and P3 medial. The mitral valve leaflets, the annulus, the chordae, the papillary muscles and the LV constitute the MV complex. Alteration of any of its components would result in MV regurgitation (MR). The MV is in a favorable location for US imaging, perpendicular to the US beam and proximal to the probe. Starting from ME 4C view with progressive increase of the scanning angle we can display all segments of both leaflets.

The mitral valve annulus antero-posterior diameter is normally smaller and is to be measured in diastole in ME LAX; the mediolateral in the mid esophageal mitral valve commissural view (ME MC).

MR is the commonest MV pathology in the developed world. It leads to volume overload resulting in LA and LV dilatation. Intraoperative TEE should aim at identifying the mechanism of regurgitation and precisely locating structural leaflet abnormalities. Assessment of MR severity is based on CFD and spectral Doppler measurements. A simple and reliable measurement is the Vena Contracta (VC), the width of the regurgitant jet at the narrowest point above the MV [7]. Given the lack of valves between the LA and the pulmonary vein (PV), the PV flow reflects the change in pressure in the LA. The blood normally flow from the PV into the LA but in case of severe MR the PV flow would be reversed in systole. Similarly to what previously described for the assessment of AI, PISA method can be applied to MV to estimate the size of the MR EROA. Knowing the EROA and multiplying it by the VTI from the tracing the CW spectral trace of the MR jet, the regurgitant Volume and fraction can be calculated. Mitral Valve stenosis (MS) is typically the consequence of Rheumatic fever. It leads to a thickening of the MV leaflets that

Mitral Valve

- **ME 4C** 2D
- **ME MC** 2D
- **ME 2C** 2D
- **ME AV LAX** 2D
- Zoom or reduce depth
- In any view assess
  - o Leaflet motion
  - o CFD (50-60cm/s)
  - o Annulus diameter
  - o PWD MV or CWD MR
- **LAA** 2D, CFD, PWD
- **RUPV/LUPV** CFD, PWD
- **ME Bicaval** 2D, CFD
- **TG Basal SAX** 2D, CFD
- **TG mid SAX** 2D
- **TG 2C** 2D **MV**

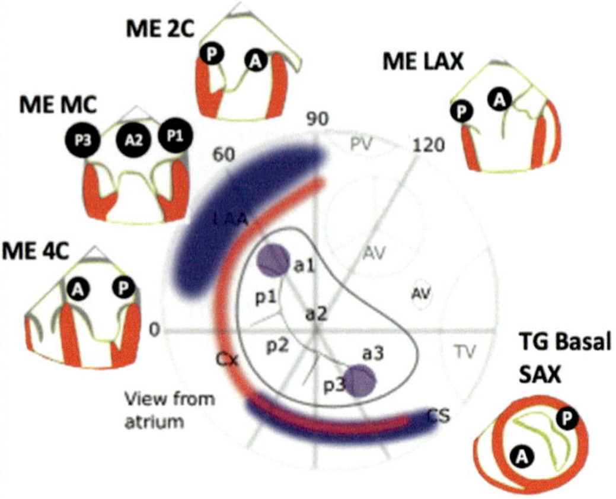

Mitral Stenosis
- ❑ **Mechanism**
  - o Rheumatic, calcific
- ❑ **Severity**
  - o PG mean
  - o MVA: planimetry, PHT, PISA
  - o PAP (RVSP)
- ❑ **Associated**
  - o LA size, SEC, thrombus
  - o PHTN, TR, RV dilated
  - o MR

MS Severity	Mild	Mod	Severe
MVA (cm^2)	>1.5	1.0-1.5	< 1.0
PG mean (mmHg)**	<5	5-10	>10
PAP (mmHg)	<30	30-50	>50

**HR dependent, values shown for HR 60-90, NSR

MVA: PISA = $\frac{2\pi r^2 \times \alpha \text{ angle}/180 \times \text{Valias}}{\text{V peak MS}}$ or = $\frac{220}{\text{PHT}}$

Mitral Regurgitation
- ❑ **Mechanism**
  - o Valve (1°)
  - o Functional (2°)
- ❑ **Severity**
  - o Vena Contracta: 2D,
  - o Flow Convergence (PISA)
  - o Pulmonary Vein Doppler
  - o Reg Volume, Reg Fraction
  - o EROA
  - o CWD: signal strength, shape
- ❑ **Associated**
  - o LV: size, function
  - o LA dilated
  - o TV annulus, TR

MR Severity	Mild	Mod	Severe
Jet Area	small	variable	large
Vena Contracta (mm)	3	3-6	≥7
Flow Convergence (cm)	<0.3	Inter	≥1.0
Pulmonary Vein	normal	blunt	reverse
Reg Volume (cc/beat)	30	30-59	≥60
Reg Fraction (%)	<30	30-49	≥50
EROA (cm^2)	<0.20	0.20-0.39	≥0.40

Reg Volume = LV stroke volume – AV SV or LVOT SV

Reg Fraction = Reg Volume/LV SV

EROA: PISA = $\frac{2\pi r^2 \times \alpha \text{ angle}/180 \times \text{Valias}}{\text{V peak MR}}$ or = $\frac{\text{Reg Volume}}{\text{VTI MR}}$

Fig. 10 Assessment of the Mitral Valve. ME: Mid Esophageal; 4C: Four Chambers; MC: Mitral Commissural; 2C: Two Chambers; AV: Aortic Valve; LAX Long Axis, TG: Transgastric; SAX: Short Axis. A: Anterior; P: Posterior; CFD: Color Flow Doppler; MV: Mitral Valve; MR: Mitral Regurgitation; MS: Mitral Stenosis; PWD: Pulsed Wave Doppler; CWD: Continuous Wave Doppler; LAA: Left Atrial Appendage; RUPV: Right Upper Pulmonary Vein; LUPV: Left Upper Pulmonary Vein; MVA: Mitral Valve Area; PHT: Pressure Half Time; PISA: Proximal Isovelocity Surface Area; PAP: Pulmonary Artery Pressure; RSVP: Right Ventricular Systolic Pressure; TR: Tricuspid Regurgitation, RV: Right Ventricle; PG: Peak Gradient; MVA: Mitral Valve Area; PHTH: Pulmonary Hypertension; EROA: Effective Regurgitant Orifice Area; Reg: Regurgitant; VTI: Velocity Time Integral

won't be fully opening and assume a hockey stick appearance in Diastole. It is always associated with a severe LA dilatation and slow flow in the LA, especially in presence of atrial fibrillation that appears as spontaneous echo contrast (smoke-like). MS severity grading is based on the diastolic pressure gradient through the MV measured using CW and estimation of MV area (MVA) [6]. MVA can also be estimated by tracing the diastolic MV flow steep and calculating the time needed to decrease the pressure to half (pressure half time) (automatically calculated by the echo machine). 220 divided by the pressure half time give an estimation of the MVA. Alternatively, we can use the PISA method using the hemisphere of flow acceleration that can be seen above the MV in diastole.

In case of hypovolemia, especially in presence of LV hypertrophy the anterior leaflet of the LV is pulled into the LVOT in systole and result into MR. This phenomenon is called Systolic Anterior Motion (SAM), can also be observed after MV repair and it is best displayed in the ME LAX. LA dilatation almost invariably results into atrial fibrillation which leads to thrombus formation in the LA appendage that needs to be carefully inspected in case of MR and MS.

Tricuspid and Pulmonic Valve

The tricuspid valve (TV) (Fig. 11) comprises three leaflets (anterior, posterior and septal) and is the biggest of all valves. Assessment of the TV consists in the assessment of valve size and leaflet morphology. Precise leaflet identification with standard TEE views is difficult and one of the two leaflets cannot be clearly identified. The TV annulus is measured at end diastole in the ME 4C view. A normal TV annulus is <4 cm. The most common TV pathology is functional TV regurgitation (TR) which is the result of TV dilatation. TV annular dilatation result in the lateral displacement of the anterior and posterior leaflets that will no longer get in contact with the septal leaflet in Systole and therefore leave a gap. Assessment of TR severity is done in a similar fashion as for MR [7]. TR results invariably into RA dilatation and the increased systolic RA pressure, in case of severe TR, will result in a reverse systolic hepatic vein flow. The measurement of peak MR jet flow velocity squared and multiplied by four (simplified Bernoulli equation) added to the central venous pressure provides an estimate of RV systolic pressure which, in absence of pulmonary valve (PV) pathology, corresponds to the systolic pulmonary pressure. TV stenosis (TS) is a rate pathology and can also be caused by rheumatic fever. TS is identified by measuring the TV diastolic pressure gradients, with the continuity equation or dividing 190 by the TV pressure half time [6].

The PV (Fig. 12) is the most anterior of all cardiac valves. Its annulus is adjacent to that of the AV and it is normally rotated 90 degree from it. The PV comprises three cusps (anterior, left and right), the PV annulus is measured in the ME RV in–out and the flow can be measured either in the Transgastric RV inflow outflow view (TG RV in–out) or in the upper esophageal Aortic arch short axis view. PV stenosis (PS) and PV insufficiency (PI) are quantified in a similar fashion as AS and AI [6, 7].

Tricuspid Valve

- **ME 4C** 2D
- **ME RV In/Outflow** 2D
- **ME Bicaval mod TV** 2D
- **ME CS LAX** 2D
- Zoom or reduce depth
- In any view assess
  - o Leaflet motion
  - o CFD (50-60cm/s)
  - o CWD TR
  - o Annulus diameter (0°)
- **IVC LAX:** 2D, CFD
  - o PWD hepatic vein
- **TG Basal SAX** 2D, CFD
- **TG RV Inflow** 2D, CFD

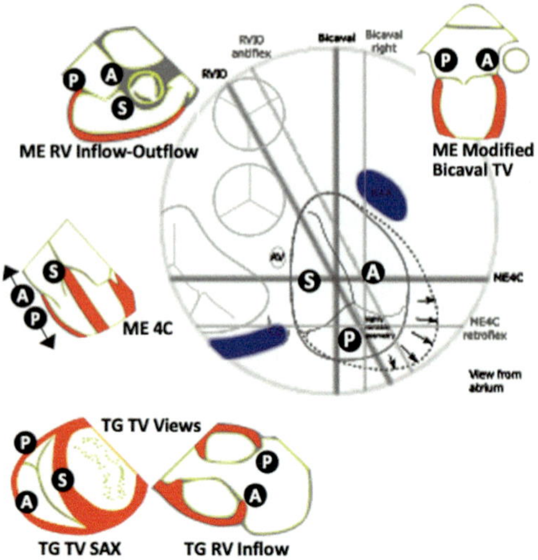

Tricuspid Stenosis
- ❑ **Mechanism** (2D)
  - o Rheumatic, congenital
- ❑ **Severity**
  - o PG mean
  - o TV inflow VTI
  - o TV Area (PHT, continuity)
  - o PHT
- ❑ **Associated**
  - o TR
  - o RA size, SEC, thrombus
  - o IVC dilated

TS Severity	Significant
PG mean (mmHg)*	≥ 5
TV Inflow VTI (cm)	> 60
PHT (msec)	≥ 190
TVA (cm^2)	≤ 1.0

*NSR 70-80bpm
TVA: Continuity = $\frac{\text{AV VTI} \times 0.785(\text{AV diam})^2}{\text{TV VTI}}$ **or** = $\frac{190}{\text{PHT}}$
Supportive: dilated RA, IVC

Tricuspid Regurgitation
- ❑ **Mechanism** (2D SAX/LAX)
  - o Functional (2°):
    - ▪ Annulus: 2D
  - o Valve (1°)
- ❑ **Severity**
  - o TR CWD density
  - o Jet area
  - o Vena Contracta: 2D
  - o PISA radius
  - o EROA: 2D
  - o Reg Volume
  - o Hepatic Vein S wave PWD
- ❑ **Associated**
  - o RV: size, function
  - o RA size
  - o IVC dilated

TR Severity	Mild	Mod	Severe
CWD TR	soft	dense	dense
Jet Area (cm^2)	<5	5-10	>10
Vena Contracta (mm)	NA	<7	>7
PISA radius (mm)	<5	6-9	>9
EROA (cm^2)	NA	NA	>4
Reg Volume (cc/beat)	NA	NA	>50
Hepatic Vein S wave	Norm	Blunted	Reverse

Reg Volume = TV VTI x TVA – RV (or LV) stroke volume
EROA: PISA = $\frac{2\pi r^2 \times \alpha\ \text{angle}/180 \times \text{Valias}}{\text{Peak V TR}}$ **or** = $\frac{\text{Reg Vol}}{\text{VTI TR}}$

Fig. 11 Assessment of the Tricuspid Valve. ME: Mid Esophageal; 4C: Four Chambers; AV: Aortic Valve; LAX Long Axis, TG: Trans gastric; SAX: Short Axis; mod: modified; CS: Coronary Sinus; IVC: Inferior Vena Cava, A: Anterior; P: Posterior; S: Septal CFD: Color Flow Doppler; TV: Tricuspid Valve; TR: Tricuspid Regurgitation; TS: Tricuspid Stenosis; RA: Right Atrium; PWD: Pulsed Wave Doppler; CWD: Continuous Wave Doppler; PHT: Pressure Half Time; PISA: Proximal Isovelocity Surface Area; PAP: Pulmonary Artery Pressure; RV: Right Ventricle; PG: Peak Gradient; TVA: Tricuspid Valve Area; NSR: Normal Sinus Rhythm; EROA: Effective Regurgitant Orifice Area; Reg: Regurgitant; VTI: Velocity Time Integral

Pulmonic Valve

- **ME RVIO** 2D
- **UE Ao Arch SAX** 2D
- **TG RV Basal** 2D
- Zoom or reduce depth
- In any view assess
  - Leaflet motion
  - CFD (50-60cm/s)
  - Annulus diameter
  - PWD/CWD PV Inflow
- **ME 4C** 2D
  - TV: CFD, CWD, annulus
  - RV: size, function

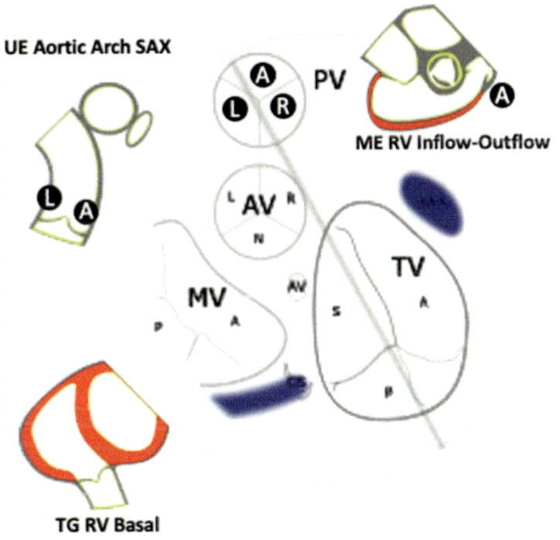

Pulmonic Stenosis

- ❑ **Mechanism** (2D)
  - Calcific, congenital
  - Previous surgery
- ❑ **Severity**
  - Velocity peak
  - PG peak
- ❑ **Associated**
  - RV size, RVH
  - RV function
  - PI
  - TV morphology
  - TR (RVSP)
  - PA morphology

PS Severity	Mild	Mod	Severe
Leaflets	N	Abn	Abn
RV Hypertrophy	N	Mild	Mod
Velocity peak (m/s)	<3	3-4	>4
PG peak (mmHg)	<36	36-64	>64

Pulmonic Insufficiency

- ❑ **Mechanism** (2D)
  - Valve
    - Previous surgery
  - Functional (PHTN)
- ❑ **Severity**
  - Jet length
  - Jet width (JW)/RVOT
  - CWD density
  - PV annulus
- ❑ **Associated**
  - RV size: EDD, ESD
  - RV function
  - RA size
  - TR (RVSP)
  - TV morphology
  - PA morphology

PI Severity	Mild	Mod	Severe
Leaflets	N	± Abn	Abn
RA/RV/annulus (mm)	N	± Abn	Dilated
Jet length (mm)	<10	10-20	>20
JW/RVOT diam (%)	<34	35-74	>75
CWD signal Deceleration rate	Soft Slow	Dense Variable	Dense Steep
Other Indicators Severe PI			
• PI jet deceleration time < 100ms • Ratio PI jet width/pulmonary annulus > 0.7 • Pressure half-time of PI jet <100 msec • Short deceleration time PI spectral Doppler <260 msec			

◂**Fig. 12** Assessment of the Pulmonic Valve. ME: Mid Esophageal; 4C: Four Chambers; RVIO: Right Ventricular Inflow-outflow; AV: Aortic Valve; MV: Mitral Valve; TV: tricuspid Valve; Ao Arch: Aortic Arch; TG: Trans gastric; SAX: Short Axis; mod: modified; CS: Coronary Sinus; IVC: Inferior Vena Cava, A: Anterior; R: Right; L: Left; CFD: Color Flow Doppler; TV: Tricuspid Valve; TR: Tricuspid Regurgitation; PA: Pulmonary Artery; PV: Pulmonic Valve; RV: Right Ventricle; PWD: Pulsed Wave Doppler; CWD: Continuous Wave Doppler; PS: Pulmonary Stenosis; PI: Pulmonary Insufficiency; PHT: Pressure Half Time; PISA: Proximal Isovelocity Surface Area; RA: Right Atrium; PG: Peak Gradient; TVA: Tricuspid Valve Area; NSR: Normal Sinus Rhythm; JW: Jet Width; RVOT: Right Ventricular Outflow Tract; Reg: Regurgitant; VTI: Velocity Time Integral; PHTN: Pulmonary Hypertension; EDD: End Diastolic Diameter; ESD: End Systolic Diameter; RSVP: Right Ventricular Systolic Pressure; Abn: Abnormal

Thoracic Aorta and Pleura

The Esophagus is located right next to the Thoracic aorta (TA). From the ME 4C, rotation of the probe would display the short axis of the TA. The TA can be scanned from the stomach to the arch by advancing and withdrawing the probe. A TA dissection would be easily identified with this view. Next to the TA the left pleural space can be clearly displayed at zero degrees as a crescent opening to the left. Rotation of the probe to the Right allows display of the right pleural space. These can only be clearly displayed in presence of pleural effusion.

Reporting and Storage

Digital storage of TEE examination is mandated by most guidelines [1, 2, 8]. TEE views are usually saved as two beat loops in the echo machine as DICOM files. They can be copied to a DVD, a memory medium or stored in a cloud or network server. Server storage allows retrieval and review of studies, off-line measurements and electronic reporting. Given the high cost this remains in many centers a limiting factor specially for non-cardiac surgical examinations. The availability of cloud storage may allow storage at lower costs and may be available for more centers. Reporting of TEE examination is recommended, and it is required in many countries for billing and medico-legal purposes. The European Association of Cardiothoracic anesthesiologists has recommended a standard template with the purpose of allowing standardization and quality control (Fig. 13).

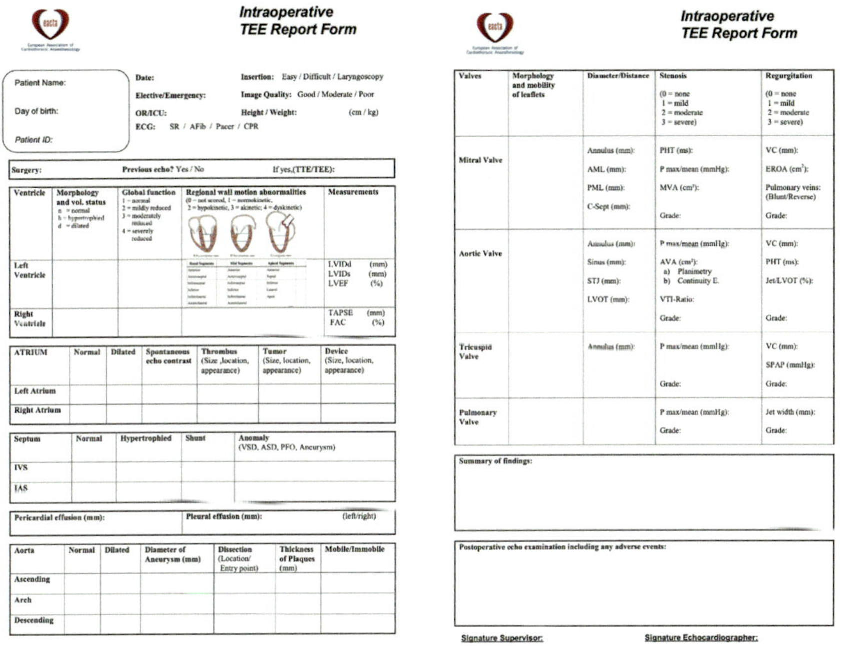
Intraoperative TEE Report Form

Patient Name:
Day of birth:
Patient ID:

Date: | Insertion: Easy / Difficult / Laryngoscopy
Elective/Emergency: | Image Quality: Good / Moderate / Poor
OR/ICU: | Height / Weight: (cm / kg)
ECG: SR / AFib / Pacer / CPR

Surgery: | Previous echo? Yes / No | If yes,(TTE/TEE):

Ventricle	Morphology and vol. status (n = normal, h = hypertrophied, d = dilated)	Global function (1 = normal, 2 = mildly reduced, 3 = moderately reduced, 4 = severely reduced)	Regional wall motion abnormalities (0 = not scored, 1 = normokinetic, 2 = hypokinetic, 3 = akinetic; 4 = dyskinetic)	Measurements
Left Ventricle				LVIDd (mm) LVIDs (mm) LVEF (%)
Right Ventricle				TAPSE (mm) FAC (%)

ATRIUM	Normal	Dilated	Spontaneous echo contrast	Thrombus (Size ,location, appearance)	Tumor (Size, location, appearance)	Device (Size, location, appearance)
Left Atrium						
Right Atrium						

Septum	Normal	Hypertrophied	Shunt	Anomaly (VSD, ASD, PFO, Aneurysm)
IVS				
IAS				

Pericardial effusion (mm): | Pleural effusion (mm): (left/right)

Aorta	Normal	Dilated	Diameter of Aneurysm (mm)	Dissection (Location/ Entry point)	Thickness of Plaques (mm)	Mobile/Immobile
Ascending						
Arch						
Descending						

Intraoperative TEE Report Form

Valves	Morphology and mobility of leaflets	Diameter/Distance	Stenosis (0 = none, 1 = mild, 2 = moderate, 3 = severe)	Regurgitation (0 = none, 1 = mild, 2 = moderate, 3 = severe)
Mitral Valve		Annulus (mm): AML (mm): PML (mm): C-Sept (mm):	PHT (ms): P max/mean (mmHg): MVA (cm^2): Grade:	VC (mm): EROA (cm^2): Pulmonary veins: (Blunt/Reverse) Grade:
Aortic Valve		Annulus (mm): Sinus (mm): STJ (mm): LVOT (mm):	P max/mean (mmHg): AVA (cm^2): a) Planimetry b) Continuity E. VTI-Ratio: Grade:	VC (mm): PHT (ms): Jet/LVOT (%): Grade:
Tricuspid Valve		Annulus (mm):	P max/mean (mmHg): Grade:	VC (mm): SPAP (mmHg): Grade:
Pulmonary Valve			P max/mean (mmHg): Grade:	Jet width (mm): Grade:

Summary of findings:

Postoperative echo examination including any adverse events:

Signature Supervisor: Signature Echocardiographer:

Fig. 13 European Association of Cardiothoracic Anesthesiologists' intraoperative TEE reporting Template

References

1. Flachskampf FA, Badano L, Daniel WG, Feneck RO, Fox KF, Fraser AG, et al. Recommendations for transoesophageal echocardiography: update 2010. Eur J Echocardiogr. 2010;11(7):557–76.
2. Hahn RT, Abraham T, Adams MS, Bruce CJ, Glas KE, Lang RM, et al. Guidelines for performing a comprehensive transesophageal echocardiographic examination: recommendations from the American Society of Echocardiography and the Society of Cardiovascular Anesthesiologists. J Am Soc Echocardiogr. 2013;26(9):921–64.
3. Reeves ST, Finley AC, Skubas NJ, Swaminathan M, Whitley WS, Glas KE, et al. Basic perioperative transesophageal echocardiography examination: a consensus statement of the American Society of Echocardiography and the Society of Cardiovascular Anesthesiologists. J Am Soc Echocardiogr. 2013;26(5):443–56.
4. Arntfield R, Pace J, Hewak M, Thompson D. Focused Transesophageal Echocardiography by Emergency Physicians is Feasible and Clinically Influential: Observational Results from a Novel Ultrasound Program. J Emerg Med. 2016;50(2):286–94.
5. Lang RM, Badano LP, Mor-Avi V, Afilalo J, Armstrong A, Ernande L, et al. Recommendations for cardiac chamber quantification by echocardiography in adults: an update from the American Society of Echocardiography and the European Association of Cardiovascular Imaging. Eur Heart J Cardiovasc Imaging. 2015;16(3):233–70.

6. Baumgartner H, Hung J, Bermejo J, Chambers JB, Evangelista A, Griffin BP, et al. Echocardiographic assessment of valve stenosis: EAE/ASE recommendations for clinical practice. J Am Soc Echocardiogr. 2009;22(1):1–23; quiz 101–2.
7. Zoghbi WA, Adams D, Bonow RO, Enriquez-Sarano M, Foster E, Grayburn PA, et al. Recommendations for Noninvasive Evaluation of Native Valvular Regurgitation: A Report from the American Society of Echocardiography Developed in Collaboration with the Society for Cardiovascular Magnetic Resonance. J Am Soc Echocardiogr. 2017;30(4):303–71.
8. Feneck R, Kneeshaw J, Fox K, Bettex D, Erb J, Flaschkampf F, et al. Recommendations for reporting perioperative transoesophageal echo studies. Eur J Echocardiogr. 2010;11(5):387–93.

Cardiopulmonary Bypass

Pablo Motta and Sean P. Walker

Background

The first heart lung machine (HLM) was used by Gibbon 1953 for an atrial septal defect closure. HLM was developed as an alternative to cross circulation. The disc oxygenator was one of the first generation oxygenators and increase the time cardiac surgery could be performed safely. The initial HLM were bulky requiring up to 7 L for priming. Hypothermia was used topically and the heart was allowed to fibrillate for extended periods of time.

Pre Bypass Stage

Perfusion Equipment

Heart lung machines components include one arterial head, three sucker pumps, and one cardioplegia pump for a total of five. Mandatory alarms contain: level alarm, bubble sensor alarm, arterial and cardioplegia pressure line alarm. Battery back up system is also necessary in case of emergency (Fig. 1).

There are two main types of arterial pump heads which are centrifugal and roller head. Centrifugal pumps contain a cone that uses centrifugal force to propel blood forward. It is pre load and after load dependent that delivers a characteristic laminar

P. Motta (✉)
Perioperative and Pain Medicine Baylor College of Medicine, Texas Children's Hospital, Houston, TX, USA
e-mail: pmotta@bcm.edu

S. P. Walker
Texas Children's Hospital, Houston, TX, USA
e-mail: spwalker@texaschildrens.org

M. Vives and A. Hernandez (eds.), *Cardiac Anesthesia and Postoperative Care in the 21st Century*, https://doi.org/10.1007/978-3-030-79721-8_8

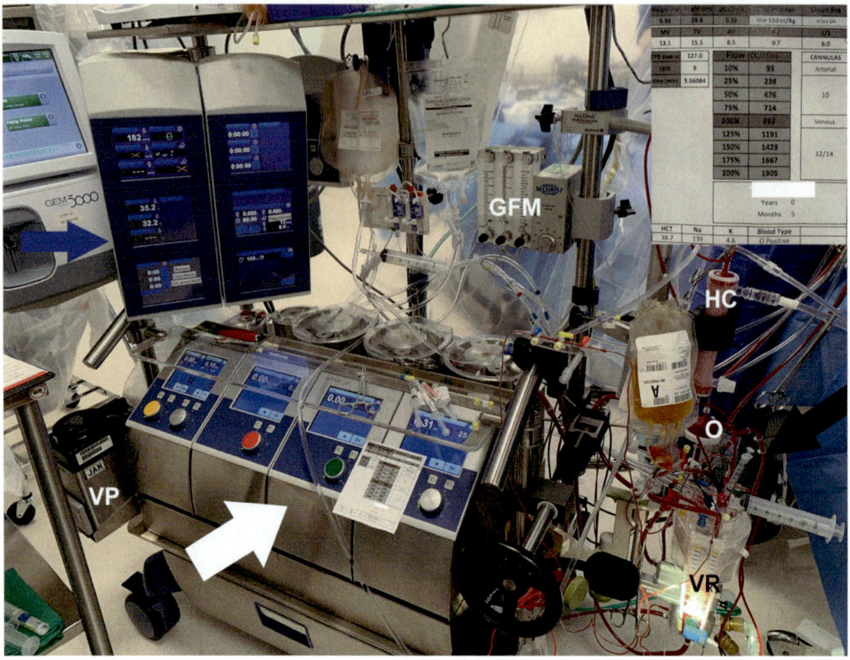

Fig. 1 Picture of a heart and lung machine. The black arrow shows the venous reservoir (VR), the oxygenator (O), and the hemoconcentrator (HC). The white arrow shows the roller head arterial pump (right grey knob), three sucker pumps (green, red, and yellow), and one cardioplegia pump (left grey knob). The blue arrow shows the alarm panel with pressure, volume, and temperature alarms. In addition, the gas flow meter (GFM) and the vaporizer (VP) can be seen. Finally in the right upper corner customized patient information with cannulas used and target cardiopulmonary bypass flows is visualized

flow. The pro for this pump is safety. A cardiopulmonary bypass (CPB) circuit with a centrifugal pump may be clamped anywhere and the pump will not explode. The con is that the pumps run at very high speeds creating heat which can lead to hemolysis and platelet dysfunction. The characteristic non pulsatile delivered by centrifugal pumps is not the preferred flow for end organ preservation. Centrifugal pumps are almost exclusively used in adults. Roller head pumps are positive displacing occlusive pumps that deliver a pulsatile flow. The amount of pulsatility is small usually only approximately 4 mmHg. However any amount of pulsatility is viewed as beneficial and more physiologic. The other advantage of roller head pump are not load dependent and are very accurate. The set flow by the perfusionist is what is delivered not being affected by downstream resistance or any other factors. Its accuracy makes it the most popular system among pediatric centers in which precise flows is a mandatory requirement.

The selection of the CPB circuit is based on patient size and the amount of flow needed. The circuit selection is detailed in Table 1. Patients who are greater than 75 kg have a 1/2 inch pump head boot to decrease the RPM's of the arterial head

Table 1 CPB circuit selection by patient size

Patient size (kg)	Arterial cannula size (Fr)	Arterial line (inches)	Venous line (inches)	Single RA cannula (Fr)	Bicaval cannulae (Fr)	Flow (mL/min)
0–7	6	3/16	1/4	16	8/10	0–350
	8			18	10/12	350–650
7–25	10	1/4	3/8	20	12/14	650–1000
	12			24	12/16	1000–1250
					14/16	1250–1800
25–45	14	3/8	3/8	28	14/18	1800–2000
					16/18	2000–2400
	16			32	18/20	2400–3000
					20/24	3000–4000
>45–75	18	3/8	1/2	36	24/24	4000–4500
					24/28	4500–5000
	20				28/28	5000–6500
>75	22	3/8	1/2	36	28/28	6500

Abbreviations: kg, kilograms; Fr, French; mL, milliliters; min, minutes

when using a roller pump. All the tubing packs include three 1/4 inch suction lines that are color coded for ease of differentiation at the surgical table as well as in the selected pump heads on the pump. A variety of connectors are included in the tubing packs as to accommodate different cannulation possibilities.

Several cannulation techniques are used based on the type of procedure being performed. Cannula size is determined by the amount flow need for each patient. The general guideline for cannula size and selection is detailed in Table 1. Typically bicaval cannulation is used on any procedure that requires intracardiac repair. For example atrial septal defect repair, ventricular septal repair and/or auriculoventricular valve repair or replacement. A single atrial venous cannula is used predominately on "closed procedures" where the heart does not have to be opened. (e.g. coronary artery bypass graft (CABG) and pulmonary valve repairs or replacement). Innominate and subclavian arterial graft cannulation is employed when antegrade cerebral perfusion (ACP) is going to be used in lieu of deep hypothermic circulatory arrest (DHCA). This technique is used to establish and maintain flow to the brain while the rest of the arch vessels are snared so an aortic arch reconstruction may be preformed.

The venous reservoirs and oxygenators are sold by many manufactures and most CPB oxygenators are microporous hollow fiber. When selecting a product careful consideration must be paid to the volume of the reservoir to insure it will accommodate the volume of a given size patient. The oxygenator size must also be considered since they have limited ability to oxygenate and flow. One must again insure that the oxygenator selected will be able to meet the needs of the patients given size (see Table 1).

A variety of filters are used during CPB to avoid emboli. Pre-bypass 5 microns filter is used in the bypass circuit to dispose the circuit of any particulate from the manufacturing process. Once the circuit is crystalloid primed and circulated this filter is removed before any blood is added. Pall filters (40 micron) are used for the addition of blood products. The venous reservoir has an internal "sock" filter (47 microns) is used to ensure any clot or bone chips sucked through the pump suckers is not reintroduced to the patient. The arterial line filter is primarily used as a last line of defense to catch any air that may have passed though the oxygenator. It is usually placed at the highest point in the circuit.

The cooler heater is used to cool and warm the patient and the cardioplegia circuit. Water lines from the cooler heater are connected to both the oxygenator and cardioplegia circuits. Water is pumped through both units at a high rate of speed to raise and low the temperature as so desired by the team.

Continuous ultrafiltration also known as Zero Balance Ultrafiltration (ZBUF) is the practice of adding a set amount of volume into the circuit and removing the same amount of volume via the hemoconcentrator during the bypass run. This practice has proven to remove inflammatory mediators such as inteleukins 6 and 8 and decrease the inflammatory response. ZBUF has been linked to shortened ventilator, ICU and hospital length of stay. Continuous ultrafiltration is also utilized to manipulate electrolytes as well as lowering the lactate. Modified ultra filtration (MUF) is a technique used after bypass completion to hemoconcentrate. Blood is pulled off the arterial limb of the circuit and pumped through the hemoconcentrator and returned to the patient via the venous line.

A pre-bypass checklist is an essential tool to insure the safety of the patient. Similar to a pre-flight safety checklist used in the aviation industry. It should go over all the major systems and components of the CPB system. Careful inspection of all system components, settings, connections and alarms must be checked and assured they are correct before bypass may being. The check list we use at Texas Children's Hospital is presented in Table 2.

Bypass Prime

While most institutions we employ a strategy of a crystalloid priming with 5000 units of heparin in the adult population. The type of prime depends on the size of the patient, underlying cardiac lesion (e.g. cyanotic vs non cyanotic) and type of bypass circuit. Institutionally we try and maintain a haematocrit > 25% in acyanotic patients and > 30% in cyanotic patients and/or comorbitidities. Research has shown that hematocrits under 24% during hypothermic cardiopulmonary bypass in infant heart surgery are associated with lower psychomotor development index scores and increased lactate levels. In our practice will tolerate lower hematrocirts in selected situations (e.g. to avoid blood transfusion) as long as it is clinically acceptable guided by cerebral oxymetry at or above baseline values and no increase in the arterial lactate. Hemodilution calculation is preformed in all the patients and if the

Table 2 Texas children's hospital perfusion checklist

I. Equipment inspection	II. Assembly of perfusion circuit per TCH protocol
A. Pump 1. Visual inspection of electrical plugs and components 2. Roller assembly and modes checked 3. Hand cranks functional	1. Gas flow initiated if indicated 2. CO_2 flush if indicated 3. Sterile connection of circuit components 4. Fluid paths are correct with the lines loaded in the pump housing correctly 5. Cardiotomy reservoir is vented 6. Oxygenator and heat exchanger integrity 7. Proper pharmacological agents added to the prime (double check with anesthesiologist) 8. Prime is heparinized 9. Circuit is debubbled 10. Check for leaks in the circuit 11. Final occlusions are properly set
B. Safety devices 1. Air bubble detector operating correctly 2. Level sensor operating correctly 3. Check blender alarms	
C. Heater–cooler 1. Operational modes operating correctly 2. Visual inspection of electrical plug and components 3. Proper connections are made	
D. Gas inspection 1. Flow meters operating correctly 2. Tubing and connections checked for leaks/obstruction 3. Blender is operational	
E. Brackets 1. Oxygenator 2. Cardiotomy reservoir 3. Arterial filter	
F. Disposables 1. Package integrity (each item) 2. Observe for manufacturer defects (each item) 3. Sterilization is current (each item) 4. Spare disposables are available	
G. Accessories 1. Tubing clamps, scissors/sterile blade and tape are available 2. Heparin available (check expiration date) 3. Coagulation monitoring equipment available and operational 4. Arterial blood gas machine available and operational	

predicted hematocrit value is borderline a collegial conversation between the surgeon, anesthesiologist and the perfusionist will take place about the decision to use blood or not in the prime. The use of plama however is not a clearly defined. Plasma may be used in the prime in selected situations such as cyanotic patients with a high hematocrit (> 45%), multiple redo chest, and/or suspected ATIII deficiency. The neonate or infant circuit is primed with 0.45% NaCl (350 mL) before blood products are added. In the toddler or pediatric the circuits is primed with 0.45% NaCl (500 mL) and Plasmalyte-A (150 mL) before blood products are added. Older patients the prime consist of plasmalyte A, 0.45% NaCl, 25% Albumin and 5% Dextrose. Detailed examples of cardiopulmonary bypass primes are presented in Table 3.

Pharmacology of Bypass

CPB involves extreme changes in physiologic conditions incluing hypothermia, hemodilution, lung isolation, non pulsatile blood flow, low flow and even situation with no flow (deep hypothermic circulatory arrest – DHCA). CPB provides non-pulsatile blood flow which reduces hepatic blood flow by 20–50% depending on the concurrent presence of hypothermia and/or low CPB flow and tiggers the inflammatory cascade. Inflammation results from hemolysis, ischemia, reperfusion, and exposure to foreign CPB surface material. All these factors of affects drug pharmacokinetis and pharmacodynamics. Hydorfilic drugs suffer dilution on initation of CPB decreasing plasma levels. The amount of dilution in direct relationship between the patient blood volume and the prime volume. The hemodilution effect is more pronounced in neonates and infants in which there is an 100% dilution. It can be calculated using this formula:

$$\Delta \mathbf{C}_{\mathbf{D''}} = \mathbf{C}_{\mathbf{D'}}\mathbf{x}\left(\mathbf{V}_{\mathbf{prime}}/\mathbf{V}_1 + \mathbf{V}_{\mathbf{prime}}\right)$$

where:

$\Delta C_{D''}$ Drug change in concetration
V_{prime} prime volume
$C_{D'}$ drug concentration before hemodilution
V_1 central compartment volumen of distribution.

To compensate the hemodilution effect hydrophilic drugs (e.g. non depolarizing muscle relaxants or antibiotics) need to be redosed on initiation of CPB. In addition the CPB circuit is not inert and adsorption of drugs by CPB circuit materials occurs. Lipophilic drugs have a higher volume of distribution and trend to accumulate in the tissues while on CPB. The isolated lung works as a drug reservoir for basic drugs (i.e. fentanyl, propofol or lidocaine) and plasma levels of these type of drugs may increase after weaning of CPB. Hypothermia decreases the activity of microsomal hepatic metabolism system. Furthermore, hypothermia preferentially shifts blood flow to the coronary and cerebral circulation decreasing blood flow to the liver and kidney favouring drug accumulation. In addition hypothermia affects the affinity of opiod agonist with its receptors and decreases MAC requirements.

Table 3 Examples of CPB primes varying with age

	Priming volume (mL)	Arterial line (inches)	Venous line (inches)	PRBC (mL)	FFP or 25% Albumin (mL)	0.45% NaCl	Plasmalyte A (mL)	Heparin (U)	$NaHCO_3$ (mEq)	$CaCl_2$ (mg)	5% Dextrose (mL)
Neonate/ infant	350	3/16	1/4	175	125[a]	50		1500	8	350	
Toddler/ pediatric Blood prime	650	1/4	3/8	300	100[b]	150	100	3000	15	400	
Toddler/ pediatric clear prime	650	1/4	3/8		100[b]	150	400	3000	20	200	15
Adolescent	1000	3/8	3/8		150	250	600	4000	30	300	25
Adult	1250	3/8	1/2		200	300	700	5000	40	450	50

[a]Infant prime always uses FFP
[b]FFP used in place of albumin when clinically indicated (e.g. cyanotic heart disease)
Abbreviations: PRBC, packed red blood cells; FFP, fresh frozen plasma

During rewarming the opposite process occurs making the patient prone to light anesthesia and recall unless provisions are taken.

Anticoagulation is mandatory before the initation of CPB to avoid bypass circuit clotting. Unfractioned intravenous heparin is used to accomplish anticoagulation at a dose of 300 U/kg. Achieving adecute anticoagulation is confirmed with an activate clotting time (ACT) > 480 seconds. Neonates and infants due to a large volume of distribution secondary to increase water content require higher doses of heparin (400 U/kg). Heparin resistance is seen in patient with low levels of antithrombin III (AT III) (heparin cofactor) such as patients previously exposed to heparin. These may require recombinant AT III administration (50 U/kg) to achieve the desire level of anticoagulation. Fresh frozen plasma has low levels of AT III (1 U/mL) so its administration to correct AT III is not recommended in neonate and infants to avoid fluid overload. Reversal of anticoagulation is achieved with protamine in a relationship of 1.2 mg per 100 units of heparin.

Heparin induced thrombocytopenia (HIT) is dangerous complication to heparin administration which makes CPB management very challenging. The clinical presentation is characterized by rapid decline of platelet count (>50%) but manifest with arterial and/or venous thrombosis. Patient with confirmed diagnosis of HIT that need to undergo cardiac surgery on CPB require a careful pharmacologic management with direct thrombin inhibitors (i.e. argatroban or bivalirudin).

Antifibrinolytic drugs are effective in reducing bleeding and transfusion associated with cardiac surgery involving CPB in adults and children. The lysine analogs ε-aminocaproic acid (EACA) and tranexamic acid (TXA) competitively inhibit the binding of plasminogen to fibrin. The EACA concentration of required to inhibit fibrinolysis varies with age. In neonates the concentration of EACA needed is (50 mg/l) due to the immaturity of the fibrinolytic system at birth. In adults and children the recommended concentration of EACA is 130 mg/l. EACA is mostly cleared by renal filtration. Due to the decrease glomerual filtration rate in the neonatal period ($\sim$30% of the adults) the recommended dose is about half those required in adult and children see Table 4. TXA is likewise mostly excreted by the kidney and dose adjustments are needed in renal impairment. Both antifibrynolitcs carry the risk of increase thromobisis so its administration (bolus and infusion) should be delayed until CPB has been initiated in patients with shunt dependent pulmonary circulation. In addition TXA use has been associated with four fold increase incidence of postoperative seizure. Its use should be avoided in patiens with seizure disorders. Comparative studies between EACA and TXA have heart surgery, there was no statistically significant difference according to postoperative blood loss.

Antibiotics are used in all cardiac surgery cases to decrease the incidence of surgical site infections (SSI). The majority of SSI are caused by staphylococcus aureus and coagulase-negative staphylococci, including staphylococcus epidermidis. Cephalosporins are the first line prophylactic antibiotic used in cardiac surgery. The antibiotic plasma concentration should be therapeutic all through out the procedure to be effective and is continued for 48 hours. CPB affects the antibiotic level due to several pharmacokinetic changes mentioned above.

Table 4 EACA dose and age

	Bolus (mg/kg)	Infusion (mg/kg)	Prime dose (μg/ml of prime volume)
Neonate	30	40	100
Children	75	75	250
Adult	50	50	250

Abbreviations: EACA, ε-aminocaproic acid

In addition CPB compromises humoral defenses, reduces phagocytosis and affects the activations of white blood cells imparing natural defense against infections. Hypothermia and coagulopathy also increase the risk for SSI. The first dose of antibiotics should be administered 30 minutes or less before skin incision and every two half-lives of the antibiotic while the chest is open. An additional dose is given to the bypass prime to elude the effect of hemodilution.

The pharmacokinetics of intravenous anesthetics is also affected by CPB initiation, cooling and rewarming. Changes are detailed in Table 5. Inhalatory anesthetics (IA) solubility changes with the start of CPB. Decrease temperature increases IA solubility where as hemodilution decreases IA solubilty. There is also potential sequestration of IA by the oxygenator. It is important to monitor the IA concentration beyond the oygenator to confirm and adequate delivery of IA. Deep of anesthesia by spectral analysis should be monitored too. Finally non depolarizing muscle relaxant (NDMR) agents due to its hydrophilic nature and intravascular distribution are affected initially by hemodilution requiring a dose on the CPB prime. During cooling requirements for NDMR decrease so interval dosing should be prolonged. Neuromuscular monitoring is important to avoid under and/or over dosing. Currently with the availability of sugamedex overdosing has become less of a problem since complete neuromuscular blockage can be achieved at any level of neuromuscular relaxation.

Table 5 CPB pharmacokinetics of anesthetic agents

	CPB initiation (Dilution)	Hypothermia (↓ metabolism)	Rewarming (↑ metabolism)
Propofol	↓	↑	↑[a]
Benzodiazepine	↓	↑	↓
Dexmedetomidine	↓	↑	↓
Etomidate	↓	↑	↓
Ketamine	↓	↑	↓
Narcotics	↓	↑	↑[a]

Abbreviation: CPB, cardiopulmonary bypass; Drug plasma concentration↓ decrease; ↑ increase; ↔ unaffected

[a]Plasma concentration might increase due to release from lung reservoir upon restarting lung ventilation

Conduct of Bypass

The initiation of CPB begins by opening the venous line to drain and then starting the arterial head. As venous drainage increases, the arterial flow increases until full flow is reached (100% flow). The ideal flows are calculated by body surface area (BSA) and are age specific (See Table 6). This commencement should be done in a manner and rate that maintains a reasonable perfusion pressure. If initiation is done too slowly the patient blood volume will be drained and not enough forward flow will be present to maintain blood pressure. If done too fast the patient would not be fully drained and the cannulas would overflow the patient. If the appropriately sized positioned cannulas and optimal drainage is still not achieved vacuum assisted venous drainage (VAVD) can be implemented. The negative pressure on the vacuum must never exceed negative 60 mmHg to avoid hemolysis and/or air emboli. VAVD must be discontinued before the termination of bypass air as may draw across the membrane.

At the beginning of bypass the temperature set on the cooler/heater should be the same of the patient nasal temperature. Often times especially on redo operations the patients temperature may drift down a few degrees. If the patient naturally drifted to 34 °C and CPB is initiate bypass at 37 °C the patient will be warmed, worsening the hypotension caused by the clear prime. The temperature gradient between the cooler/heater and the nasal temperature should be maintained at 8 °C or less on both cooling and warming phases. Every 7 °C of cooling the oxygen demand of the decreses by 50%. The degree of hypothermia required varies with the complexity and duration of the procedure (see Table 7). Any procedure that requires antero-grade cerebral perfusion or DHCA, a target nasal temperature of 18 °C should be achieved.

The blood gas management on bypass at Texas Children's e employs the strategy of permissive hypercapnia with target a CO_2 of 48–55 to improve cerebral perfusion. This is the PH stat technique where all blood gas values are temperature corrected. Other institutions employ alpha stat where all values are calculated at 37 °C. The mixed venous saturation is used as a determination of optimal perfusion

Table 6 Recommended CBP flow by weight and BSA

Patients weighing < **10 kg**	Flow = Wt (kg) × 150 ml/min
Patients weighing > **10 kg**	Flow = BSA × Cardiac Index (Age Specific)

$BSA = \sqrt{\frac{Ht(cm) \times Wt(kg)}{3600}}$
0–2 yr 3.0–3.2 × BSA
2–4 yr 2.8 × BSA
4–6 yr 2.6 × BSA
6–10 yr 2.5 × BSA
>10yr 2.4 × BSA
Abbreviations: BSA, body surface area

Table 7 Classification of degree of cooling

	Temperature °C	Type of procedure
Mild	37–32	Closed procedures i.e. CABG, BDG, or Fontan
Moderate	31–28	Open procedures i.e. VSDs, MVR, TOF, etc
Deep	28–18	Complex open procedures i.e. TOF with extensive PA reconstruction
Profound	18–0	Aortic reconstruction procedures
		(i.e. Norwood, arch advancement, etc.)
		TAPVR

Abbreviations: CABG, coronary artery bypass graft; BDG, bidirectional Glenn shunt; VSD, ventricular septal defect; MVR, mitral valve repair or replacement; TOF, tetralogy of Fallot and TAPVR, total anomalous pulmonary vein return

and a value 75% is sought. Blood gas should be monitored at least every 15–20 min.

After CPB cooling is underway, preparation for cross clamp (XC) and cardio plejia (CPG) administration follows. Once the surgeon is ready to apply the XC the CPB flow is decreased (~ 20% of full flow values) and then XC is applied. Once the XC is on CPG administration begins. Anti-grade flow rates 250 mL/min and a pressure target of at least the patient's baseline diastolic blood pressure or slightly higher (5–10 mmHg) is administered. Severe aortic insufficiency is particularly challenging situation because CPG preferentially flows into the left ventricle (LV) and not into the coronaries. This causes LV distension and fails to arrest the heart in timely maner. In these situation aortotomy is needed with direct ostial CPG injection. Anti-grade administrations is preferable to retrograde as it protects the right side of the heart. Adults with coronary artery disease will require retrograde however and usually given at 150 ml/min near baseline diastolic pressures. There are many types of CPG solutions that are given at different time intervals and temperatures. The dosing interval is also determined by the type of solution used. At Texas Children's Hospital we use the Del Nido CPG which after the initial arresting dose of 20 mL/kg (maximum dose of 1000 mL for patients > 50 kg) is delivered the subsequent maintenance doses are given every 60 min. If the XC time is expected to be < 30 min, a half dose can be used (e.g. ASD closure). Another alternative is to use the Buckburg dextrose based solution which is administered as an induction arresting dose, maintenance doses (every 15–20 min) and reperfusion normothermic dose ("hot shot") just before aortic unclamping (Table 8).

The target mean arterial pressure (MAP) is discussed between during surgical time out before the procedure begins. Careful and frequent monitoring of all pre-determined physiologic parameters should be performed constantly throughout the bypass run. The cerebral oxymetry is monitored and kept at baseline levels (e.g. patient awake ventilating in room air). A step wise approach to cerebral desaturation on bypass is used, similar to the one proposed by Denault et al. Unilateral desaturations are usually related to cannula malposition and position needs to be

Table 8 Comparison between the modified buckberg CPS and del Nido CPS*

	Modified Buckberg CPS		del Nido CPS
Base solution	Induction	D5 1/4 NS 392 mL	Plasma-Lyte A 1000 mL
	Maintenance	D5 1/4 NS 798 mL	
	Reperfusion	Sterile water 235 mL	
Total volume (approximate)	Induction	500 mL	1100 mL
	Maintenance	1000 mL	
	Reperfusion	500 mL	
KCL	Induction	36 mEq/500 mL	26 mEq
	Maintenance	36 mEq/L	
	Reperfusion	15 mEq/500 mL	
Tromethamine 0.3 M	Induction	60 mL/500 mL	None
	Maintenance	123 mL/L	
	Reperfusion	56 mL/500 mL	
C-P-2-D	Induction	30 mL/500	None
	Maintenance	61 mL/L	
	Reperfusion	113 mL/L	
$NaHCO_3$	None		13 mEq
Mannitol 20%	None		16 mL

Abbreviation: CPS, cardioplegia
Adapted with authorization from Kim K, Ball C, Grady P, Mick S. Use of del Nido Cardioplegia for Adult Cardiac Surgery at the Cleveland Clinic: Perfusion Implications. J Extra Corpor Technol. 2014;46(4):317–323

verified by the surgeon. Bilateral desaturations which are the majority are treated initially by increasing CPB flow to increase MAP. In addition the FiO_2, hematocrit and/or CO_2 may need to be optimized too. Monitoring of the lactate level is done with every arterial blood gas during the bypass run (every 15 min).

Upon the conclusion of the surgical procedure after rewarming has been completed weaning from CPB will ensue. All electrolytes should be corrected and a predetermined target hematocrit achieved. To wean off CPB all shunts should be closed and vacuum assisted drainage terminated if in use. Ventilation should be resumed fully and that the depth of anesthesia should be adequate. In close communication with the surgical and anesthesia teams weaning begins by partially occluding the venous line transferring volume from the reservoir to the patient. The patient will begin to show ejection in the arterial tracing and the central venous pressure (CVP) should be closely monitored to avoid over distension of the heart. Once ejection has commenced weaning of the pump flow should begin while maintaining ejection and a targeted CVP. Reduce the flow to 75%, then 50, then 25 and finally turning the pump off and fully clamping the venous line.

Deep hypothermic circulatory arrest (DHCA) is a technique that is employed to achieve a completely bloodless field (e.g. TAPVR repair). Basically is achieved by cooling the patient to 18 °C and shutting the pump off. Cooling to 18 °C must take at least 20 min to ensure even and effective cooling. Once instructed to shut the pump off the arterial line must be clamped and the venous line should be clamped either at the field or at the perfusion end. Selective anti-grade cerebral perfusion (ACP) is a technique that is usually employed when aortic arch work must be done. Performed at 18 °C by cannulating the innominate or subclavian artery (directly or with a graft) and snaring the other head vessels so the flow is directed anti-grade only to the head. A flow rate of approximately 30% is used at this time with careful monitoring of cerebral oximetry to ensure the circle of Willis is intact. The TCH ACP protocol is detailed in Table 9.

Table 9 Texas children's hospital infant antegrade cerebral perfusion technique

1. Heparinization	• 100 units/kg heparin
2. Graft placement	• PTFE graft to right innominate artery[a]
3. Aortic cannulation	• 10 Fr standard aortic cannula to distal end of graft
4. Venous cannulation	• Single atrial or bicaval cannulation
5. Neuromonitoring	• Bilateral cerebral oximetry and TCD through anterior fontanelle for cerebral physiological monitoring • Establish baseline mean cerebral blood flow velocity using TCD, and rSO2 (18–22° C at full flow CPB: 150 ml/kg/min)
6. Conduct of CPB	• Goal MAP 30–35 mm Hg (α-receptor blockade if necessary) • rSO2 90–95% bilaterally—mean CBFV normally 18–25 cm/sec • Target hematocrit 30–35% • Use pH stat management during all phases of CPB
7. Conduct of ACP	• ACP initiated after brief DHCA for atrial septectomy for Norwood • All brachiocephalic vessels and descending thoracic aorta snared • Temperature at 18° C • Begin at 37.5 ml/kg/min • Adjust ACP flow using TCD to achieve CBFV within ± 10% of baseline at full CPB flow • rSO2 should be within ± 10% of baseline, or 90–95% bilaterally • If left rSO2 falls to more than 10% below right, increase ACP flow
8. Rewarming	• Once repair completed full flow CPB is resumed and ACP stopped • Rewarming has to be cautious to avoid cerebral hyperthermia

Abbreviations: PTFE, polytetrafluroethylene; NIRS, near-infrared spectroscopy; TCD, transcranial Doppler; rSO2, regional brain oxygen saturation; CPB; cardiopulmonary bypass; MAP, mean arterial pressure; CBFV; cerebral blood flow velocity; ACP, antegrade cerebral perfusion; DHCA, deep hypothermic circulatory arrest

[a]3.0 to 4.0 mm shunt depending on patient size with 8–0 prolene sutures

Complications

There are several potential complications during a CPB run. Some are related to equipment failure, cannulation difficulties, transfusion and/or medication related. A "run away" pump is the situation in which the arterial pump head rapidly accelerates spontaneously. This can result in draining the venous reservoir and introducing air into the circuit. With a roller head pump the corrective action is to power down the individual pump head and hand crank until a replacement pump head can be implemented. With a centrifugal pump the outflow needs to be clamped, the cone removed and hand crank until a replacement pump is available. In the event of a line disconnection in either the arterial or venous lines the first action step must be to isolate and protect the patient by clamping that side of the line. Then re-priming and reconnecting the line or lines and reestablish CPB flow. Presently with increased popularity of vacuum assisted venous drainage, negative pressure air emboli are more common than in the past. Thankfully with today's microporous hollow fiber membrane oxygenators and venous purge lines (most micro) gross air can be eliminated by the reservoir antifoam sock. Careful attention must be placed on not allowing the negative venous pressure to exceed −60 mmHg. In the event of a power outage most hospitals have generators that will back up critical areas. The majority of current HLM are equipped with battery backups as well. However in the scenario of total lack of power the only option is to hand crank until power is resorted.

Surgical cannulation problems include aortic dissection, preferential blood flow and superior and/or inferior vena cava obstruction. Transesophageal echocardiography and pressure differente between the extremities can aid in the diagnosis of aortic dissection. Preferential blood flow and superior vena cava obstruction can be detected by asymmetric cerebral oxymetry readings. During cannulation there is also potential for massive blood loss in case of tearing a mayor vessel so the anesthesiologis and perfusionist should be ready to massively transfuse and cell save. Atrial arrhythmias can develop during heart manipulation. Usually this arrhytimias are self limited but measures need to be taken to be able to internally cardiovert if poorly tolerated hemodynamically. Finally clerical mistakes during drug and blood product administration should be avoided by double checking by two providers.

Finally the systemic inflammatory reaction syndrome (SIRS) inflammatory response to CPB is a fairly common (incidence of ~30%) and feared complications of a bypass run. SIRS increases morbiborbidity and mortality after cardiac surgery. In adults the SIRS is inversely related with age and extracardiac arteriopathy, and directly related with preoperative white blood cell count. In infants SIRS is associated with the CPB duration and the use of fresh frozen plasma on the prime. Neonates seem to be less prone to develop SIRS.

Recommended Reading

1. Kunst G, Milojevic M, Boer C, et al. EACTS/EACTA/EBCP guidelines on cardiopulmonary bypass in adult cardiac surgery. Br J Anaesth. 2019; 123 (6):713e757.
2. Wypij D, Jonas RA, Bellinger DC et al. The effect of hematocrit during hypothermic cardiopulmonary bypass in infant heart surgery. Results from the combined Boston hematocrit trials. J Thorac Cardiovasc Surg 2008; 135:355–60.
3. Denault A, Deschamps A, Murkin JM. A proposed algorithm for the intraoperative use of cerebral near-infrared spectroscopy. Seminars in Cardiothoracic and Vascular Anesthesia 2007; 11:274–281.
4. Martin K, Breuer T, Gertler R et al Tranexamic acid versus e-aminocaproic acid: efficacy and safety in paediatric cardiac surgery. Eur J Cardio-Thorac Surg 2011; 39:892–897.
5. Paruk F, Sime FB, Lipman J et al Dosing antibiotic prophylaxis during cardiopulmonary bypass—a higher level of complexity? A structured review. Int J Antimicrob Agents 2017; 49:395–402.
6. Kim K, Ball C, Grady P et al Use of del Nido Cardioplegia for adult cardiac surgery at the Cleveland clinic: perfusion implications. JECT. 2014; 46:317–323.

Critical Incidents During Cardiopulmonary Bypass

Filip De Somer

Since the introduction of cardiopulmonary bypass (CPB) over 60 years ago there has been a major evolution in both CPB components as perfusion techniques. In opposition to many other extracorporeal therapies such as dialysis where these innovations resulted in standard circuit configurations this did not happen in CPB. The heterogeneity and complexity of circuits and perfusion techniques makes CPB potentially prone to incidents.

Risk for incidents depends not only on the equipment and supplies used but also on training and education of the perfusionist as well as on the use of correct communication with other specialties during the procedure.

Several retrospective surveys were conducted over the last 20 years to investigate the occurrence of critical incidents and accidents during CPB procedures. Reported incident rates varied between 1:16 and 1:198 whereas the number of incidents resulting in serious injury or death were reported as 1:1236 to 1:3220.

A problem with all published surveys is that although all of them were retrospective in nature, the questionnaires and definitions of incidents were not similar what in part explains the reported differences.

In this chapter we will discuss some of the more common incidents during CPB.

Aortic Dissection During Cannulation

Intraoperative aortic dissection is a rare but potentially fatal complication. Although the incidence rate is low, this complication frequently lead to catastrophic results with high operative mortality. The most common sites of aortic injury are the ascending aorta cannulation site, cross-clamp site, partial occlusion clamp, proximal

F. De Somer (✉)
Chief Perfusionist, Ghent University Hospital, Ghent, Belgium
e-mail: Filip.DeSomer@ugent.be

M. Vives and A. Hernandez (eds.), *Cardiac Anesthesia and Postoperative Care in the 21st Century*, https://doi.org/10.1007/978-3-030-79721-8_9

anastomosis site and the cardioplegia cannula site. Femoral artery cannulation has a higher risk for dissection, compared to ascending aorta cannulation.

Prevention

Optimal blood pressure during cannulation with systolic blood pressure (SBP) around 100 mmHg. Too high SBP increases the risk of Aortic dissection. If SBP is too low (< 80 mmHg), aorta tend to collapse making more difficult to make the incision and having greater risk of tear too.

Diagnosis

Intraoperative recognition of aortic dissection is not straightforward. Suspicious clinical signs are sudden disappearance of radial arterial pressure, a sudden drop in cerebral oxygenation as measured by NIRS or a major change in EEG pattern. However, none of these signs is uniquely related to the occurrence of aortic dissection and differential diagnosis remains vital. Differential diagnosis can be made by Transesophageal Echocardiography (TEE) which has a high specificity and sensitivity or by epiaortic scanning.

Management

Once aortic dissection is confirmed it is key to know whether it is a type A or type B dissection. For type A, the aortic cannula should be replaced towards another insertion site most often the femoral artery or axillary artery. The patient is then cooled to 22–24 °C in order to stop the circulation and head cooling is applied. The use of selective cerebral perfusion should be considered. Perfusion techniques used during cooling down such as pH-strategy, flow rate and perfusate temperature will all influence outcome. A type B dissection can be often treated medically or with an endograft.

Aortic Cannula Malposition

Proper position of the aortic cannula tip is important. 1 to 2 cm into the aorta, directed toward the middle of transverse arch. The cannula might be inserted too much or misdirected, entering the cannula to the left carotid artery or misdirecting the flow to the innominate artery. The diameter of the aortic cannula can be too small causing a jet effect redirecting the flow to the brain. Intramural placement of the cannula is another potential complication.

Diagnosis

- High systemic line pressure plus facial edema and a sudden increase of cerebral oxygenation by NIRS.
- Intramural placement of the cannula may be diagnosed by the absence of noting pulse flow in the systemic line pressure.

Treatment

Repositioning the cannula or changing to longer or shorter one.

Aortic Cannula Outlet Bleeding

Diagnosis

In some cases, blood loss is observed at the arterial cannula insertion site.

Management

- Maintain mean arterial pressure low.
- Place an additional suture string around the cannula.

Cerebral Edema Caused by Venous Cannula Obstruction

Vascular access remains a challenge during CPB procedures. Optimal venous drainage is essential for the prevention of tissue edema in organs. So, correct positioning of the venous cannula is important in preventing cerebral edema. The tip of the venous cannula might be malpositioned into the hepatic vein or the coronary sinus or the azygos or into the left atrium (LA) across the atrial septal defect.

Diagnosis

- Sudden rise in central venous pressure (CVP) and excessive flow resistance e.g. when the purse string is placed around the cannula. A sudden rise in CVP may cause RV dilatation and contractility impairment.
- Sudden or continuous drop in cerebral oxygenation.
- TEE may play an important role to detect malpositioning of the venous cannula.

Management

Reposition the cannula as soon as possible.

Misplacement of Venous Cannula

Over the years the use of minimally invasive cardiac surgery (MICS) has expanded. There is no questions that MICS is technically more demanding for the cardiac team. In most cases vascular access is done through the femoral blood vessels. Especially the insertion of the venous cannula towards the right atrium can pose difficulties. In rare cases the cannula tip might be positioned in the coronary sinus or hepatic vein (20). Prevention of malpositioning is done by TEE monitoring of the guide wire until it is at the level of the right atrium.

Diagnosis

- Difficulty in obtaining full flow with scattering of the venous line.
- TEE observation of the cannula positioned in the coronary sinus or hepatic vein.

Management

- Control with TEE volume status and cannula position.
- Replace the cannula.

Coronary Sinus Rupture During Retrograde Cardioplegia Administration

Retrograde cardioplegia offers several advantages such as avoidance of coronary ostium injury, more effective cooling of the myocardium in the case of distal coronary lesions, no interruption of surgery, diminished atrial rewarming and effective cardioplegia delivery in case of aortic regurgitation. Disadvantages are inadequate preservation of the right ventricle, delayed cardiac arrest and injury to the coronary sinus (CS). Typical CS injuries are hematoma, perforation and laceration of the CS or right ventricle. They can be caused by traumatic insertion of the catheter with stylet, overinflation of the CS catheter balloon, elevated CS infusion pressure, excessive flow during cardioplegia delivery, or excessive retraction of the heart when the catheter is in place or with the balloon inflated.

Prevention

When administering retrograde cardioplegia maintain:

- Delivery pressure between 0–40 mmHg
- Start delivery slowly, 125 mL/min/m^2, or approximately 200–250 mL/min
- Observe the pressure wave during inflation of the balloon and maintain pressure below 40 mmHg

Diagnosis

Any sudden increase or decrease in delivery pressure is suspicious and the surgeon should be immediately informed.

Management

In case of hematoma stop retrograde cardioplegia delivery and choose an alternative delivery site (aortic root or coronary ostium).

In case of a perforation perform a direct suture repair.
- In case of laceration a pericardial patch is mostly used.
- Use TEE for follow up during the operation and the immediate postoperative period.

New Left Persistent SVC (LSVC) Diagnosis During Retrograde Cardioplegia Administration

- LSVC is present 0.3–0.5% of the population.
- LSVC usually drains into coronary sinus and then into the Right Atrium.
- In some cases, LSVC drains into the LA.
- LSVC should be rule out when large coronary sinus is observed on TEE.
- Suspect LSVC when Right SVC is small and left innominate vein is small or absent.

Diagnosis

Observing saline in the coronary sinus and then entering the RA on TEE when saline administered through a vein in the left arm.

Management

Use cardiotomy suction in the coronary sinus and Cannulate LSVC.

Circuit Thrombosis

According to all surveys coagulation disorders occur regularly during CPB. Circuit thrombosis can be caused by low heparin sensitivity, antithrombin III deficiency, platelet activation, diffuse intravascular coagulation (DIC), heparin induced thrombocytopenia (HIT) and in rare situations by erroneous administration of protamine.

Diagnosis

The detection of ongoing thrombosis is done by:

- Controlling ACT, a normal or marginally prolonged ACT value is a strong indicator of inadequate anticoagulation.
- Measuring the pressure drop over the oxygenator: an increase in pressure drop over the oxygenator is an indicator of beginning thrombosis in the hollow fiber bundle. The need for continuous increase of the revolutions per minute (RPM) of a centrifugal pump to maintain the desired blood flow without any changes in patient hemodynamics can also be a first sign of beginning thrombosis in the fiber bundle.

- Check if there is breakthrough of blood above the blood level in the venous reservoir as this represents partial filter obstruction in the defoamer/filter sock.

Management

- Administer immediately a bolus of 300 IU/kg unfractionated heparin (UFH) in case of a normal ACT or a bolus of 100 IU/kg UFH in case of a marginal prolonged ACT in the CPB circuit.
- Inform the other members of the cardiac surgical team and check whether clots are present in the surgical field.
- Check the circuit for visible clots and or fibrin deposits.
- Check the mass transfer of the oxygenator by taking a blood sample before and after the oxygenator.
- Order a spare CPB circuit.
- In case of severe thrombosis, check if it is possible to wean the patient from CPB. If not, cool down the patient and prepare for circuit/component exchange.

Oxygenator Failure

The term oxygenator failure can have different meanings. It can be defined as the inability of an oxygenator to transfer oxygen and to remove carbon dioxide, but also as a mechanical failure such as a blood or water leak. Exchange of a failing oxygenator is a technical demanding task and not without risk for the patient.

Diagnosis

A mechanical failure is relatively easy to diagnose as in most cases blood or water will be dripping out of the unit. Minor blood leaks should not be cured by exchanging the unit as the risk does not outweighs the benefit. Failure to oxygenate is mostly witnessed by dark colored blood leaving the oxygenator.

Management

Mechanical failure

Analyze where the leak is localized. A leak in a low pressure area such as the venous reservoir can often be cured by putting some bone wax over the fracture. The loss of small amounts of blood out of the gas exhaust can be caused by damage to one or two hollow fibers and can be tolerated as it almost never will jeopardize gas transport. Larger leaks will necessitate component exchange.

Mass transfer failure

- This is witnessed by dark blood leaving the oxygenator eventually combined with a drop in cerebral oxygenation and low arterial oxygen saturation.
- Put the patient on 100% oxygen and check the complete gas circuit for lose connections.
- Warn the team that you experience an oxygenator failure.
- Take a blood gas before and after the oxygenator and calculate the oxygen transfer. If the oxygen transfer equals maximum oxygen transfer for the unit discuss with the anesthesiologist to deepen anesthesia level and check muscular relaxation.
- If venous saturation is low increase blood flow and check the calibration of the arterial pump.
- Check if foam is coming out of the gas exhaust. This indicates that plasma is leaking through the microporous oxygenation membrane. In patients on ECMO before undergoing cardiac surgery it is advisable to use a dense membrane instead of a microporous membrane.
- Take new blood gases before and after the oxygenator, if low oxygen transfer persist exchange the oxygenator.

Oxygenator exchange

- Mention loud and clear to the cardiac team that an oxygenator replacement is required.
- When available ask for a second perfusionist
- Bring a spare unit into the operating theatre
- If the aorta is not yet clamped, wean the patient from CPB and replace the unit afterwards.
- If the aorta is clamped, cool the patient down to at least 25 °C.
- Prime the spare oxygenator with an auxiliary pump.
- Once cooled exchange the oxygenator according to the hospital protocol. Each hospital should have an internal protocol for oxygenator exchange.
- After exchanging the oxygenator carefully check the circuit for remaining air.
- Restart CPB and check the functioning of the oxygenator by taking an arterial blood gas.
- Slowly rewarm the patient to the desired temperature.

Massive Air Embolism

Massive air embolism is a potential lethal complication that requires an immediate response. Causes of massive air embolism are (1) inattention to reservoir level, (2) reversal of pump head tubing or direction of pump head rotation, (3) unexpected resumption of heartbeat, (4) inadequate steps to remove air after cardiotomy, (5) high-flow suction deep in a pulmonary artery, (6) defective oxygenator, (7) use of a pressurized cardiotomy reservoir, defective low level alarm (8) and (9) inadvertent detachment of oxygenator during bypass.

Diagnosis

Visual air passing through the arterial line. Once noticed immediately warn the whole team and look for the cause of the air embolism.

Management

- Stop CPB, clamp arterial and venous line.
- Place the patient in Trendelenburg position (Head down).
- Remove the aortic cannula and de-air the aorta by using a pump sucker.
- De-air the CPB circuit including arterial line and aorta cannula.
- Start retrograde venous cerebral flow over the superior vena cava at 2 L/min until no air is observed in the aortic root.
- Intermittent compression of the carotid arteries during retrograde cerebral perfusion will improve de-airing of the vertebral arteries.
- Induce hypertension by means of vasoconstrictor drugs.
- Ventilate the patient and the oxygenator with 100% oxygen.
- Administer steroids.
- Barbiturate anesthesia to decrease the cerebral metabolic rate of oxygen (CMRO2).
- After completing the de-airing of the patient re-establish full antegrade flow and maintain hypothermia (20 °C) for 45 min in order to optimize gas absorption.
- Slowly rewarm the patient to 35 °C and wean the patient from bypass
- When available the use of a hyperbaric chamber is advisable.

Summary

Although the number of incidents resulting in serious adverse effects or death remain low during CPB, vigilance of the cardiac team is important. Well trained perfusionists, use of check lists and simulation training sessions are all necessary in the prevention of incidents during CPB (Table 1).

Table 1 Summary of most common critical incidents its diagnosis and treatment

Incident	Diagnosis	Management
Aortic dissection during cannulation	– Sudden disappearance of radial arterial pressure – Sudden drop in cerebral oxygenation as measured by NIRS or a major change in EEG pattern – Differential diagnosis can be made by TEE which has a high specificity and sensitivity or by epiaortic scanning	– For a type B dissection can be often treated medically or with an endograft – For type A, the aortic cannula should be replaced towards the femoral artery or axillary artery and Asc Aorta and/or aortic arch replaced – The patient should be cooled to 22–24 °C in order to stop the circulation and head cooling is applied – Selective cerebral perfusion should be considered
Aortic cannula malposition	– High systemic line pressure plus facial edema and a sudden increase of cerebral oxygenation by NIRS – Intramural placement of the the cannula may be diagnosed by the absence of noting pulse flow in the systemic line pressure	– Repositioning the cannula or changing to a longer or shorter one
Aortic cannula outlet bleeding	– Blood loss is observed at the arterial cannula insertion site	– Maintain mean arterial pressure low – Place an additional suture string around the cannula
Cerebral edema caused by venous cannula obstruction	– Sudden rise in CVP and excessive flow resistance – Sudden rise in CVP may cause RV dilatation and contractility impairment – Sudden or continuous drop in cerebral oxygenation	– Reposition the cannula as soon as possible
Misplacement of venous cannula	– Difficulty in obtaining full flow with scattering of the venous line – Observing the the cannula positioned in the coronary sinus or hepatic vein by TEE	– Control volume status and cannula position by TEE – Replace the cannula
Coronary sinus rupture during retrograde cardioplegia administration	*Prevention* – Delivery pressure between 0–40 mmHg. Start delivery slowly, 125 mL/min/m^2, or approximately 200–250 mL/min. Observe the pressure wave during inflation of the	– In case of hematoma stop retrograde cardioplegia delivery and choose an alternative delivery site (aortic root or coronary ostium) – In case of a perforation perform a direct suture repair

(continued)

Table 1 (continued)

Incident	Diagnosis	Management
	balloon and maintain pressure below 40 mmHg *Diagnosis* – Any sudden increase or decrease in delivery pressure is suspicious and the surgeon should be immediately informed	– In case of laceration a pericardial patch is mostly used – Use transesophageal echography for follow up during the operation and the immediate postoperative period
LSVC diagnosis during retrograde cardioplegia administration	– Observing saline in the coronary sinus and then entering the RA on TEE when saline administered through a vein in the left arm	– Use cardiotomy suction in the coronary sinus – Cannulate LSVC
Circuit thrombosis	– A normal or marginally prolonged ACT value is a strong indicator of inadequate anticoagulation – An increase in pressure over the oxygenator is an indicator of beginning thrombosis in the hollow fiber bundle. The need for continuous increase of the RPM of a centrifugal pump to maintain the desired blood flow without any changes in patient hemodynamics can also be a first sign of beginning thrombosis in the fiber bundle – Check if there is breakthrough of blood above the blood level in the venous reservoir as this represents partial filter obstruction in the defoamer/ filter sock	– Administer immediately a bolus of 300 IU/kg unfractionated heparin (UFH) in case of a normal ACT or a bolus of 100 IU/kg UFH in case of a marginal prolonged ACT in the CPB circuit – Inform the other members of the cardiac surgical team and check whether clots are present in the surgical field – Check the circuit for visible clots and or fibrin deposits – Check the mass transfer of the oxygenator by taking a blood sample before and after the oxygenator – Order a spare CPB circuit – In case of severe thrombosis, check if it is possible to wean the patient from CPB. If not cool down the patient and prepare for circuit/component exchange
Oxygenator Failure	– A mechanical failure is relatively easy to diagnose as in most cases blood or water will be dripping out of the unit. Minor blood leaks should not be cured by exchanging the unit as the risk does not outweighs the benefit – Failure to oxygenate is mostly witnessed by dark colored blood leaving the oxygenator	– Analyze where the leak is localized – A leak in a low-pressure area such as the venous reservoir can often be cured by putting some bone wax over the fracture – The loss of small amounts of blood out of the gas exhaust can be caused by damage to one or two hollow fibers and

(continued)

Table 1 (continued)

Incident	Diagnosis	Management
		can be tolerated as it almost never will jeopardize gas transport. Larger leaks will necessitate component exchange Mass transfer failure: Dark blood leaving the oxygenator eventually combined with a drop in cerebral oxygenation and low arterial oxygen saturation – Put the patient on 100% oxygen and check the complete gas circuit for lose connections - Warn the team that you experience an oxygenator failure – Take a blood gas before and after the oxygenator and calculate the oxygen consumption. If the oxygen consumption equals maximum oxygen transfer for the unit discuss with the anesthesiologist to deepen anesthesia level and check muscular relaxation – If venous saturation is low increase blood flow and check the calibration of the arterial pump – Check if foam is coming out of the gas exhaust. This indicates that plasma is leaking through the microporous oxygenation membrane. In patients on ECMO before undergoing cardiac surgery it is advisable to use a dense membrane instead of a microporous membrane – Take new blood gases before and after the oxygenator, if low oxygen transfer persists exchange the oxygenator – Oxygenator exchange (see text)

Recommended Reading

1. Charriere JM, Pelissie J, Verd C, Leger P, Pouard P, de Riberolles C, et al. Analysis of incidents, monitoring and safety devices of cardiopulmonary bypass for cardiac surgery for the year 2005 in France. Ann Fr Anesth Reanim. 2007;26(11):907–15.
2. Williams ML, Sheng S, Gammie JS, Rankin JS, Smith PK, Hughes GC, Richard E, Clark Award. Aortic dissection as a complication of cardiac surgery: report from the Society of Thoracic Surgeons database. Ann Thor Surg. 2010;90(6):1812–6; discussion 6–7.
3. Winiszewski H, Perrotti A, Chocron S, Capellier G, Piton G. Malposition of the extracorporeal membrane oxygenation venous cannula in an accessory hepatic vein. J Extra Corpor Technol. 2018;50(3):167–9.
4. Kurusz M, Girouard MK, Brown PS Jr. Coronary sinus rupture with retrograde cardioplegia. Perfusion. 2002;17(1):77–80.
5. Mills NL, Ochsner JL. Massive air embolism during cardiopulmonary bypass. Causes, prevention, and management. J Thorac Cardiovas Surg. 1980;80(5):708–17.
6. Authors/Task Force M, Kunst G, Milojevic M, Boer C, De Somer F, Gudbjartsson T, et al. EACTS/EACTA/EBCP guidelines on cardiopulmonary bypass in adult cardiac surgery. British J Anaesth. 2019.

Pacemaker and Other Implantable Devices

Paula Trucco and Emilce Trucco

Introduction

In surgery settings, it is common to encounter patients with cardiac implantable electronic devices (CIEDs). These devices perform many functions, including bradycardia pacing, arrhythmias monitoring, cardiac resynchronization in case of heart failure, and defibrillation and anti-tachycardia pacing in case of tachyarrhythmias. CIEDs have been used for many years. During this time, the clinical efficacy has been proven in terms of improvement of quality of life and decrease of morbidity and mortality.

Although the devices available nowadays are complex, the vast majority of procedures can be safely performed in patients who carry them. Safe surgical planning requires familiarity with these devices. The anesthesiology must be aware of possible complications and be able to coordinate a multidisciplinary approach to ensure a safe management of patients with CIEDs during the perioperative period, in order to decrease the possibility of adverse events.

P. Trucco
Anaesthesiology Department, Hospital Universitario de Canarias, Santa Cruz de Tenerife, Spain

E. Trucco (✉)
Arrhythmia Section, Cardiology Department, Hospital Universitari Doctor Josep Trueta, Girona, Spain
e-mail: metrucco.girona.ics@gencat.cat

M. Vives and A. Hernandez (eds.), *Cardiac Anesthesia and Postoperative Care in the 21st Century*, https://doi.org/10.1007/978-3-030-79721-8_10

Types of Cardiac Implantable Electronic Devices

Cardiac rhythm management devices include pacemakers (PM), implantable cardioverter defibrillators (ICDs), cardiac resynchronization devices (CRDs) and implantable loop recorders (ILR) Table 1.

Pacemakers

These devices produce and deliver electrical impulses to stimulate the heart. They are indicated in patients with different types of bradyarrhythmia. The permanent forms of bradyarrhythmia are caused by an intrinsic disease of the sinus node or AV conduction system. There is a strong consensus that patients with symptomatic sinus node disease will benefit from cardiac pacing for symptom relief. Also, permanent cardiac pacing is indicated in patients with third or second degree type 2 AV block to improve mortality.

Table 1 Types of cardiac implantable devices and their functions. CRT- P: Cardiac resynchronization therapy with pacing, CRT-D: Cardiac resynchronization therapy with defibrillator, S-ICD: Subcutaneous implantable cardioverter defibrillator

Device	Function	
Pacemaker	Bradycardia pacing Rhythm monitoring	Transvenous or leadless pacing
Defibrillator	Bradycardia pacing Defibrillation Antitachycardia pacing Rhythm monitoring	Fast pacing to terminate the arrhythmia (not in S-ICD) Shock delivery to restore normal heart rhythm
Cardiac resynchronization therapy	Cardiac resynchronization Bradycardia pacing (CRT-P/CRT-D) Defibrillation (CRT-D) Rhythm monitoring	Biventricular pacing to improve systolic function in electrical desynchronize heart (wide QRS)
Implantable loop recorder	Rhythm monitoring (no therapies)	Detects bradycardia, pauses and tachycardia

Some patients may be entirely dependent on their PM and have no underlying rhythm, while others may only pace intermittently.

The chamber of the heart where the pacing electrodes sit may also vary from single lead in one chamber to three leads in cardiac resynchronization therapy (CRT).

Depending on the indication and the patient's underlying rhythm, the PM may be programmed in different ways. The nomenclature uses three to five letters. The first letter refers to the chamber paced (A—atrium, V—ventricle, D—dual), the second to the chamber sensed, and the third to the response to a sensed event (O—none, I—inhibit, T—trigger, D—dual). A fourth letter (R) is often used if the pacemaker has rate-modulation capability, whereby the PM increases the patient's heart rate with exercise. A fifth letter relates to the presence and location of multisite pacing.

By applying a magnet, pacemakers automatically reprogram in asynchronous mode of pacing (AOO, VOO, DOO), which means 'neglecting' impulses that are being sensed and deliver pacing at a programmed magnetic rate.

Defibrillators

They produce and provide fast pacing or shock to interrupt tachyarrhythmias.

These devices are indicated in prevention of sudden death due to malignant arrhythmias in populations at risk. The first detection mode is cardiac heart rate (instead cardiac frequency). However, they also have another screening method to classify cardiac arrhythmias in supraventricular or ventricular origin, such as stability of the rhythm, sudden onset of the episode and morphology comparable to normal QRS.

In the interrogation of the device, the programmed anti-tachycardia therapy, rhythm disorders presented by the patient, as well as the therapies received (whether appropriate or inappropriate), are evaluated.

Patients who receive a single shock should communicate with the cardiology service by telephone. In case of receiving multiple shocks, the scenario must be treated as a medical emergency. These patients must be admitted with access to an external defibrillator, being necessary to assess reversible causes such as metabolic or electrolyte abnormalities. Electrical storm is defined as the presence of 3 or more episodes of arrhythmias requiring the intervention of the device in a 24 h period. Ventricular arrhythmia storm leading to heart failure is the most frequent cause of multiple shocks.

Nevertheless, in some situations, the shocks are inappropriate. The most common causes of inappropriate shocks are supraventricular tachycardias, including atrial fibrillation. Another less frequent cause is complex detection other than QRS. Electromagnetic interference is also a reason for inappropriate therapies. In these cases, we can avoid therapies by approaching a magnet. The use of magnet in patients with ICDs inhibits the detection and therapy of ventricular arrhythmias (antitachycardia and shock function), but does not inhibit the antibradycardia pacing function. However, most patients do not need pacing.

Loop Recorders

These devices only function is to monitor for cardiac arrhythmias. They are implanted as a diagnostic tool, but do not provide cardiac therapies.

Cardiac Devices Complications

Concerns regarding potential device-related complications should be discussed with the implanting physician Tables 2 and 3.

Cardiac Devices Malfunctions

When a patient carrying a CIED is attending the preanesthesia consultation, anesthesiologist should determine the likelihood of that symptoms being related to a device malfunction.

Undersensing

It occurs when the device cannot detect the intrinsic cardiac activity. The conditions that can cause this are ischemia, new branch block, hydroelectrolytic disorders,

Table 2 Pocket complications

Pocket complications	
Hematoma	It may be due to residual bleeding. More frequent in patients on treatment with antiplatelets or anticoagulants. 1 to 2% of cases require evacuation. Never perform needle puncture
Infection	It causes local inflammation and fluctuation. Can lead to endocarditis and sepsis. Prolonged antibiotic therapy and complete removal of the device may be required
Pacemaker migration	The main cause is the bad fixation of the device. It causes pain and can cause erosion, requiring surgical debridement and relocation. Syndrome of Twiddler: It is the rotation of the generator with possible displacement of the electrodes

Table 3 Electrodes complications

Electrodes complications	
Pneumothorax/ Hemothorax	It can manifest immediately or in the days following the implant. The symptoms consist of breathlessness, pain, and subcutaneous emphysema. The incidence is 1.6–2.6%. In severe cases a pleural drainage must be implanted
Venous thrombosis	Produced by venous endothelial injury, cause pain and inflammation of the ipsilateral arm. May also produce superior vena cava syndrome. Nevertheless, asymptomatic thrombosis is common. The ultrasound confirms the diagnosis and treatment is anticoagulation
Tricuspid insuficiency	Symptoms depend on the degree of valve failure. It is usually accompanied by right heart failure
Cardiac perforation	Pericardial commitment can occur during electrode placement, but also in days following the implant. Electrode implant in coronary sinus may cause cardiac perforation. The incorrect position of the lead is observed in the ECG as a right bundle branch block, since the stimulation takes place in the left ventricle. It may cause diaphragmatic stimulation

ventricular extrasystoles or supraventricular arrhythmias. Displacement or electrode rupture are also a possible cause for undersensing; however, these conditions are usually associated to capture problems too.

Oversensing

It is due to improper device inhibition. There are signals that should not be detected that can cause stimulation failures. The T wave, noise from electromagnetic fields or skeletal muscle activity can be misinterpreted as intrinsic activity, inhibiting the device stimulation function. Emergency treatment consists on the application of a magnet, this will set the device on asynchronous stimulation (stimulating at fixed heart rate). This maneuver should be performed on monitored patients.

Stimulation Failure

It may be due to the lack of stimulus generation or the inability to capture. The first case can be caused by damage or depletion of the battery of the generator. The second scenario occurs when the impulse is insufficient to effectively depolarize the myocardium. Cable displacement or rupture and cardiac perforation should be ruled out. Electrolyte abnormalities could also affect the threshold for capturing. PM dependent patients may require external temporal stimulation.

Pacemaker Mediated Tachycardia

PM-mediated tachycardia may occur secondary to a closed loop reentry produced in bicameral pacesmakers. The mechanism consist on the use of the electrode as an aterograde route and the normal electric system as a retrograde route.

It can be produced by a ventricular extrasystole, or by atrial over or under sensing. Retrograde P waves can be detected in the twelve leads electrocardiogram (ECG). Current devices have algorithms to prevent or terminate PM mediated tachycardia, a widely used option is the prolongation of the post atrial refractory period.

Pacemaker Syndrome

It is caused by the loss of atrioventricular synchrony. This syndrome is observed mostly in single-chamber PM. The atrial contraction is lost, hence, a decrease in cardiac output and blood pressure occur. Patients usually show signs of hypoperfusion (fatigue, confusion, headache, dyspnea, and syncope).

Electromagnetic Interference

The most frequent sources of interference are large magnets such as resonances, speakers, airport security arches. In the operating room, the surgical electrocautery unit and other electronic procedural equipment can behave as intraoperative electromagnetic interference (EMI). These may alter the stimulation, leading to an inhibition by oversensing. Permanent damage of the device is rare, although it may occur during exposure to high sources of energy, such as external defibrillation and electrocautery.

Surgical Planning

Before Surgery

The purpose of preoperative planning is to gather information on the CIED and patient conditions. The clinical and physical exam should include a review of vital signs, cardiovascular examination and the complete inspection of the implant area.

The ECG is the first diagnostic tool. On its analysis, the intrinsic rhythm, the position of the stimulation electrode and the correct functioning of the device can be assessed. The ECG of a patient carrying a CIED must be interpreted with caution, since the new automatic pacemaker`s algorithms can be mistaken and identified as malfunction.

Radiologically we can determine which CIED type is implanted. On chest x-ray, ICD electrodes are clearly differentiated from PM electrodes by visible thickness, which corresponds to the high energy delivery part of the electrode.

In some cases, a complete interrogation of the device is mandatory. This is performed by the implant physician. It will give us crucial information, through the record of arrhythmias or malfunctions.

It is also necessary to determine the type, model, and manufacturer of the CIED, since each device has its own programmer. Usually, patients carry a card with identification and information regarding the device and electrodes. Some CIED even have telemonitoring, so the patient may have sent information through the website to the center where the implant was performed and subsequent monitored. Implant date, battery status, programming data and parameters of electrodes should be checked.

Immediate preoperative interrogations are not likely necessary in patients who are compliant with routine periodic interrogations by their pacemaker physician, nevertheless it is consider a good practice to do it (Table 4).

During Surgery

In addition to the usual care during surgery, there are a few specific requirements for patients with CIEDs. Continuous monitoring of heart rhythm and availability of external defibrillator with transcutaneous pacing and self-adhesive electrodes are essential. A magnet must also be available in the operating room.

Electromagnetic interference during surgery is frequent. The American Society of Anesthesiologist (ASA) Task Force states that electromagnetic interference could be minimized by different actions. These include positioning the cautery tool and current return pad away from the implant area; avoiding proximity of the cautery's

Table 4 Check list before surgery

Before surgery	
Patient interrogation and physical examination	Vital signs, cardiovascular exam, and implant area inspection
Check X-Ray and ECG	Normal positioning of device and cardiac rhythm assessment
Device type and brand, implant date and last follow-up	Information about device
Location of the device and surgery area	Possible interference surgery area—implant area
Type of the surgery	Emergency or programmed

Table 5 Check list during surgery

During surgery	
Pacemaker dependence	Does the patient still have intrinsic rhythm?
Arrhythmia density	Does the patient have arrhythmias and need therapy?
Electromagnetic interference	It is possible to minimizes electrical noises?

electrical field to the pulse generator and leads; using short, intermittent, and irregular bursts at the lowest feasible energy levels and using bipolar electrocautery whenever possible.

To prevent interferences during surgery, the behavior of a CIED can be temporarily altered with magnet application or permanently altered with a manufacturer-specific programming device.

Magnet application, apart from being simple and for most patients safe, it is also the preferred way of perioperative care, as it avoids repeated, incorrect, or incomplete reprogramming. This technique improves workflows in the perioperative period.

Absolute indications for CIED testing or reprogramming before surgery are suspicion of device malfunction, PM dependent patients with surgery performed in the area of the CIED (impossibility of magnet application) and patients with an ICD dependent on anti-bradycardia pacing (Table 5).

After Surgery

It is necessary to monitor patients until the function of the CIED is recovered. If the CIED has been reprogrammed preoperatively, monitoring is mandatory until new CIED testing and reprogramming to the previous mode is performed. If the CIED has not been reprogrammed, postoperative interrogation is indicated only in clinical situations where there is a suspicion that the device function may had been altered (Table 6).

Table 6 Check list after surgery

Afther surgery	
Check normal device function	If the CIED was reprogramed before surgery
Check ECG	Electrical normality

Conclusions

The recent advances in CIEDs function have greatly improved survival and the quality of life of patients. The preoperative assessment is mandatory to detect device complications or malfunctions. Surgical planning includes device last follow up and minimize of electrical interferences. With few exceptions, magnet application is the preferred way of perioperative care, as it avoids repeated, incorrect or incomplete reprogramming of the devices.

Recommended Readings

1. Epstein AE, Dimarco JP, Ellenbogen KA, Estes NA 3rd, Freedman RA, Gettes LS, Gillinov AM, Gregoratos G, Hammill SC, Hayes DL, Hlatky MA, Newby LK, Page RL, Schoenfeld MH, Silka MJ, Stevenson LW, Sweeney MO. A report of the American college of cardiology foundation/American heart association task force on practice guidelines and the heart rhythm society. J Am Coll Cardiol. 2013;61(3):e6-75.
2. Gillis A, Russo AM, Ellenbogen KA, Swerdlow CD, Olshansky B, Al-Khatib SM, Beshai JF, McComb JM, Nielsen JC, Philpott JM, Shen WK. HRS/ACCF Expert consensus statement on pacemaker device and mode selection. Heart Rhythm. 2012;9:1344–65.
3. Pavlović N, Manola S, Vražić H, Vučić3 M, Brusich S, Radeljić V, Zeljković I, Matasić R, Anić A, Benko I, Gavranović Z, Glogoški M. Recommendations for preoperative management of patients with cardiac implantable electronic devices. Acta Clin Croat 2018; 57:383.
4. Feldman JB, Stone ME. Anesthesia teams managing pacemakers and ICDs for the perioperative period: enhanced patient safety and improved workflows. Rev Curr Opin Anesthesiol. 2020;33:441–7.

Hemostasis and Coagulation Monitoring: Thromboelastogram, ROTEM and Platelet Mapping

Gerhardus J. A. J. M. Kuiper and Keyvan Karkouti

Introduction

Many processes during cardiac surgery contribute to coagulopathy, which can lead to increased blood loss and necessitate the transfusion of blood components. During surgery, prompt diagnosis and management of coagulopathy together with good communication among the members of the operative team, the diagnostic laboratory, and blood bank is imperative for effective bleeding control. This chapter will expand on the diagnostics of perioperative coagulopathy in cardiac surgery.

Management Approach to Bleeding

During cardiac surgery, particularly when cardiopulmonary bypass (CPB) is prolonged, coagulation is prone to many potential disturbances (Table 1). This table, which is not comprehensive, uses prior knowledge of the possible threats to coagulation in order to narrow it down to specific goals for managing the coagulopathy. The many examples included illustrate the complexity of the pathophysiology of coagulopathy during cardiac surgery and why management may not be conducive to a bottom-up approach.

The use of flowcharts may provide a more practical means for managing coagulopathy in the peri-operative period. Various flowcharts can be found in the

G. J. A. J. M.Kuiper
Department of Anesthesia and Pain Management, Peter Munk Cardiac Centre, Toronto General Hospital, University Health Network, University of Toronto, Toronto, ON, Canada

K. Karkouti (✉)
Department of Anesthesia and Pain Management, Toronto General Hospital, 200 Elizabeth Street 3EN-460, Toronto, Canada
e-mail: Keyvan.karkouti@uhn.ca

M. Vives and A. Hernandez (eds.), *Cardiac Anesthesia and Postoperative Care in the 21st Century*, https://doi.org/10.1007/978-3-030-79721-8_11

Table 1 Coagulopathy during cardiac surgery

Attributable to	Threat	Pathophysiology	Possible solutions
Patient characteristics	Known coagulopathies	Inherited (hemophilia or Von Willebrand Disease (VWD)) or acquired coagulopathy (VWD in aortic valve stenosis)	Pre-operative consultation with hematologist for peri-operative strategy
	Pre-operative anemia	Multiple: iron deficiency anemia, chronic kidney disease, diagnostic phlebotomy, etc	Timely pre-operative diagnosis and optimization
	Patients on (multiple) antiplatelet drugs	Part of the treatment strategy of acute myocardial infarction	Planning of surgery, pre-operative platelet transfusion, future reversal agents for antiplatelet drugs
	Cannot use certain transfusion products	Jehovah's Witnesses; Previous allergies or reactions to transfusion products	Pre-planned strategy: pre-operative optimization, off-pump surgery, etc.
CardioPulmonary Bypass	Large non-endothelial surface area of CPB circuit	Activation of coagulation	High dose of anticoagulation with heparin, coating of CPB circuit
	Large non-endothelial surface area of CPB circuit	Excessive fibrinolysis	Use of antifibrinolytics
	Large non-endothelial surface area of CPB circuit	Platelet activation	Prevention of platelet activation by using acetylsalicylic acid
	Roller/centrifugal pumps	Platelet destruction	Platelet transfusion
	Extravascular reservoir	Dilution of coagulation factors, platelets and red blood cells	Minimized circuit
Coagulation monitoring	Platelet dysfunction	Platelet count gives no information on platelet function	Point-of-care platelet function tests
	Caveats in platelet function tests	Inaccurate in conditions of thrombocytopenia and anemia	Normalize results from point-of-care platelet function tests
	Repeated diagnostic phlebotomies	Mean daily loss over 40 ml of blood, exceeds the normal healthy replacement rate	Reduce amount and volume of withdrawals

(continued)

Table 1 (continued)

Attributable to	Threat	Pathophysiology	Possible solutions
	Delay between bleeding, diagnosis and treatment	Long turnaround times: traditional monitoring can have a minimum of 30 min for first results	Use of point-of-care coagulation devices
Anticoagulation on CPB	Heparin overdose	Coagulation shutdown by heparin via ATIII anticoagulation effect on thrombin and FX	Reversal with protamine
	Protamine overdose	Inhibition of FV, FVII, and FX. Platelet dysfunction	Titration of protamine to heparin
Surgery	Overt bleeding due to surgery	Surgical incisions, large wound bed	Surgical hemostasis with sutures and hemostatic wound dressings
	Overt bleeding due to reduced coagulation factors and platelets	Consumption of coagulation factors and platelets while keeping up with coagulation	Transfusion of FFP, cryoprecipitate, PCC, fibrinogen concentrate
	Overt bleeding with red blood cell loss	Loss of red blood cells results in reduced lateral dispersion of platelets under flow	Optimize hematocrit by red blood cell transfusion
	Overt bleeding with red blood cell loss	Loss due to surgical suction and sponges	Cell saver usage
	Overt bleeding with loss of circulating volume	Hypoperfusion and hypoxia leads to anaerobic metabolism and acidosis and thereby worsening coagulation	Prevent acidosis by optimizing perfusion
	Thrombosis	Prothrombotic, inflammatory response in a bedridden patient	Prophylactic anticoagulation postoperatively
	Deep cooling with circulatory arrest	Hypothermia induced coagulopathy	Re-warming
Massive transfusion	Reduced calcium levels	Citrate overdose from transfusion products	Measure calcium levels and treat accordingly
	Autologous donated transfusion products	Non-standardized contents in each transfusion product; high volume with risk of overload; scarce commodity	Use of concentrated procoagulant medication
…	…	…	…

literature, but examples provided in Figs. 1 and 2 illustrate the basics of this approach. As a first step, the goal should be to achieve a 'coagulation friendly environment,' which is a state of normothermia, normal pH, normocalcemia, and optimized hematocrit. The coagulation proteins function optimally at close to normal body temperature, with major dysfunction occurring when temperature drops below 33 °C. For acidemia, little protein dysfunction occurs if pH levels are kept above 7.20; however, bleeding can be increased if pH levels are below 7.35 in the presence of hyperlactataemia. Multiple steps in the coagulation cascade are calcium dependent, and transfusion of blood products with citrate-based preservative solutions can cause hypocalcemia. Optimizing hematocrit is important because red cells, being the larger components of blood, displace the smaller components such as circulating platelets towards vascular endothelium, where they can be activated at the site of injury. This is called the 'Fåhraeus-Vejlens' or 'margination effect'.

Next, coagulation assays should be used to determine the cause of coagulopathy. It is important to note that all laboratory assays have false positives; thus, patients should not be treated if they are not bleeding, irrespective of what the assays show. The ideal coagulation assay would rapidly and accurately identify the coagulation defect at the bedside. Traditional coagulation assays, such as prothrombin time, partial thromboplastin time, and fibrinogen levels, are far from this ideal as they generally cannot be conducted at the bedside, require time consuming sample preparation, and do not provide information on the overall coagulation process as they are plasma-based. Whole-blood based assays are now available that can rapidly provide a global assessment of coagulation at the bedside using only small amounts of blood. Coagulation management algorithms that use these assays have been shown to reduce allogeneic blood component transfusions, and the use of these assays it is now recommended by major guidelines.

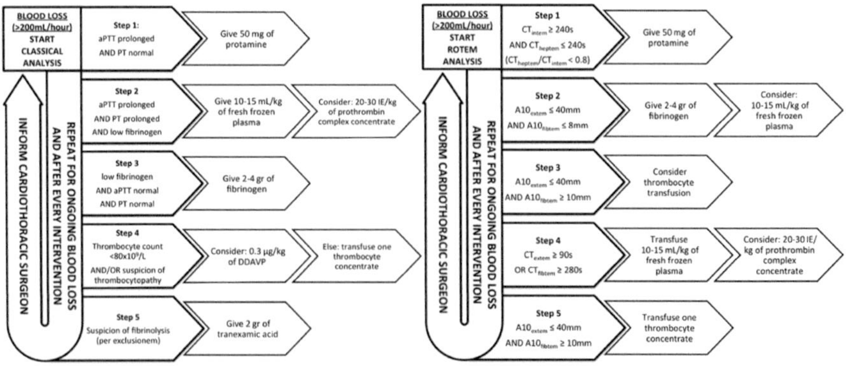

Fig. 1 Two peri-operative cardiac surgery flowcharts of managing coagulation based on traditional laboratory and ROTEM approaches from Maastricht UMC+, the Netherlands. Reprinted by permission from G. J. A. J. M. Kuiper (Gerhardus J. A. J. M. Kuiper. Haemostasis monitoring: pinpointing using point-of-care. Maastricht: Datawyse/Universitaire Pers Maastricht; 2018. ISBN 9789462958869), copyright 2018

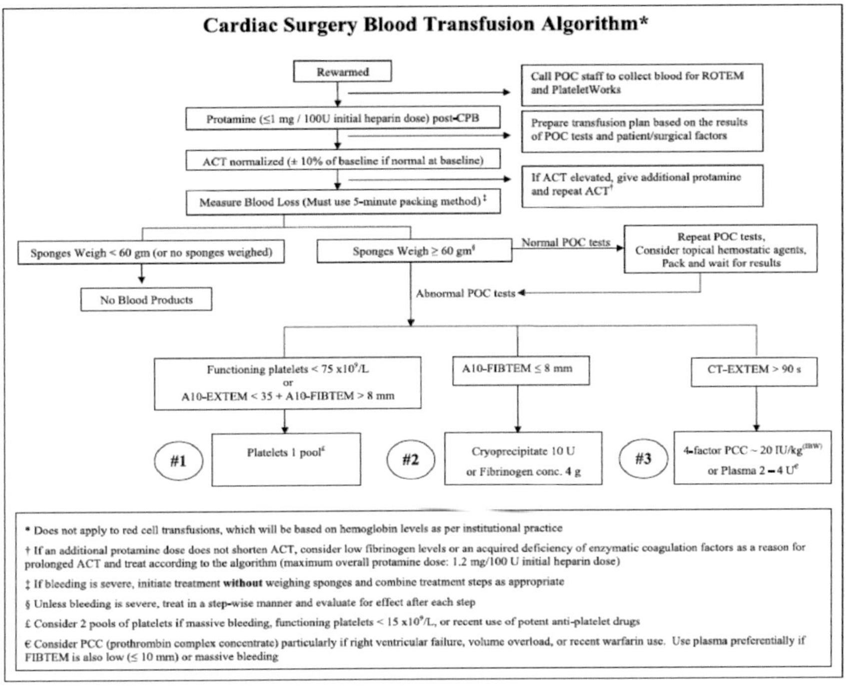

Fig. 2 Perioperative cardiac surgery flowchart of managing coagulation based on a POC approach using ROTEM and PlateletWorks from Toronto General Hospital, Canada. Reprinted by permission from Wolters Kluwer Health, Inc.: Circulation (Keyvan Karkouti, Jeannie Callum, Duminda N. Wijeysundera, et al. Point-of-Care Hemostatic Testing in Cardiac Surgery, Circulation. 2016; 134(16): 1152–62. https://www.ahajournals.org/journal/circ), copyright 2016

ROTEM

One of the more commonly used whole-blood based assays is rotational thromboelastometry (ROTEM, Instrumentation Laboratory, Bedford, MA, USA), which measures the viscoelastic properties of coagulation. There are several different types of viscoelastic assays on the market, but the basis for all current methods was laid out in 1948 by Hellmut Hartert. In his paper he described his method of '*Thrombelastographie*' and gave a first graph of a normal curve (Fig. 3). Modern assays include more parameters and tests that provide additional information using one small tube of citrate anticoagulated whole blood (Table 2). The inner workings of ROTEM do not differ much from Hartert's method that later became the commercially available TEG 5000 device (Haemonetics Corporation, Braintree, MA, USA). Another well-known viscoelastic system is the Sonoclot Analyzer (Sienco Inc., Boulder, CO, USA). The focus of this chapter is on ROTEM.

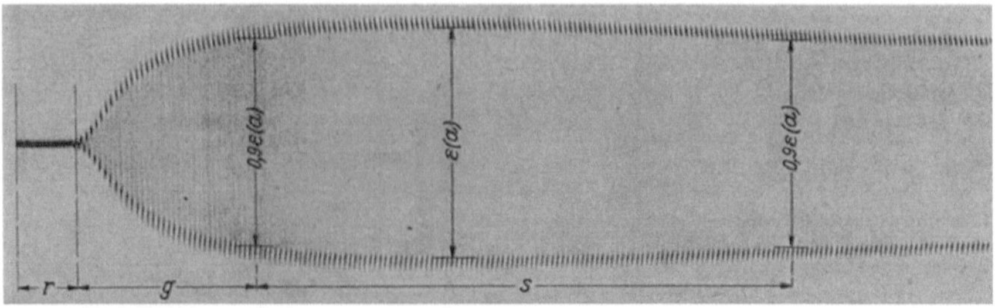

Fig. 3 Depicted is the '*Thrombelastographische Normalkurve*' from Hartert's 1948 publication. *r* = '*Reaktionszeit*' or 'reaction time'; *g* = '*Gerinnselbildungszeit*' or 'clot building time'; *s* = '*Retraktionszeit*' or 'retraction time'; ε = '*lineare Gesamtelastizität*' or 'linear combined elasticity'. Reprinted by permission from Springer Nature: Klinische Wochenschrift (Hartert Hellmut. Blutgerinnungsstudien mit der Thrombelastographie, einem neuen Untersuchungsverfahren, Klinische Wochenschrift. 1948; 26(37–38): 577–83. https://link.springer.com/journal/109), copyright 1948

Modern Thromboelastogram

The ROTEM technique to produce the thromboelastogram is as follows (Fig. 4). Citrated anticoagulated blood is put in a small cup. The blood is recalcified, an activator from either the extrinsic or intrinsic pathway is added, and a measuring pin is put in the mixture (more activators can be found in Table 2). While this pin starts rotating (±4.75°), the blood starts to clot. The stronger the clot, the more restricted is the pin's ability to rotate. A light beam is reflected off a mirror on the pin. Rotation is recorded and a graph is plotted over time (Fig. 5). The graphs portray three different colors: green, pink and blue. By convention, the graph starts off green until an amplitude of 2 mm has been reached (this is the clotting time or CT). From this point on the graph is colored pink until an amplitude of 20 mm has been reached. The pink part is the clot formation time (CFT). After the 20 mm point the graph remains blue. After the maximum clot firmness (MCF) has been reached a slow decline of the graph towards zero is seen. This decline is part clot retraction and part fibrinolysis.

Correlation Between ROTEM Parameters and Traditional Laboratory Assays

Since viscoelastic assays are whole-blood based and standard traditional laboratory coagulation assays are plasma-based, correlation between the two assays is not perfect. The timed parameters (CT) correlate well with the timed parameters in traditional coagulation studies (PT and aPTT) depending on the activator used (i.e. EXTEM-CT vs. PT and INTEM-CT vs. aPTT). The amplitude parameters (A5, A10, and MCF) correlate well with concentration parameters in traditional

Table 2 Nine different ROTEM tests. The first seven are original ROTEM tests, while the last two are externally validated adaptations (1, 2)

	Activators	Route	Goal
NATEM	Non-activated	Intrinsic pathway by contact activation of the cup and pin	Non-activated, recalcified coagulation profile. This is a non-boosted version of INTEM
EXTEM	Tissue factor	Extrinsic pathway	Coagulation profile through activation via extrinsic pathway
INTEM	Ellagic acid	Intrinsic pathway by ellagic acid	Coagulation profile through activation via intrinsic pathway
FIBTEM	EXTEM + Cytochalasin D	Extrinsic pathway Breakdown of platelet cytoskeleton	Coagulation profile of fibrinogen without platelet contribution
HEPTEM	INTEM + Heparinase	Intrinsic pathway Heparin neutralizer	If the INTEM CT is prolonged due to heparin, the CT HEPTEM will be shortened back to normal ranges
APTEM	EXTEM + Aprotinin	Extrinsic pathway Fibrinolysis blocker	If ML in EXTEM is >15% and it is due to excessive fibrinolysis, the APTEM test will block the fibrinolysis and revert it back to normal
ECATEM (2)	Ecarin	Conversion of prothrombin to meizothrombin	Like thrombin, meizothrombin is also able to convert fibrinogen into fibrin, but it is not affected by heparin. In the presence of thrombin inhibitors, clotting times will be prolonged by the inactivation of meizothrombin
'PLTEM' (1)	EXTEM FIBTEM	Extrinsic pathway Without fibrinogen contribution	Subtract the FIBTEM amplitude results from the EXTEM amplitude results. This yields the coagulation profile of platelets without fibrinogen contribution
'TPATEM' (1)	EXTEM + recombinant TPA	Extrinsic pathway Fibrinolysis promoter	By actively breaking down the clot with rTPA, fibrinolysis occurs earlier. Used in order to diagnose occult hyper- and overt hypofibrinolysis

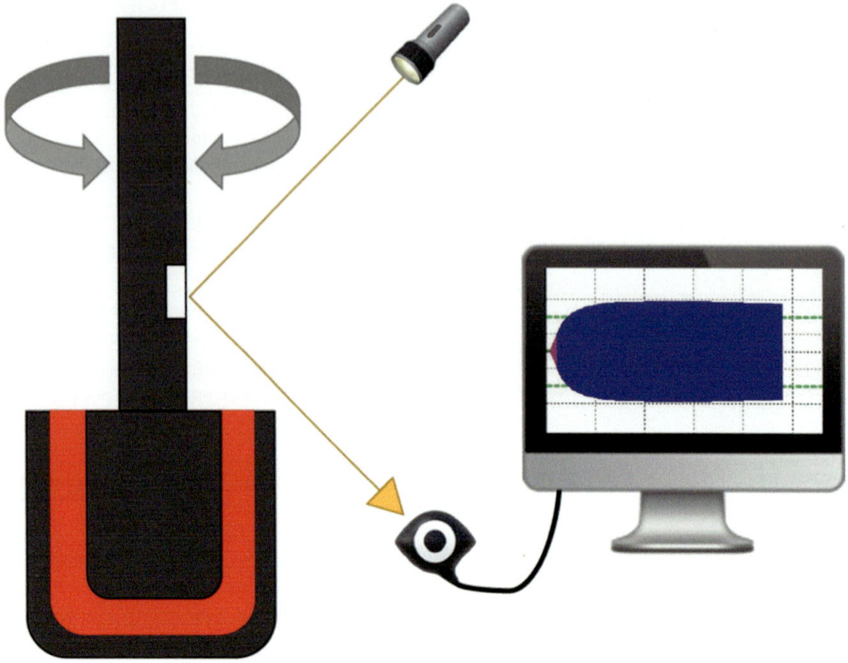

Fig. 4 ROTEM measuring technique. The main components of a the ROTEM device are a rotating axis (back-and-forth by 4.75°), which holds a pin and a stationary cup for the blood and reagents. Once all fluids are injected in the cup, the rotating pin will be placed into the mixture. Coagulation will start and the stronger the clot, the more the pin is restricted in its movement. The rotational movement is sensed by reflecting light of a mirror on the rotating axis onto a light sensitive cell. This signal is transmitted to a processor and the thromboelastogram is being produced on screen with all its parameters

laboratory results (platelet count and fibrinogen levels). FIBTEM-A5, FIBTEM-A10, and FIBTEM-MCF correlate with Clauss-based fibrinogen levels and 'PLTEM-A5' (EXTEM-A5 minus FIBTEM-A5) correlates with platelet count.

Interpreting the Thromboelastogram

Several ROTEM assays are available that assess different components of coagulation (Table 2), but since each ROTEM device only has 4 channels, only 4 assays can be conducted simultaneously. Usually EXTEM, INTEM and FIBTEM are performed as the standard 3 assays, and Table 3 has an overview of the abnormal results of these assays. The HEPTEM assay, which contains heparinase to reverse the action of heparin, can be used as the 4th assay in patients who have received heparin to determine any residual heparin effect. In patients with residual heparin

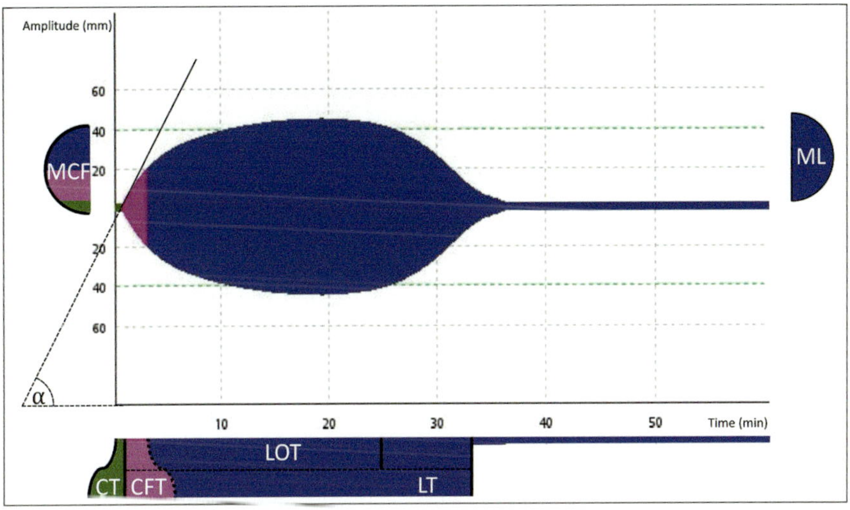

Fig. 5 Thromboelastogram with parameters *(actual patient data from an EXTEM assay)* CT: Coagulation Time (s). Time from start of coagulation till 2 mm of amplitude *(CT = 51 s)*. CFT: Clot Formation Time (s). Time from 2 mm till 20 mm of amplitude *(CFT = 135 s)*. α: Alpha angle (°). Angle between baseline and a tangent to the ROTEM curve going through the 2 mm point and *(α = 69°)*. A(x): Amplitude at x minutes (mm). At any time point the amplitude is given. Standard parameters are given for A5 to A30 in intervals of 5 min after CT *(A5 = 31 mm)*. MCF: Maximum Clot Firmness (mm). Maximum amplitude reached *(MCF = 45 mm)*. LOT: Lysis Onset Time (min). Time from CT till 85% is left of MCF *(LOT = 25 min 28 s)*. LT: Lysis Time (min). Time from CT till 10% is left of MCF *(LT = 33 min 55 s)*. ML: Maximum Lysis (%). The amount of lysis percentage between the MCF and the lowest amplitude after MCF *(ML = 100%)*

effect, INTEM CT will be prolonged and a shortening of the CT in the HEPTEM assay relative to the INTEM CT would confirm the presence of heparin effect. If hyperfibrinolysis is suspected, then the APTEM assay (which contains the antifibrinolytic aprotinin) can be used to confirm the diagnosis by comparing the amount of clot lysis to that observed in the EXTEM assay (Table 2).

As a rule, the graphs should have smooth lines. Jagged lines with abnormal results are likely due to device faults or other errors. Although rare, the automatic pipetting setting could still lead to erroneous results by human error (mixing up the reagents order or contaminating the reagents themselves).

Medication Effects

The influence of medication (antiplatelet medication, vitamin K antagonists (VKA's) and direct oral anticoagulants (DOAC's) on viscoelastic tests is well described in the literature. In case of the DOAC dabigatran (a direct thrombin inhibitor), a modified ecarin activated ROTEM assay (ECATEM) can be used to measure dabigatran levels (Table 2). In patients with heparin induced thrombocytopenia (HIT) needing cardiopulmonary bypass, alternative direct thrombin inhibitors, like the anticoagulants hirudin, argatroban or bivalirudin, can be monitored with ecarin based viscoelastic modifications as well.

Platelet Mapping

"For effective primary haemostasis, a sufficient number of functional platelets need to be present in vivo. Likewise, this applies to in vitro assays of platelet function." A simple platelet count (or the ROTEM derivative PLTEM to estimate platelet count) is a good start, but this does not provide information on platelet function. Furthermore, typical viscoelastic assays have activators that mask the effects of platelet dysfunction in clotting, meaning that patients may have normal ROTEM measures despite having significant platelet dysfunction. This is of concern in cardiac surgery as platelet dysfunction is a common cause of bleeding due to the frequent use of antiplatelet drugs and the effects of cardiopulmonary bypass on platelets. Thus, measuring platelet function is crucial for managing bleeding during cardiac surgery.

Multiple devices haven been developed for measuring platelet function, but there is limited data on their clinical utility. Platelet mapping was developed in order to give insight in the contribution of platelets to hemostasis using TEG. Three to four tests are compared: a normal kaolin activated (KA) TEG (comparable to INTEM) for maximum coagulation due to the thrombin burst; a heparinized sample, which is activated by reptilase and crosslinked by activated factor XIII (FXIIIa), that would give a fibrin specific curve without the thrombin influence; and finally, a platelet activator (either adenosine-diphosphate (ADP) or arachidonic acid (AA)) is added to the previously described sample condition. Herein, platelet contribution can be measured on top of the fibrin specific assay in the absence of thrombin as the strongest activator of platelets. The % platelet aggregation and inhibition would then be calculated by using the maximum amplitude (MA) of these curves and the following formulas:

$$\%\,platelet\,aggregation = \left(\frac{MA_{ADP\,or\,AA} - MA_{FIB}}{MA_{KA} - MA_{FIB}}\right) \times 100\%$$

$$\%\,platelet\,inhibition = 100\% - \%\,platelet\,aggregation$$

Newer versions of the ROTEM *delta* devices can also have a platelet function method incorporated: ROTEM *platelet*. It is essentially a hybrid of a regular ROTEM viscoelastic device with a Multiple Electrode Aggregometry (MEA or Multiplate Analyzer by Roche Diagnostics, Indianapolis, IN, USA) technique for measuring platelet function added. This bundled machine has the features of both assays for POC hemostasis monitoring. The MEA technique acts by analyzing

Table 3 Common ROTEM abnormalities of the three standard tests with differential diagnosis during/after cardiac surgery

ROTEM finding	Differential diagnosis	Strengthening diagnosis
EXTEM-CT prolonged	Isolated factor VII deficiency	Measure FVII level, PT prolonged
	Thrombocytopenia	Measure 'PLTEM' and/or platelet count
	Hypofibrinogenemia	Measure regular fibrinogen levels
	Extreme hyperfibrinolysis	APTEM test normal, lysis after MCF
	Low coagulation factor levels or factor inhibitors	Measure traditional lab: PT, aPTT, etc.
	Erroneous test	Normal re-test
EXTEM-CFT prolonged	Thrombocytopenia	Measure 'PLTEM' and/or platelet count
	Hypofibrinogenemia	Measure regular fibrinogen levels
	Hyperfibrinolysis	APTEM test normal, lysis after MCF
	Low coagulation factor levels or factor inhibitors	Measure traditional lab: PT, aPTT, etc.
EXTEM-alpha reduced	Thrombocytopenia	Measure 'PLTEM' and/or platelet count
	Hypofibrinogenemia	Measure regular fibrinogen levels
	Hyperfibrinolysis	APTEM test normal, lysis after MCF
	Low coagulation factor levels or factor inhibitors	Measure traditional lab: PT, aPTT, etc.
EXTEM-MCF reduced	Thrombocytopenia	Measure 'PLTEM' and/or platelet count
	Hypofibrinogenemia	Measure regular fibrinogen levels
	Hyperfibrinolysis	APTEM test normal, lysis after MCF
INTEM-CT prolonged	Intravenous heparin therapy	HEPTEM-CT is shorter
	Protamine overdosing	HEPTEM-CT is similar
	Thrombocytopenia	Measure 'PLTEM' and/or platelet count
	Hypofibrinogenemia	Measure regular fibrinogen levels
	Extreme hyperfibrinolysis	APTEM test normal, lysis after MCF
	Erroneous test	Normal re-test

(continued)

Table 3 (continued)

ROTEM finding	Differential diagnosis	Strengthening diagnosis
INTEM-CFT prolonged	Thrombocytopenia	Measure 'PLTEM' and/or platelet count
	Hypofibrinogenemia	Measure regular fibrinogen levels
	Hyperfibrinolysis	APTEM test normal, lysis after MCF
	Low coagulation factor levels or factor inhibitors	Measure traditional lab: PT, aPTT, etc.
INTEM-alpha reduced	Thrombocytopenia	Measure 'PLTEM' and/or platelet count
	Hypofibrinogenemia	Measure regular fibrinogen levels
	Hyperfibrinolysis	APTEM test normal, lysis after MCF
	Low coagulation factor levels or factor inhibitors	Measure traditional lab: PT, aPTT, etc.
INTEM-MCF reduced	Thrombocytopenia	Measure 'PLTEM' and/or platelet count
	Hypofibrinogenemia	Measure regular fibrinogen levels
	Hyperfibrinolysis	APTEM test normal, lysis after MCF
FIBTEM-CT prolonged	Hypofibrinogenemia	Measure regular fibrinogen levels
	Extreme hyperfibrinolysis	EX-/APTEM test normal, lysis after MCF
	Erroneous test	Normal re-test
FIBTEM-MCF reduced	Hypofibrinogenemia	Measure regular fibrinogen levels
	Hyperfibrinolysis	EX-/APTEM test normal, lysis after MCF

platelet function by immersing two pairs of rods into hirudin anticoagulated whole blood; activating the platelets using one of various platelet agonists; and then measuring the impendence between the rods. Activated platelets adhere to the rods altering the impendence between the rods and as such platelet function can be measured. The MEA method is again susceptible to low platelet counts. Many other whole blood platelet function measuring technique are available each with its pros and cons.

Guidelines

A survey conducted for the 2015 American Society of Anesthesiologists guideline on perioperative blood management showed consensus of viscoelastic testing together with a platelet count in bleeding patients. If such viscoelastic testing is not available, standard laboratory testing is recommended. They stated that multimodal protocols and/or algorithms should be employed for effective patient blood management. However, they did not recommend a specific protocol and/or algorithm, as there seems to be no superiority of one over the other.

In 2018 a taskforce from the European Association for Cardio-Thoracic Surgery (EACTS) and the European Association of Cardiothoracic Anaesthesiology (EACTA) published specific guidelines for patient blood management in adult cardiac surgery patients. The following are their recommendations of the role of viscoelastic testing: "Routine use of viscoelastic […] testing is not recommended to predict bleeding in patients without antithrombotic treatment." "Perioperative treatment algorithms for the bleeding patient based on viscoelastic POC tests should be considered to reduce the number of transfusions."

Advances in Viscoelastic Testing

Newer viscoelastic systems are fully automated and cartridge based. The ROTEM *sigma* uses the same methodology of ROTEM *delta* but uses a cartridge that is inserted into a slot in the device. The cartridge houses multiple cup-and-pin combinations with freeze-dried reagents including EXTEM, INTEM, and FIBTEM. On top of the cartridge there is an aspiration needle where an inverted citrate anticoagulated whole blood tube can be placed for the initiation of testing. The ROTEM *sigma*, however, does not come with an integrated platelet function analyzer.

The automated version of TEG is the TEG 6s. Similar to ROTEM *sigma*, the TEG 6 s uses preloaded cartridges with a slot at the top for patients' blood. The measuring technique is significantly changed in the TEG 6s compared to the TEG 5000. The TEG 6s uses a resonance technique where blood is subjected to a range of audible soundwaves. Blood droplets at the end of microfluidic channels vibrate differently based on their viscoelastic properties. The sound induced up-and-down motion of the blood meniscus is detected by changes in light transmission. In comparison to the ROTEM *sigma*, the TEG 6s does have a platelet mapping cartridge available. Downsides of both machines are that they have only one slot, thereby limiting the user in measuring multiple cartridges at the same time, and the cartridge-based systems cost more than the older versions of the assays.

Another company, Hemosonics (Charlottesville, VA, USA; https://hemosonics.com), has released the Quantra device. This compact device uses Sonic Estimation of Elasticity via Resonance (SEER) ultrasound technology. Similar to TEG 6s, resonance is measured in preloaded cartridges, but this time ultrasound is used for detection. Results are depicted in units of time (seconds) or shear modulus (hecto Pascal). One of the results is the Platelet Contribution to Clot Stiffness (PCS) which employs a similar concept to platelet contribution in PLTEM.

All these machines have evolved from laboratory-based hemostasis devices to POC easy to use tests. Some of the bulkiness of the machines persists and we are still far removed from portable finger prick POC viscoelastic hemostasis testing.

Final Remarks

Whole blood viscoelastic hemostasis monitoring offers many advantages over traditional coagulation assays. The techniques are well validated, they can be used at the bedside, and provide results on the entire coagulation pathway within minutes. Their use has been shown to improve the management of coagulopathy and is recommended by current guidelines.

Recommended Readings

1. Boer C, Meesters MI, Milojevic M, Benedetto U, Bolliger D, von Heymann C, et al. 2017 EACTS/EACTA Guidelines on patient blood management for adult cardiac surgery. J Cardiothorac Vasc Anesth. 2018;32(1):88–120.
2. American society of anesthesiologists task force on perioperative blood management. Practice guidelines for perioperative blood management: an updated report by the American society of anesthesiologists task force on perioperative blood management. Anesthesiology. 2015;122 (2):241–75.
3. Wikkelsø A, Wetterslev J, Møller AM, Afshari A. Thromboelastography (TEG) or thromboelastometry (ROTEM) to monitor haemostatic treatment versus usual care in adults or children with bleeding. Cochrane Emergency and Critical Care Group, editor. Cochrane Database Syst Rev [Internet]. 2016 Aug 22 [cited 2019 Aug 6]. https://doi.org/10.1002/14651858.CD007871.pub3.

Intraoperative Management

General Principles of Anaesthesia for Adult Cardiac Surgery

Fabrizio Monaco, Ambra Licia Di Prima, and Giovanni Landoni

Intraoperative Management

The intraoperative management has a major impact on the perioperative course of patients undergoing cardiac surgery. Although a proficient surgical technique and a short surgical time are a relevant component of an uneventful course, an adequate preoperative assessment, a skillful anesthetic technique, and meticulous intraoperative monitoring, are all necessary measures to avoid potentially fatal complications.

Preoperative Counselling

The intraoperative management of patients undergoing cardiac surgery starts before the operating theatre with a preoperative counselling (Table 1).

F. Monaco · A. L. Di Prima · G. Landoni (✉)
Department of Anesthesia and Intensive Care, IRCCS San Raffaele Scientific Institute, Via Olgettina 60, 20132 Milan, Italy
e-mail: landoni.giovanni@hsr.it

F. Monaco
e-mail: monaco.fabrizio@hsr.it

A. L. Di Prima
e-mail: diprima.ambralicia@hsr.it

G. Landoni
Vita-Salute San Raffaele University, Via Olgettina 58, 20132 Milan, Italy

M. Vives and A. Hernandez (eds.), *Cardiac Anesthesia and Postoperative Care in the 21st Century*, https://doi.org/10.1007/978-3-030-79721-8_12

Table 1 Preoperative counselling

History	
Cardiac symptoms, significant comorbidities, previous anesthetic experiences, surgical procedures, allergies, medications and recent use of steroids	
Medical therapy	
Antihypertensive and antianginal medications	Continue up to and including the morning of surgery
Angiotensin-converting enzyme (ACE) inhibitors and angiotensin receptor blockers (ARBs)	Stop (eg the morning of surgery) to reduce the risk of low systemic resistance in the perioperative period
Insulin or oral hypoglycemic medications	Stop the morning of surgery. Check frequently blood glucose during surgery
Warfarin	Stop at least 4 days before surgery to have INR normalized before surgery
Aspirin (little impact on perioperative bleeding)	• In elective CABG or valvular surgery without coronary disease Stop 3–5 days before surgery • In symptomatic coronary patients Continue
Clopidogrel and prasugrel	• Stop 5–7 days before elective surgery • Continue or stop for a shorter period of time in patients with recently placed drug-eluting stents
Unfractionated heparin	• stop about 4 hours before surgery • continue into the operating room for patients with critical coronary disease
Low molecular-weight heparin	• Last dose should be given 18–24 hours before surgery • Fondaparinux stop at least 48 hours before surgery
IIb/IIIa Inhibitors (Eptifibatide and Tirofiban)	Stop at least 4 hours prior to surgery

Premedication

Premedication decreases the sympathetic tone and usually induces vasodilatation and bradycardia which may lead to cardiogenic shock in poorly compensated patients (e.g. critical aortic stenosis, congestive heart failure). In these patients premedication, should be given with caution due to the risk of cardiocirculatory collapse (Table 2).

The prophylactic antibiotics (usually a cephalosporin) must be administered within 1 hour of skin incision. In patients allergic to β-lactam, vancomycin giving in 1 h is the antibiotic of choice.

Table 2 Anesthetic premedication for cardiac surgical patients

• Temazepam 10–20 mg or diazepam 5 mg P.O the night before surgery
• Midazolam 1–4 mg IV or fentanyl 50–100 μg IV under monitoring

Monitoring

Before anesthesia induction, a peripheral venous access and a full monitoring are required. A 5-leads electrocardiography (E.C.G) with a continuous visualization through DII and V5 leads, an arterial line usually placed in the radial artery for invasive blood pressure, pulse oximetry, urinary Foley catheter for urine output, and core body temperature are the standards for basic Anesthetic monitoring in cardiac surgery it is common practice to defer central lines placement after anesthetic induction to avoid discomfort and anxiety in awake patients. In fact, tachycardia and hypertension increase myocardial oxygen consumption. Only in patients with low cardiac output (CO) or hemodynamic instability would need a pre-induction central line placement to start vasoactive drugs.

Cannulation of the right or alternatively left jugular vein under ultrasound guidance is achieved with a 7 Fr 3 lines catheter to measure central venous pressure (CVP) and in some hospitals with a 8.5 F pulmonary artery catheter (PAC) introducer. Usually, PAC is placed after the induction only in high risk patients with pulmonary hypertension, low ejection fraction or when a difficult weaning from the CPB is anticipated. Possible complications associated with PAC are summarized in the Table 3. There is no evidence showing that the routine use of PAC improve outcomes. However, data from observational cohorts in selected high-risk patients show that might be of benefit. Literature shows that TEE is a cost-effective tool impacting the surgical planning. The probe is inserted before heparinization and after intubation. It provides information on ventricular function, valve pathology or intracardiac masses by Bright mode, 3D, M-Mode, flow Doppler (continuous, pulse, color and tissue) (Table 4). TEE has few contraindications and in less than 0.1% of cases it is associated with severe complications (Table 5).

General Anesthetic Considerations

Cardiac surgery patients are fragile, and no single protocol can guarantee hemodynamic stability during induction. Hemodynamic changes depends on patient's pathophysiology and on the administered pharmacological agents. A reduction in sympathetic tone, due to inhalation and I.V agents is associated with vasodilatation, cardiac depression, and relative hypovolemia, which acting together may lead to hypotension and cardiogenic shock if not promptly treated. Thus, the use of small dose of vasoconstrictor for induction (e.g. etilefrine 1–4 mg iv), in rapid succession

Table 3 Complications associated with pulmonary artery catheter

During positioning	Post positioning
• Arterial puncture	• Thrombosis and venous embolism
• Tricuspid valve traumatism	• Infections—Endocarditis
• Arrhythmias	• Transient Right Bundle Branch Block
• Pulmonary artery disruption	
• Mechanical damage to cardiac structures	

Table 4 Role of transesophageal echocardiography

Before surgery	During surgery	Post surgery
Confirming diagnosis and feasibility of surgical correction	Modifying and targeting anesthetic management	Evaluation of RV/LV systolic and diastolic function
Helping in choice of surgical technique correction	Check placement of CPB cannulas	Verification of surgical correction
	Weaning from CPB	Detection of regional wall motion abnormalities
	De-airing after CPB	
	Check for IABP position	

CPB: cardiopulmonary bypass; IABP: Intra-aortic balloon pump

Table 5 Complication and contraindications of transesophageal echocardiography

Complication of TEE	Contraindications of TEE
Esophageal rupture/perforation	Esophageal pathologies
Upper GI bleeding	Large diverticulum
Laryngospasm or bronchospasm	Obstruction, stricture
Arrhythmias	Recent upper GI bleeding

TEE: transesophageal echocardiography; GI: gastrointestinal

after the administration of sedative drugs may be useful in preventing the "lethal triade" hypotension, ischemia and ventricular fibrillation.

The following cardiovascular medications should be available before induction:

a. Atropine (bolus)
b. Epinephrine (bolus or continuous infusion)
c. Calcium chloride (bolus)
d. Ephedrine or Etilefrine (bolus)
e. Lidocaine (bolus)

Laryngoscopy can lead to hypertension and cardiac decompensation and opioids do attenuate the hemodynamic response. The administration of IV lidocaine 1.5 mg/kg 1–3 min before laryngoscopy is also effective in blunting the sympathetic effected triggered by direct laryngoscopy (and can also reduce propofol-related pain). However, given its vasodilatation and myocardial depression effects, it is not recommended in patients with moderate to severe LV impairment or severe aortic stenosis. Recommended anesthesia induction doses are shown in Table 6.

Since almost all fasted patients are are associated with relative hypovolemia, a careful augmentation of the intravascular volume in the preinduction period with crystalloids may be useful. It is important to avoid overload and hemodilution especially in patients with congestive heart failure. A precocious initiation of inotropes in patients with low cardiac index sometimes helps to maintain a stable perfusion pressure and cardiac output during the preinduction period. In Table 7, an hemodynamic responses to surgical stimuli is shown.

Precardiopulmonary Bypass Period

In patients undergoing cardiac surgery, even if an intraoperative anesthetic regimen including volatile agents is associated with a reduced postoperative cardiac dysfunction when compared to a total intravenous drug anesthesia, no differences in postoperative and long term survival are detectable. During the pre-CPB period the maintenance of a sufficient myocardial oxygen supply/consumption can be achieved with an adequate analgesia plan and administration of short-acting agents to manage blood pressure (norepinephrine as vasoconstrictor and nitroglycerine as vasodilator) is seldom required (Fig. 1). Monitoring anesthesia depth should be

Table 6 Suggested anesthesia induction doses

Hypnotics	
Propofol	1–2 mg/kg or
Thiopental	2–4 mg/kg or
Etomidate	0.15–0.3 mg/kg or
Ketamine	0.5–1.5 mg/kg
Opioids	
Fentanyl	3–10 μg/kg or
Sufentanyl	0.1–1 μg/kg or
Remifentanyl	0.1–0.75 μg/kg/min
Muscle relaxants	
Cisatracurium	70–100 μg/kg or
Rocuronium	0.3–1.2 mg/kg or
Succinylcoline	1–2 mg/kg

Table 7 Hemodynamic responses to surgical stimuli

	Pre-incision	Incision	Sternotomy	Cannulation
Surgical stimulation	↓	↑	↑↑	↓
Heart rate	↓↓	= or ↑	↑↑	= or ↓
Blood pressure	↓↓	↑	↑↑↑	↑ or ↓
Preload	= or ↓	= or ↑	= or ↑	↓
Afterload	= or ↓	↑↑	↑↑	= or ↓
O_2 Myocardial demand	↓	= or ↑	↑↑↑	↓

encouraged as it allows to avoid over sedation, hypotension and burst suppression, associated with the excess of hypnotic drugs.

Dysrhythmias are associated with intraoperative ischemia and it is therefore very important to preserve the sinus rhythm when present or to guarantee at least rate control with short-acting β-blockers (esmolol or landiolol). Consider to place sticky patches on the chest in case arrhythmias occur (atrial fibrilation, ventricular tachicardia, etc).

Specific Anesthetic Considerations

Different cardiac procedures requires specific considerations during the pre-bypass time.

Coronary Artery Bypass Grafting

Since patients undergoing coronary artery bypass grafting (CABG) have a low coronary reserve, tachycardia, hypertension and hypotension may lead to ischemia before the CPB institution. Patients with coronary disease are more vulnerable to the increase of myocardial oxygen consumption due to inability to increase

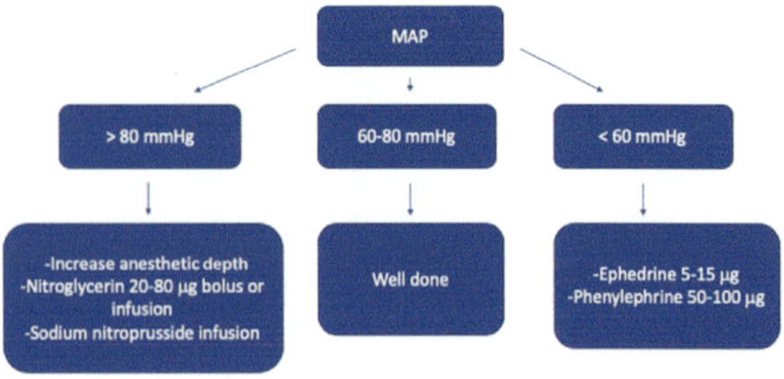

Fig. 1 Management of intraoperative blood pressure before cardiopulmonary bypass. MAP: mean arterial pressure

coronary reserve flow. In light of this, anemia should also be carefully avoided. ECG (ST alteration) and TEE (new regional wall motion abnormalities, alteration of the diastolic function) allow a prompt detection of ongoing ischemia.

Nitroglycerin, α agents vasopressors, short acting β-blockers should be considered in the event of hypertension, hypotension or to improve the consumption/delivery oxygen ratio respectively. If not sufficient, early CPB institution is required.

In off pump CABG the surgical manipulation of the heart can be associated with hypotension and suboptimal hemodynamics. Trendelemburg position, careful fluid expansion, use of α-agent vasopressors, inotropes or intraortic balloon pump should be considered on the base of blood pressure and cardiac function. A switch to CPB without aortic crossclamp (beating heart) or with aortic clamp is required in the event of persistent hemodynamic instability. Normothermia with warming systems is recommended to avoid arrhythmias.

Aortic Stenosis

Anesthesia induction of aortic stenosis patients is at high risk of complication and suggestions for the management of this period are reported in Table 8. It is crucial to avoid atrial fibrillation before CPB as it is associated with hypotension. Prompt electrical cardioversion is usually needed.

Transcatheter Valve Implantation

Transcatheter valve implantation, usually performed in sedation and local anesthesia, is an alternative to standard open cardiac surgery in selected patients with aortic stenosis at high or intermedium risk.

Nevertheless, in order to prevent malposition and embolization of the prosthesis during aortic valve ballooning and balloon prosthesis implantation, a transient partial cardiac standstill, avoiding pulsatility, and usually targeting a systolic BP below 60 mmHg, is induced by rapid pacing.

Table 8 Hemodynamic management goals in aortic stenosis

	Pre-load	Heart Rate	Contractility	SVR	PVR	Drugs to avoid
AS	LV↑	↓ (SR)	Keep normal	↑	Keep normal	Artero/venodilators β-blockers

AS: aortic stenosis; LV: left ventricle; SR: sinus rhythm; SVR: systemic vascular resistance; PVR: pulmonary vascular resistance

Aortic Regurgitation

The hemodynamic management for aortic regurgitation is summarized in Table 9.

Obstructive Hypertrophic Cardiomyopathy

Patients with obstructive hypertrophic cardiomyopathy are at risk of hemodynamic instability in the pre-CPB period. Hypovolemia or a drop in afterload may increase LV outflow tract (LVOT) gradient and trigger the systolic anterior motion. Fluid therapy, alfa 1- agonists and B-blockers may mitigate or revert the hemodynamic impairment. On the contrary, inotropes and inodilators should be avoided since they increase gradient and left ventricle (LV) obstruction.

Mitral Valve

The measures able to guarantee a good hemodynamic profile for mitral regurgitation (MR) are reported in Table 10.

Intraoperative TEE is particular useful in describing mitral anatomy and can significantly affect the surgical plan.

Percutaneous mitral repair with MITRACLIP allows treating patients with MR and at prohibitive perioperative risk. The procedure requires general anesthesia and a continuous TEE monitoring.

Mitral Stenosis

Patients with mitral stenosis should be treated following the criteria reported in Table 11.

In patients with high pulmonary pressure and/or right ventricular impairment, the insertion of PAC is recommended. Particular caution should be paid in minimising

Table 9 Hemodynamic management goals in aortic regurgitation

	Pre-load	Heart rate	Contractility	SVR	PVR	Avoid
AR	LV↑	↑	Normal or ↑ (in case of ↓ EF use inodilators)	↓	Normal	Venodilators

AR: aortic regurgitation; LV: left ventricle; EF: ejection fraction; SVR: systemic vascular resistance; PVR: pulmonary vascular resistance

Table 10 Hemodynamic management goals in mitral regurgitation

	Pre-load	Heart rate	Contractility	SVR	PVR	Avoid
MR	LV↑ (risk of augmentation MR due to annular dilatation) or ↓	↑ (Frequently AF)	Normal or ↑ (inotropes in case of ↓EF)	↓	↓	Vasopressors increasing LV afterload with caution. Hypoxia, hypercapnia, acidosis ↑ sPAP

MR: mitral regurgitation; LV: left ventricle; AF: atrial fibrillation; sPAP systolic pulmonary artery pressure; SVR: systemic vascular resistance; PVR: pulmonary vascular resistance

the number of inflations of the PAC balloon, to get the pulmonary wedge pressure. To inflate only when is needed (if low CO syndrome) and not routinely, in order to minimise the risk of PA rupture.

Tricuspid Valve Surgery

The induction of patients with tricuspid stenosis or regurgitation requires a manipulation of the pre-load, afterload and contractility as reported in Table 12. In this setting, the estimation of the CO with thermodilution is not reliable. On the contrary, echocardiography and arterial pulse wave contour analysis are more effective in the assessment of the forward stroke volume.

The correction of tricuspid regurgitation may lead, in RV dysfunction due to an increase of RV strokework. A prompt support with inotropes, vasopressors, agents able to decrease the pulmonary vascular resistances (nitric oxide), and mechanical circulatory supports is recommended.

Tricuspid diseases, increasing the central venous pressure, may affect hepatic and renal function. Thus, a subclinical coagulopathy may further worsen the effect of CPB on the coagulation system.

Table 11 Hemodynamic management goals in mitral stenosis

	Pre-load	Heart rate	Contractility	SVR	PVR	Avoid
MS	LV↑	↓	Keep normal	Normal	↓	Hypoxia, hypercapnia, acidosis ↑ sPAP

MS: mitral stenosis; LV: left ventricle; sPAP: systolic pulmonary artery pressure; SVR: systemic vascular resistance; PVR: pulmonary vascular resistance

Table 12 Hemodynamic management goals in tricuspid regurgitation

	Pre-load	Heart rate	Contractility	SVR	PVR	Avoid
TR	RV↑	Normal or ↑	Keep normal	Normal	↓	Pulmonary hypertension

TR: tricuspid regurgitation; RV: right ventricle; SR: sinus rhythm; SVR: systemic vascular resistance; PVR: pulmonary vascular resistance

Aortic Aneurysm

Ascending aortic aneurysms are usually treated surgically with CPB and aortic cross clamping. When the aortic arch is involved, a deep hypothermic circulatory arrest is necessary. If a selective perfusion of the supra-aortic vessels is required anterogradely (Kazui) or retrogradely, target temperature ranges between 24–28 °C. Without supra-aortic perfusion, a temperature of 18–20 °C allows a period of no flow of 45 min minimizing the risk of neurological injury.

Right and left radial artery, EEG/NIRS, BIS, and core temperature monitoring are mandatory during surgery involving the aortic arch. For cerebral protection, head wrapping with ice (regional cooling), methylprednisolone (30 mg/kg), thiopental or pentobarbital (5–10 mg/kg) may be considered, although there are no clear evidences.

Aortic Dissection

Since dissection requires emergency surgery, a rapid sequence induction should be applied to minimize the risk of gastric aspiration when the stomach is full. Moreover, hypertension must be treated aggressively with short term β-blocker or nitroprussiate/nitroglycerin.

TEE gives invaluable information on intimal tear, extent of dissection, degree of aortic regurgitation, involvement of the aortic root, presence of a hemopericardium and regional wall motion abnormalities secondary to the involvement of coronary arteries from the dissection, and hemothorax.

Preparation for Cardiopulmonary Bypass (CPB)

Unfractionated heparin (300 units/kg) administered directly into a central vein is the preferred anticoagulation agent for CPB. An activated clotting time (ACT) of at least 300 s is safe for cannulation, and > 480 s for CPB institution. In patients with heparin induced thrombocytopenia (HIT) bivalirudin (a thrombin direct inhibitor) is used (Table 13).

Table 13 Bivalirudin

Half time life: 25–30 min
Metabolism: 20% renal + proteolysis
Posology: 1 mg/Kg
Infusion during CPB: 2,5 mg/kg/h and up to 0,25 mg/kg/h
Stop 30 min before cardiopulmonary bypass weaning

Cannulation

CPB provides oxygenated systemic non pulsatile blood flow to organs when the heart and the lung are not functioning. With standard cannulation, an aortic cannula is positioned in the ascending aorta and a venous cannula in the right atrium (atrial cannulation) or in the superior and inferior vena cava (bicaval cannulation). In some circumstances (i.e. Type A aortic dissection), the axillary artery is the site of choice for arterial cannulation. A peripheral cannulation with the arterial and venous cannulae positioned in the femoral artery and vein may be required during some cardiac surgeries (i.e. mitral valve surgery through mini-thoracothomy, aortic valve replacement through mini-sternotomy and selected high-risk redo surgeries). During arterial cannulation a systolic blood pressure lower than 90 mmHg reduces the risk of aortic dissection.

Cardiopulmonary Bypass Period

Since the majority of CPB machines provides non pulsatile flow, mean arterial pressure (MAP) is used in order to guide the hemodynamic status (target 50–70 mmHg), combined with monitoring of urine output and lactate through seriate blood gasses analysis.

The use of CPB inevitably leads to an high degree of hemodilution owing to the use of a non-sanguineous prime. A hemoglobin value below 6.5–7 g/dl (Hct 22–24%) is usually enough to avoid oxygen delivery impairment (Table 14).

The route of anesthesia administration in cardiac surgery deserves some considerations:

1. In the event of bicaval cannulation total endovenous anesthesia must be provided in a peripheral vein because the heart is bypassed and the drugs administered in the central line can be lost in the surgical field.
2. In the pre CPB period, if the anesthesia is maintained with a volatile agent, the halogenated is usually suspended and replaced by an infusion of intravenous anesthetic (e.g. propofol) as soon as the CPB is started and the ventilator is stopped.
3. When propofol is used, an infusion rate of 3 to 6 mg/kg/h or a target plasma concentration of 2–4 μg/ml is usually enough. In fact, anesthetic requirement falls with temperature drops and hemodilution. The opposite happens during rewarming.

Table 14 On pump targets

Systemic flow rates	• 2–2,5 L/min/m2 at 37 °C • 1.8–2.5 at 30 °C
Systemic blood pressure	50–80 mmHg[a]
Arterial blood gases	PO_2 > 250 mmHg; PCO_2 35–45 mmHg; pH 7.40 and avoidance of hyperchloraemic acidosis
ACT	>480 s (can be less if heparin coated circuit)
SvO_2	>65%
Hematocrit	>22%

ACT: activated clotting time; SvO_2: mixed venous oxygen blood saturation; PO_2: pressure of oxygen; PCO_2: pressure of carbon dioxide

[a]Recently a cerebral autoregulation monitoring has been advocated to set the best MAP during CPB (J Thorac Cardiovasc Surg 2017;154:1590–8)

Cardiopulmonary Bypass Weaning

Before starting CPB weaning, heart de-airing is crucial through venting the aortic root and right superior pulmonary vein prior to cross-clamp release. Manually inflating the lungs for few seconds allows to fill in the left ventricle facilitating the de-airing process (Valsalva maneuver). TEE helps to detect residual air. The criteria to start the weaning from CPB are summarized in Table 15.

CPB weaning is the progressive reduction of the venous return from the extracorporeal circulation to a spontaneous and normal mechanical heart activity. This process is considered completed after the administration of protamine and the removal of the venous and arterial cannulae.

TEE is crucial in promptly checking ventricles' preload and contractility, detecting overdistension and dysfunction.

CPB flow is progressively reduced (500 ml per time) until the systemic circulation is totally sustained from the heart. A flow chart on the hemodynamic management during CPB is reported in Fig. 2.

In a variable percentage of cases (10–45%), the CPB discontinuation can be complicated. Although there are no specific criteria to define the "difficult-to-wean" patient, this is a life-threatening complication associated with high perioperative mortality. In normovolemic conditions and in absence of structural or dynamic abnormalities, difficulties CPB weaning may depend on:

a. Vasoplegic syndrome (characterized by normal or elevated cardiac output with preserved ventricular function and low systemic vascular resistance) treated with vasoactive drugs (e.g. norepinephrine, phenylephrine, vasopressin). If vasoplegia is refractory refer to Table 16.
b. Right ventricular dysfunction, with or without pulmonary hypertension. The performance of the RV depends on preload, afterload and contractility.

Table 15 Checklist before CPB weaning

Temperature	Rectal/Bladder Temperature >35 °C
Rhythm	Spontaneous or paced (HR >70 bpm) Quick possible defibrillation (10–20 J)
Ventilation	Lung re-ventilation and recruitment
TEE	TEE examination under partial cardiopulmonary bypass to detect functional or structural defects
Homeostasis	pH correction: aim 7.35–7.45 Hct > 25% Normoglycemia Potassium plasma concentration control
Surgeon	De-airing cardiac cavities Aortic unclamping

FiO_2: fraction of inspired oxygen; TEE: transesophageal echocardiography; Hct: hematocrit

c. LV systolic dysfunction, characterized by left ventricle depressed contractility. Ventricular function is a major determinant of cardiac output. Global or regional dysfunction may develop after the weaning period from CPB.
d. LV diastolic dysfunction, with impairment in ventricular diastolic relaxation and restrictive filling pattern.

Flow chart of difficult CPB weaning and TEE-guided therapeutic approach is shown in Fig. 3.

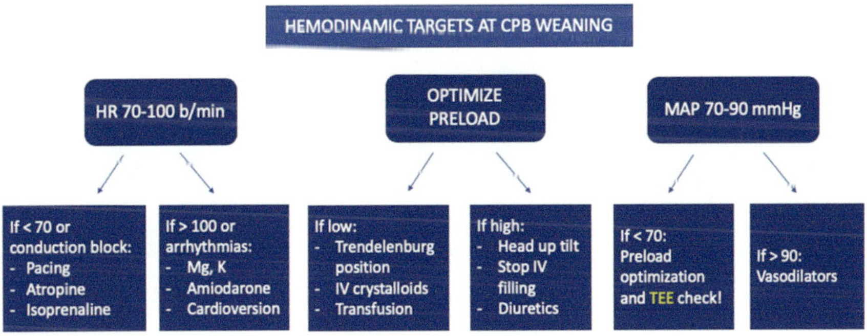

Fig. 2 Hemodynamic targets at cardiopulmonary bypass weaning. HR heart rate; MAP mean arterial pressure, Mg magnesium, K potassium, IV intravenous, TEE transesophageal echocardiograpy

Table 16 Treatment of refractory vasoplegia

First line	Transfusion (Hb target: 9 g/dL) Epinephrine infusion Steroids Diphenhydramine
Second line	If high risk of serotonin syndrome: Hydroxocobalamin IV 5–10 g If low risk of serotonin syndrome: Angiotensin II 20 ng/kg/min, up to 80 ng/kg/min (maximum dose) Bolus of Methylene Blue 1–2 mg/kg followed by a continuous infusion of 0.25 mg/kg/h for 6 hours
Rescue	Vitamin C (1.5 g every 6 hours) Consider IV Thiamine

Hb: hemoglobin; IV: intravenous

Chest Closure and Transport to Intensive Care Unit (ICU)

During chest closure, hemodynamic deterioration may ensue. Some patients with inadequate intravascular volume can experience mild hypotension, managed with fluids administration. In individuals with poor ventricular function or patients currently receiving inotropic agents, additional volume or inotropic support may be required.

After the chest is closed, the patient can be moved to ICU. Disconnect monitoring sequentially is a good way to avoid a blind period in which the patient has no vital parameter actively monitored.

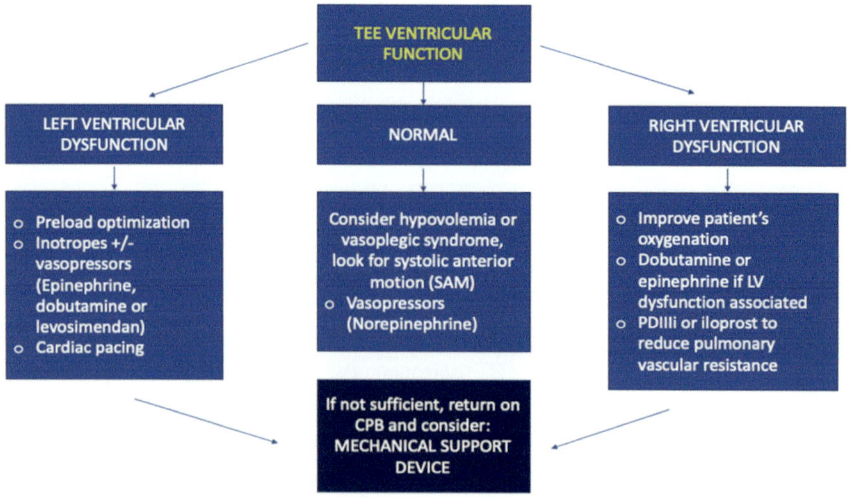

Fig. 3 TEE-guided therapeutic approach for difficult weaning. TEE transesophageal echocardiograpy, SAM systolic anterior motion, CPB cardiopulmonary bypass, LV left ventricle

Recommended Reading

1. Sousa-Uva M, Head SJ, Milojevic M, Collet JP, Landoni G, Castella M, Dunning J, Gudbjartsson T, Linker NJ, Sandoval E, Thielmann M, Jeppsson A, Landmesser U. 2017 EACTS Guidelines on perioperative medication in adult cardiac surgery. Eur J Cardiothorac Surg. 2018; 53:5–33.
2. Harrison NL, Sear JW. Barbiturates, etomidate, propofol, ketamine, and steroids. In: Evers AS, Maze M, editors. Anesthetic pharmacology: physiologic principles and clinical practice. Philadelphia, PA: Churchill Livingstone; 2004. p. 395–4126.
3. Mebazaa A, Pitsis AA, Rudiger A, Toller W, Longrois D, Ricksten SE, et al. Clinical review: practical recommendations on the management of perioperative heart failure in cardiac surgery. Crit Care. 2011; 14:201.
4. Monaco F, Di Prima AL, Kim JH, Plamondon MJ, Yavorovskiy A, Likhvantsev V, Lomivorotov V, Hajjar LA, Landoni G. Management of Challenging Cardiopulmonary Bypass Separation. J Cardiothorac Vasc Anesth. 2020; 34:1622–1635.
5. Mebazaa A, Pitsis AA, Rudiger A, et al Clinical review: Practical recommendations on the management of perioperative heart failure in cardiac surgery. Crit Care 2011; 14:201.
6. Licker M, Diaper J, Cartier V, et al Management of weaning from cardiopulmonary bypass after cardiac surgery. Ann Card Anaesth. Vol. 15:3; Jul-Sep-2012
7. McKinlay KH, Schinderle DB, Swaminathan M, et al Predictors of inotrope use during separation from cardiopulmonary bypass. J Cardiothorac Vasc Anesth. 2004; 18:404–8.
8. Landoni G, Lomivorotov VV, Nigro Neto C, et al MYRIAD Study Group. Volatile Anesthetics versus total intravenous anesthesia for cardiac surgery. N Engl J Med. 2019 Mar 28;380 (13):1214–1225. https://doi.org/10.1056/NEJMoa1816476. Epub 2019 Mar 19.

Fluid Management & Blood Transfusion

Fabio Guarracino and Rubia Baldassarri

Fluid Management

Fluid management is crucial in cardiac surgery patients. The underlying heart disease and the poor cardiovascular reserve make these patients unable to adapt to the frequent hemodynamic variations occurring during surgery. Because both positive and negative fluid balance harm organs and worsen the clinical outcome, cautious fluid management is pivotal.

Patients undergoing cardiac surgery can present with different types of cardiac dysfunction. The presence of left ventricle (LV) dysfunction, both systolic and diastolic, right ventricle (RV) failure, heart valve disease influence the response to fluid administration depending on both the severity of the illness and the surgical technique.

Although the dysfunctional heart depends on adequate preload to provide stroke volume and systemic perfusion, exceeding fluid administration can lead to pulmonary edema because the heart cannot adapt to the increasing filling pressures.

This is particularly true when RV failure and LV diastolic dysfunction occur.

At the same time, negative fluid balance can affect organ function by either reducing oxygen delivery or inducing arrhythmias, such as atrial fibrillation. For these reasons, the maintenance of stable fluid balance, ensuring proper oxygen delivery to the peripheral tissues throughout the surgical procedure, is the main purpose of intraoperative fluid management in cardiac surgery.

Some specific features of cardiac surgery, including the use of the cardiopulmonary bypass (CPB), are responsible for abnormal vascular permeability and

F. Guarracino (✉) · R. Baldassarri
Department of Anaesthesia and Critical Care Medicine, University Hospital of Pisa, Via Paradisa 2, 56L23 Pisa, Italy

M. Vives and A. Hernandez (eds.), *Cardiac Anesthesia and Postoperative Care in the 21st Century*, https://doi.org/10.1007/978-3-030-79721-8_13

altered microcirculatory function. Haemodilution, hypothermia, intraoperative bleeding, coagulation disorders, as well as surgery and anesthesia may affect the fluid distribution between the intra and extravascular space.

Impaired microcirculatory function and, as recently highlighted, endothelial glycocalyx dysfunction, harm the oxygen supply/demand balance (Fig. 1).

Thanks to the hand-held vital microscopes availability, the microcirculation can be safely investigated. Nevertheless, none of the microcirculation function indexes seem to be useful to improve the clinical outcome in cardiac surgery.

Fluid management in cardiac surgery is still a challenge. Intraoperative fluid management should be focused on the effective patient's response to fluid administration rather than on the conventional hemodynamic monitoring (mean arterial pressure, central venous pressure).

In this context, intraoperative transesophageal echocardiography (TEE) is useful to assess either the filling state or the response to fluid administration in cardiac surgery patients. Additional information about cardiac function is also fundamental to guide fluid management.

Fluid responsiveness is defined as the ability to increase the stroke volume (about 10–15%) after fluid challenge.

As aforementioned, the identification of the patients who are fluid-responder is extremely useful to manage fluid therapy during cardiac surgery. It should be kept into account that, because of the unicity of the hemodynamic pattern of the cardiac surgery patients fluids should be carefully given even in those patients who are thought to benefit from fluid therapy.

In clinical practice, dynamic indexes of fluid responsiveness, such as Stroke Volume Variation (SVV) and Pulse Pressure Variation (PVV), are useful to

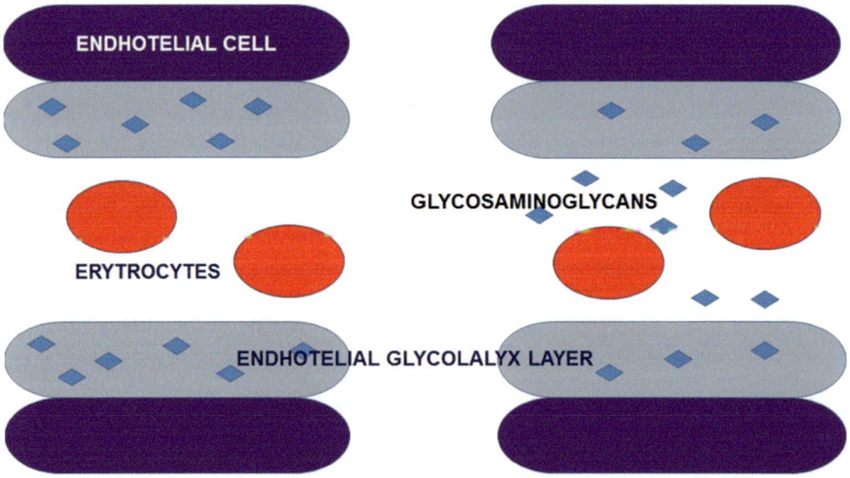

Fig. 1 Endhotelial Glycolalyx Layer. Healhty glycolalyx layer on the left and altered glycolalyx on the right where the glycosaminoglycans are shedding to the plasma

optimize the therapeutic approach in hemodynamically unstable patients. The respiratory variation of the diameters of superior and inferior vena cava are other important indicators of fluid responsiveness.

Advanced hemodynamic monitoring and intraoperative TEE are powerful tools for guiding fluid management in the cardiac surgery setting. The implementation of individualized strategies is helpful to achieve hemodynamic stabilization.

Blood Management

Perioperative bleeding, depending on both patients' predisposing risk factors and surgery-related mechanisms, is a common complication in cardiac surgery (Table 1).

In cardiac surgery, allogenic blood products, such as packed red blood cells, fresh frozen plasma, or platelets transfusion, are the usual therapeutic approach to intraoperative blood loss. Because of the strong association between blood components transfusion and adverse outcomes, any effort to prevent and minimize intraoperative bleeding should be ensured in cardiac surgery patients (Table 2).

Non-surgical intraoperative bleeding mostly depends on coagulation disorders. The cardiac surgery patients, who present with coagulopathy and/or anemia from different causes before surgery, are at high risk for major bleeding.

Several factors, including the use of CPB, systemic heparin, haemodilution, and hypothermia affect intraoperative hemostasis.

During CPB, the clot activation induced by the blood trauma in the extracorporeal circuits, as well as haemodilution and hypothermia alter the coagulation pattern by reducing and impairing the circulating coagulant factors.

The current guidelines recommend to minimize hemodilution, maintenance of normothermia (temperature > 36 °C), and pH within the physiological range (7.35–7.45) to reduce the effects of CPB on intraoperative coagulopathy. In this context, normovolaemic haemodilution, antegrade autologous priming, and retrograde autologous priming have been considered for cardiac surgery.

Table 1 Predisposing risk factors for intraoperative bleeding

Advanced age
Preoperative dual antiplatelet therapy
Poor platelet function
Preoperative anaemia
Small body surface area
Female gender
Non-elective surgery, nonisolated surgery, non-CABG surgery and redo surgery

Table 2 Adverse events associated with allogenic blood transfusion

Transfusion-associated lung injury (TRALI)
Transfusion-associated immunomodulation
Transfusion-related circulatory overload
Cellular hypoxia
Postoperative renal dysfunction
Pneumonia
Wound infections
Sepsis and septic shock
In-hospital mortality

The use of shorter, closed, and biocompatible coating extracorporeal circuits can also be helpful in patients submitted to CPB.

Patient's blood donation and cell save techniques can effectively reduce the amount of transfusion, but both of them have side effects that should be carefully considered in cardiac surgery.

Patient Blood Management

Recent Guidelines have endorsed the implementation of proper algorithms with well-defined interventional triggers to achieve adequate patient blood management (PBM) in adult cardiac surgery.

The Society for the Advancement of Blood Management has recently defined PBM as *"the timely application of evidence-based medical and surgical concepts designed to maintain hemoglobin (Hb) concentration, optimize hemostasis and minimize blood loss in an effort to improve patient outcome."*

Therefore, PBM is a global strategy for the prevention of major bleeding, including the preoperative assessment of the predisposing risk factors and the management of postoperative complications. Intraoperatively, PBM depends on interventional strategies aimed to prevent and treat blood loss (Table 3).

As recommended by the current Guidelines, the patient's history, preoperative antithrombotic/anticoagulant medicaments, anemia, and eventual congenital coagulopathy, should be therefore carefully investigated. In high-risk patients, strategies to optimize the coagulation pattern and normalize the Hb levels should be performed before surgery to reduce the perioperative risk for bleeding.

During cardiac surgery, the point-of-care (POC) coagulation tests allow the early detection of the pathophysiological mechanisms involved in the clotting formation and stabilization by analyzing the global coagulation process.

In addition to the activated clotting time (ACT), which is is used for monitoring heparin therapy and the adequacy of anticoagulation therapy during cardiac surgery, the viscoelastic coagulation tests including rotation thromboelastometry (ROTEM) and Thromboelastography (TEG) have been recommended in cardiac surgery as

Table 3 Intraoperative blood management algorithm

Surgical hemostasis	
reduce haemodilution	Retro/antegrade autologous priming, MiECC, Vaccum assisted venous return, fluid restriction
Individualized anticoagulation	Heparin/protamine tritation on ACT, heparing Monitoring System
Prevention of fibrinolysis	Tranexamic acid according to istitutional protocol
Normothermia and normal pH range	Maintain TC > 36°C and pH 7.35-7.45 by patients' warming and tissue perfusion
Cell saver, ultrafiltration	

part of the PBM. The European Society of Anesthesiology (ESA) and the European Association of Cardiothoracic Surgeon/Anesthesiology (EACTS/EACTA) guidelines on patient blood management for adult cardiac surgery, recommend the implementation of interventional algorithms based on predefined triggers. Transfusion strategies cannot be guided by solely clinical judgment; evidence-based decision-making approaches are recommended because safer and more effective in preventing perioperative adverse events.

POC testing-based interventional algorithms are effective in both the prevention and treatment of perioperative bleeding in the cardiac surgery setting. Finally, POC-test-guided algorithms are effective in reducing perioperative allogeneic blood transfusion (Tables 4 and 5).

PBM is an important part of fluid management in cardiac surgery. Intraoperative bleeding is one of the main causes of hypovolemia and major bleeding can lead to severe hemodynamic instability.

Because several causes, including intraoperative bleeding, are responsible for the hemodynamic impairment occurring in cardiac surgery, the proper diagnosis of the underlying pathogenic mechanisms is fundamental to provide adequate treatment. In this context, advanced hemodynamic monitoring is fundamental to guide fluid administration and the routine application of POC-guided interventional algorithms has been shown effective in reducing intraoperative bleeding and the requirement for blood components transfusion.

Table 4 Viscoelastic testing (VET) based perioperative management of active bleeding

CT Intem > 300 and CT Eptem < 80% CT Intem R time at TEG ® (heparinase) is 3 minutes shorter than R time standard	Protamine (25-50 mg)
Fibtem MFC < 8mm or functional fibrinogen < 6 mm Target value fibtem MFC 14 mm or Clauss firinogen 2,5 g/L	Fibrinogen concentrate (2 gr)
Fibrinogen is normalized and: platelet count < 100,000 cells/ µL or P2Y12 inhibitors not withdrawn, ADP test < 12 U	Desmopressin 0,3µg/Kg Platelet concentrate transfusion (1 U)
Hyperfibrinolysis at VET	Additional dose of tranexamic acid + fibrinogen 1 gr
CT Extem > 90 sec or R time at TEG ® (heparinase) > 15 min Consider FFp as second option only	Prothrombin complex concentrate (4 factors) 20 IU/Kg

Table 5 Management of ongoing active bleeding

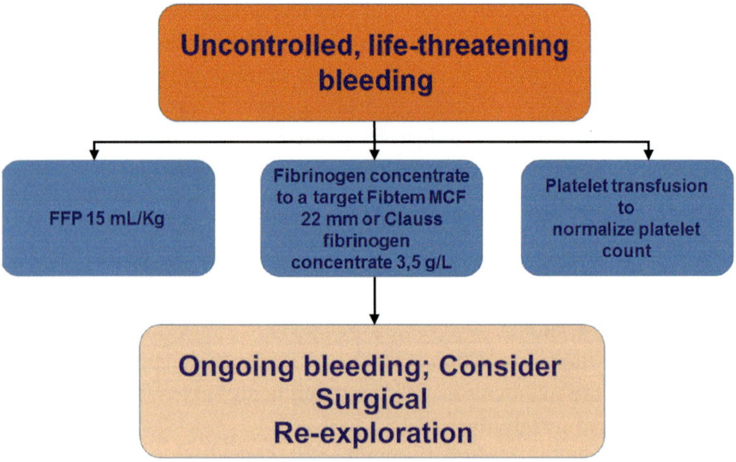

Intraoperative Coagulation

The balance between proper anticoagulation and hemostasis is crucial in cardiac surgery. The coagulation system must adequately work to prevent and stop intra-operative bleeding. Intraoperative hemostasis depends on the complex interaction of surgical and clinical strategies.

An unfavorable balance between procoagulant and anticoagulant factors can lead to hemorrhagic/thrombotic events increasing perioperative morbidity and mortality.

Heparin is commonly administered according to body weight, usually 300 IU/kg heparin with a target ACT $\geq$ 400–450 sec. The occurrence of heparin resistance and heparin rebound can affect the reliability of this tool. The implementation of interventional algorithms based on the clinical response to heparin could be effective in reducing the risk of intraoperative bleeding.

According to current Guidelines, protamine should be used to reverse the heparin-induced effects. To restore the procoagulant activity of the blood the protamine/heparin ratio 1:1 is generally adequate in cardiac surgery. An additional dose of protamine should be carefully considered because of the risk of bleeding.

In case of low blood levels of antithrombin (AT), its administration should be considered to increase heparin sensitivity when heparin resistance is shown.

Transfusion Strategies

In most cardiac surgery centers, blood transfusion is still the current strategy to treat intraoperative blood loss. Although blood transfusion can be lifesaving in some specific circumstances (major bleeding, hemorrhagic shock, ischemic complications, potential organ failure), a liberal approach to allogenic blood components transfusion is not free from risks.

Both anemia and blood transfusion affect the clinical outcome by increasing perioperative morbidity and mortality.

Therefore, the primary challenge is to understand when transfusion is appropriate and the benefits overcome the risks.

Anemia

In the cardiac surgery population, the incidence of perioperative anemia is about 30% (from 23% up to 43%). There is evidence that perioperative anemia affects the clinical outcome by increasing morbidity and mortality. Also, preoperative anemia is an independent risk factor for increased blood transfusion. Preoperative anemia should be adequately treated before surgery.

The safe transfusion threshold is still controversial and restricted versus liberal transfusion strategies have been investigated in the cardiac surgery setting.

Although the Hb value is still the main transfusion trigger, the patient's clinical conditions, as well as his/her ability to compensate for the reduction of the Hb levels, are, or should be, the main decision-making criteria when transfusion seems to be the best therapeutic option. The patient's response to either acute bleeding or the reduction of the Hb values below critical levels depends on several factors including the patient's preoperative status and the intraoperative setting. In particular, in dealing with cardiac patients the coronary perfusion plays a key role in the response to anemia by increasing the cardiac output. When coronary perfusion is suboptimal, sudden decompensation can occur in presence of low Hb levels.

The evidence of systemic hypoperfusion and reduced tissue oxygenation is pivotal to guide the transfusion strategy.

Conclusion

PBM is part of the more complex issue of fluid management in the cardiac surgery setting. Intraoperative bleeding is one of the main causes of hypovolemia and major bleeding can lead to severe hemodynamic instability.

Because the hemodynamic impairment occurring in cardiac surgery may be due to very different causes, a correct diagnose of the underlying pathogenic mechanisms is fundamental to provide an early adequate treatment. In this context, advanced hemodynamic monitoring is fundamental to guide fluid administration and the routine application of POC-guided interventional algorithms has been shown effective in reducing intraoperative bleeding and the requirement for blood components transfusion.

Recommended Readings

1. Scolletta S, et al. Patient blood management in cardiac surgery: The "Granducato algorithm." Int J Cardiol. 2019;289:37–42.
2. Pagano D, Milojevic M, et al. (2018) EACTS/EACTA Guidelines on patient blood management for adult cardiac surgery. Eur J Cardiothorac Surg. 2018;53(1):79–111. https://doi.org/10.1093/ejcts/ezx325.
3. Kozek-Langenecker SA, Ahmed AB, Afshari A, et al. Management of severe perioperative bleeding: guidelines from the European Society of Anaesthesiology: first update 2016. Eur J Anaesthesiol. 2017;34:332–95.
4. Bignami E, Guarnieri M et al (2017). Fluid management in cardiac surgery patients: pitfalls, challenges and solutions. Minerva Anestesiol. 2017;83(6):638–651. doi: https://doi.org/10.23736/S0375-9393.17.11512-9.
5. Protsyk V, Rasmussen BS, et al. Fluid management in cardiac surgery: results of a survey in European cardiac anesthesia departments. J Cardiothorac Vasc Anesth. 2017;31(5):1624–9. https://doi.org/10.1053/j.jvca.2017.04.017.
6. Raphael J, Mazer CD, et al. Society of cardiovascular anesthesiologists clinical practice improvement advisory for management of perioperative bleeding and hemostasis in cardiac surgery patients. Anesth Analg. 2019;129(5):1209–21. https://doi.org/10.1213/ANE.0000000000004355.
7. Dhir A, Tempe DK. Anemia and patient blood management in cardiac surgery-literature review and current evidence. J Cardiothorac Vasc Anesth. 2018;32(6):2726–42. https://doi.org/10.1053/j.jvca.2017.11.043.

Anaesthesia for Electrophysiology Procedures in the Cardiac Catheter Laboratory

Dan Aston and Guillermo Martinez

Introduction

The number of procedures performed for the diagnosis and treatment of cardiac arrhythmia has grown exponentially over the last two decades. The electrophysiology (EP) techniques have become more complex, more time consuming, and patients are older with more comorbidities and sedation or general anaesthesia is more often required. In addition, the presence of the anaesthetic team in the catheter laboratory (cath lab) facilitates the provision of early resuscitation in the event of complications such as ventricular perforation, embolization or pulseless arrhythmias. It is important that the anaesthetist working in the cath lab has a good understanding of the procedures performed there, and their implications for anaesthesia.

Arrhythmias can be treated pharmacologically, surgically, or with cardiovascular implantable electronic devices (CIED). A large number need to be treated in the cath lab with a permanent pacemaker, implantable cardioverter defibrillator (ICD) or ablation of the arrhythmia pathway. Common arrhythmias treated with ablation in cath lab include paroxysmal or persistent atrial fibrillation (AF), atrial flutter, other supra-ventricular tachycardias (SVTs) such as atrioventricular nodal re-entry tachycardiac (AVNRT) and atrioventricular re-entry tachycardia (AVRT), and ventricular tachycardias (VT). The ablation targets specific areas of myocardium in order to either prevent them triggering the arrhythmia or to render them electrically inert so that re-entry cannot occur and consequently the arrhythmia cannot propagate. The area to be ablated must first be mapped, and there are various methods of doing this; the actual ablation can also be performed using several different techniques.

D. Aston · G. Martinez (✉)
Department of Anaesthesia and Intensive Care, Royal Papworth Hospital NHS Foundation Trust, Papworth Road Cambridge Biomedical Campus, Cambridge CB2 0AY, England
e-mail: guillermo.martinez@nhs.net

M. Vives and A. Hernández (eds.), *Cardiac Anesthesia and Postoperative Care in the 21st Century*, https://doi.org/10.1007/978-3-030-79721-8_14

Ablation Procedures

Just as ECG electrodes placed on the skin provide vectored information about cardiac electrical activity, electrodes placed within the heart by specialised catheters can also be used to gather similar information. Standard intra-cardiac electrode positions are used to collect details about the focus and propagation pathways of arrhythmias in a process known as mapping. The intracardiac electrodes are placed in the high right atrium (HRA), the His bundle (HB), the right ventricular apex (RVA) and the coronary sinus (CS) and they are used to make recordings called electrograms which are analogous to standard ECG leads. Together with I, II, III, aVL, V1 and V6 from the standard ECG, the electrograms are used to generate a map of the arrhythmia.

In addition to the electrograms, modern arrhythmia ablation is aided by sophisticated technology that utilises magnetic fields or impedence-based systems to give the cardiologist a graphical view of the cardiac chamber being studied and the exact position of the catheter tip within it. 'CARTO' (Biosense Webster, Diamond Bar, California) is one system that utilises magnets outside the body to calculate the position of the catheter. The information from the magnetic fields and the electrograms is used to generate a three dimensional representation of the chamber being studied, which is colour coded to represent the voltage or timing of the arrhythmia at different points. The colour coding makes it easier to see the arrhythmogenic focus and the direction in which the arrhythmia is propagating (Figs. 1 and 2). Further details may also be obtained by merging these three dimensional maps with images from CT or MRI scans. Using this information the catheter can be precisely positioned to ablate the source of the arrhythmia and the tissue through which it propagates.

The origin and propagation pathways of different arrhythmias vary. The most common arrhythmias such as atrial fibrillation, usually arise on the left side of the heart while others (i.e. atrial flutter and ventricular tachycardia) mostly originate in the right-sided chambers. There are also some arrhythmias whose propagation pathway varies (e.g. AVRT that usually conducts via either the tricuspid or mitral valve annulus). Right sided arrhythmias can be treated by catheters entering the heart via the great veins while ablation of left sided arrhythmias involve catheter access to the left heart either via the aorta or via puncture of the inter-atrial septum. The placement of both intracardiac electrodes and ablation catheters can be guided by fluoroscopy or transoesophageal echocardiography (TOE).

The ablation method itself may be radiofrequency, cryoablation, laser, or direct current. The latter method allows deeper tissue penetration, but is now mostly obsolete due to complications such as barotrauma and stimulation of arrhythmias, and the development of more successful techniques. A modified version of direct current ablation—electroporation—is now available, which does not have these complications and uses a lower energy to form pores in cell membranes resulting in apoptosis. Radiofrequency ablation is the most common method, and uses alternating current between the catheter tip and a cutaneous patch to generate heat that

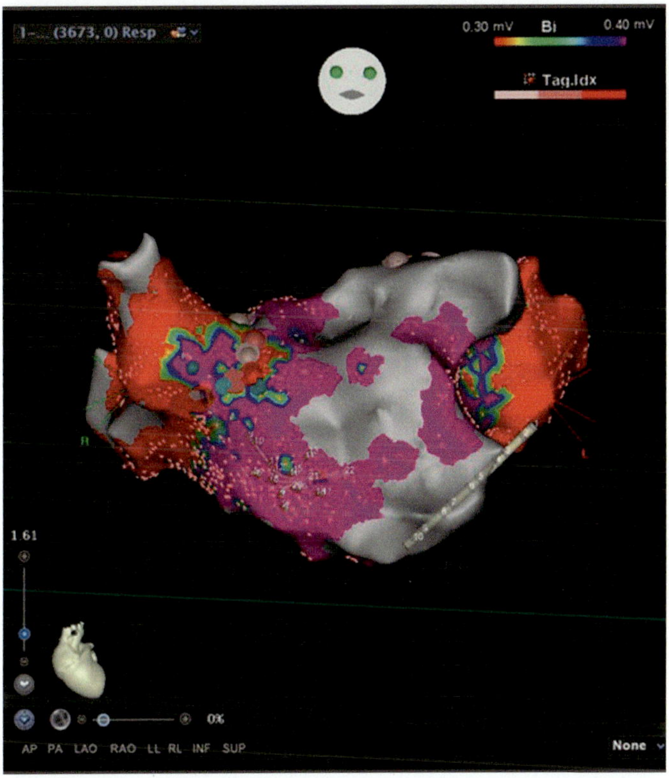

Fig. 1 Left atrial bipolar voltage mapping using CARTO (Biosense Webster, Diamond Bar, USA). Image supplied by The Royal Papworth Hospital

causes irreversible coagulation of the tissue in a small and precise area. If a more powerful ablation is required, saline may be continually flushed over the catheter tip to control the heating process ('cool flow'). Volumes of a litre or more may be infused into the patient during a single ablation procedure, and the possibility of resulting pulmonary oedema must be borne in mind if there is poor left ventricular function.

Cryoablation is used when there is concern regarding possible damage to structures surrounding the ablation site. Examples include the ablation of pathways adjacent to the AV node—which may result in complete heart block if the AV node itself is damaged—and ablation of AF originating in the right upper pulmonary vein, outside which the phrenic nerve runs and may also be damaged leading to diaphragmatic paralysis. The advantage of cryoablation is that when tissue is cooled to around 4 °C it becomes electrically inert but is not permanently damaged. If complete heart block develops or phrenic nerve conduction is impaired then the tissue can be allowed to return to body temperature and it will continue to function

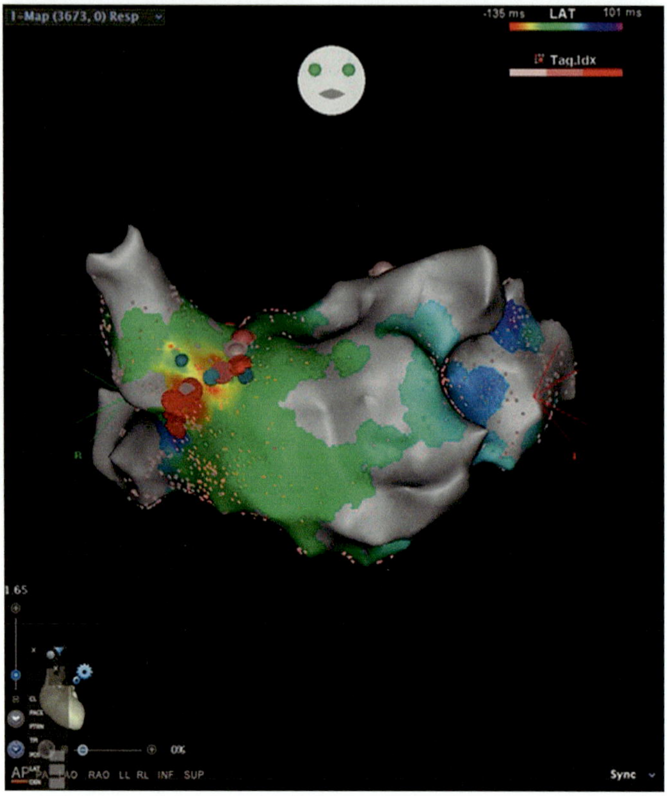

Fig. 2 Red dots indicate radiofrequency applications at the level of the right superior pulmonary vein ostium. Image supplied by The Royal Papworth Hospital

normally. Only when the correct ablation site is confirmed is the tissue then allowed to cool to –75 °C and is permanently ablated.

Cardiovascular Implantable Electronic Devices

Insertion of CIED is usually performed percutaneously, and can be carried out under local anaesthetic with or without sedation. In some cases, for example box replacement or subpectoral placement of the pacemaker, the procedure may be more painful and so a general anaesthetic is preferred. The replacement of a pacemaker does not usually require the removal of the intracardiac leads, which can simply be detached and then reattached to the new pacemaker.

Occasionally, pacemaker leads need to be removed. The exact incidence of lead extraction is currently unknown, but an estimated 10,000 – 15,000 leads are removed annually worldwide. Removal is indicated if the leads become infected, fractured, if they malfunction or in the event of a device recall. The strongest indication for removing a lead or the pacemaker itself is infection, which occurred in 1.82 to 5.32 per 1000 pacemaker-years in one study of almost 50,000 patients conducted over 25 years. It was found that infection was almost three times more likely following the replacement of a CIED than after a first-time insertion. In another study, lead failure was seen in 3.8% of cases over 15 years, most commonly due to fracture or an insulation defect. Not all of these required removal.

In the time following insertion, CIED leads can become adhered to the vascular wall or to the heart by fibrotic tissue. The likelihood that traction on the lead will cause injury to the heart or great vessels—possibly leading to massive haemorrhage, cardiac tamponade or other complications is therefore significant. Risk factors associated with a higher than average incidence of complications following lead extraction are non-elective admission, female gender, longer implant duration and the need to remove three or more leads.

Different techniques, such as the use of cutting sheaths or laser-assisted removal, may be employed to release an adhered pacemaker lead, but risks remain. The incidence of major complications of lead extraction are shown in Table 1.

Removal of pacemaker leads should be performed in a hybrid cath lab or an operating theatre where there is rapid access to cardiothoracic surgery and to cardiopulmonary bypass (CPB). The pre-procedure placement of femoral wires or catheters to facilitate emergency CPB may be necessary. Similarly, wide-bore intravenous access should be secured before the procedure and invasive monitoring should be considered.

Table 1 Incidence of complications following CIED lead extraction

Complication	Incidence (%)
Any complication	2.3
Death	0.19–1.20
Death during procedure	0.16
Cardiac arrest	0.07–0.5
Cardiac avulsion / perforation	0.19–0.96
Haemothorax	0.07–0.21
Cardiac effusion requiring drainage/cardiac tamponade	0.23–0.59
Urgent cardiac surgery required	0.36
Massive pulmonary embolism	0.08
Tricuspid valve injury requiring intervention	0.03

Cardiac Resynchronization Therapy

In 2005, the CARE-HF trial compared standard medical therapy with biventricular pacing in patients with heart failure and a prolonged QRS complex on their ECG. Eight hundred and thirteen symptomatic (NYHA III or IV) patients with a dilated left ventricle, an ejection fraction of 35% or less, and a QRS duration of greater than 150 ms (or 120 ms if dyssynchrony was apparent on echocardiography) were randomised to receive standard medical therapy or a specialized pacemaker that paced both ventricles simultaneously. These pacemakers have three leads; two in a configuration similar to a standard dual-chamber pacemaker in the right atrium and right ventricle, and the third lead passed through the coronary sinus that paces the left ventricle. After almost 30 months follow up, hospital admission or death was 39% in the resynchronization group compared with 55% in the group treated with standard medical therapy. There was also a reduction of 10% in all-cause mortality from 30 to 20% between the groups.

This cardiac resynchronization therapy (CRT) is suitable for approximately 10% of patients with heart failure, and dyssynchrony can be interventricular (a delay between contraction of the right and left ventricles) or intraventricular (where the lateral wall of the left ventricle contracts after the septum). The most common conduction abnormality present in patients having CRT is left bundle branch block (LBBB). There is no benefit to resynchronizing delay caused by RBBB or in patients who are acutely decompensated. Overall, 30–40% of patients do not respond to CRT for poorly understood reasons.

Patients presenting for CRT have symptomatic heart failure and other comorbidities, and as such are unlikely to tolerate the procedure without a general anaesthetic. Complications of CRT are similar to those of standard pacemaker insertion, but also include coronary sinus dissection which has been shown to occur in 0.28% of cases. On rare occasions due to unusual anatomy, it may not be possible to place the left ventricular lead endovascularly. In these cases, an epicardial lead may need to be placed surgically.

Biventricular pacemakers may simply pace the heart (CRT-P) or also incorporate anti-tachycardia and defibrillation functions (CRT-D). In contrast to standard pacemakers, which are usually programmed so that they start pacing when the patient's intrinsic rate falls below a set value, biventricular pacemakers are programmed to pace faster than the patient's intrinsic rate to ensure that resynchronization is maintained. An important difference between standard pacemakers and CRT devices is therefore that the former paces as little as possible, while the latter paces as much as possible. This has implications for surgery and the use of diathermy when a patient has a CRT device; interference from electrocautery will have a bigger effect than on standard pacemakers, and may cause inhibition of the device output. Similarly, stimulation or pain leading to a fast intrinsic heart rate may prevent the device pacing, although many are rate-responsive and will continue to pace at higher intrinsic rates.

Why is General Anaesthesia Required?

Some EP procedures are performed in a relatively short time in relatively fit individuals who are able to lie flat and remain motionless for the duration of the process. In these cases anaesthesia is often not required. However, ablations for AF, or patients with complex cardiac anatomy (e.g. congenital heart disease) may require the patient to remain still for many hours in order to allow accurate mapping and anaesthesia is likely to be necessary. Procedures that call for perforation of the inter-atrial septum, or ablation of left sided structures may be unpleasant for the patient. In these cases a general anaesthetic is also preferable.

Additionally, there is some evidence that the use of general anaesthesia may improve the success of ablation, particularly for AF. It is possible that this is due to better mapping and reduced movement when the patient is unconscious, which increases the accuracy of the ablation. General anaesthetics are also associated with reduced radiation exposure (reduced fluoroscopy), faster procedures, and fewer complications. There is also evidence that patients are more satisfied with their overall experience if they receive a general anaesthetic, compared with patients who do not.

Practicalities of Administering Anaesthesia in the Cath Lab

The cath lab is usually a remote site, away from the main theatre complex, and as such it could be considered a riskier place to give an anaesthetic. Help may be further away than usual, and the environment may not be well set up for anaesthesia. Space is often limited, and equipment and drugs may need to be moved into the cath lab especially for the procedure. Unlike most operating theatres, cath labs do not have anaesthetic rooms and therefore induction takes place amongst the noise and commotion of the main lab, which may be unsettling for the patient and distracting for the anaesthetic team. The lab itself is designed so that the operating cardiologist has a good view of the monitoring screens, but they may not be in a convenient position for the anaesthetist. The tables differ to those in the operating theatre and cannot manoeuvre in the same way; while they are able to move horizontally and vertically, the Trendelenburg position is not possible. For this reason, some anaesthetists prefer to induce anaesthesia on a bed or trolley and then transfer the patient after the airway is secure. An exception is in the modern hybrid cath lab, where the table may be able to adopt more positions. Staff working in cath labs are not used to caring for unconscious patients, and extra attention is needed by the anaesthetic team to protect the airway during movement and transfers of the patient, and to effectively protect pressure areas. Ankle and head supports should be used. If the arms are positioned above the head to allow optimal lateral imaging, care should be taken not to cause brachial plexus injury. Airway tubing and intravenous lines need to be positioned to avoid the C-arm as it moves and extensions may be required to ensure they comfortably reach the patient as the table moves to and fro. Extra dead-space on long intravenous lines can be significant. Positioning of TOE probes and machines is often problematic. The cath lab, like theatre, may be cold and patients require active warming and temperature monitoring to ensure they do not develop hypothermia. Emergency apparatus such as a defibrillator and equipment to perform pericardiocentesis should be immediately available.

Protection from radiation during fluoroscopy is important and lead aprons and thyroid shields are a requirement for all staff working in the lab.

Pre-op Assessment

Ablation procedures are often carried out as day cases, and are not always pre-assessed by an anaesthetist prior to their admission. Common co-morbidities accompanying cardiac disease include systemic hypertension, peripheral vascular disease, diabetes, renal dysfunction and respiratory problems. The presence and severity of each of these should be assessed to determine the likelihood of peri-procedural complications such as haemodynamic instability, adverse effects of intravenous contrast agents (e.g. worsening renal impairment), and the possibility of needing post-procedure respiratory support. A medication history should also be taken with particular attention to anticoagulants, antiplatelet agents and antiarrhythmic drugs. A thorough assessment of the airway is also made.

A baseline ECG, haemoglobin, platelet count, coagulation screen and renal function are also worthwhile. Results of a recent echocardiogram should also be reviewed and if a permanent pacemaker is in situ then it should be interrogated before the procedure.

Conduct of General Anaesthesia

Monitoring standards are as for any other general anaesthetic. Intravenous access should be acquired, and in some cases invasive arterial blood pressure monitoring may be desirable. Central venous access is not commonly required, but can be considered if the use of potent vasoactive infusions is likely to be necessary. There is no procedure for induction of anaesthesia that is specific to the cath lab. One caveat is that if cryoablation is to be performed and neuromuscular monitoring of the phrenic nerve / diaphragm is required then muscle relaxation should either be avoided or a short-acting agent used. Similarly, during CRT, the left ventricular lead is close to the phrenic nerve and may cause unintentional pacing of the diaphragm. This will be masked if a muscle relaxant is present.

The airway may be secured using an endotracheal tube or a supraglottic device depending on the patient, although the relative lack of access to the airway during the procedure should be considered when making this choice. In order to ensure that mapping is accurate, it is important that the patient does not move or cough during the procedure, even if muscle relaxation is not used. An infusion of remifentanyl reduces the likelihood of movement, and monitoring the depth of anaesthesia may also help.

If cool flow is to be used, then a diuretic may be needed and therefore a urinary catheter should be considered. An oesophageal temperature probe is sometimes used if radiofrequency ablation of the left atrium is to be performed to try to prevent overheating of the adjacent oesophageal wall and atrio-oesophageal fistula formation which occurs in 0.01–0.2% of cases.

Software used for arrhythmia mapping is often able to compensate for movement caused by respiration. However, respiration will also cause variation in the dimensions of the atria and pulmonary vessels, and it can be helpful to use low tidal volumes with higher respiratory rates or low I:E ratios (e.g. 1:4) to reduce these problems. In some cases, temporary cessation of respiration may be required or if it is important that there is no respiratory movement for a prolonged period of time then high-frequency jet ventilation (HFJV) may be employed at a rate of 100–150 breaths per minute.

Anticoagulation is required for left sided procedures to reduce the risk of stroke and other thromboembolic complications. This is usually achieved with intravenous unfractionated heparin, aiming for an activated clotting time (ACT) of 300–400 s.

Since patients having CRT will usually have LBBB, complete heart block should be anticipated if there is manipulation of the right bundle branch during lead placement. As such, external defibrillation pads should be placed to allow pacing if necessary. Similarly, if a CRT-D device is to be inserted, the defibrillation function is usually tested at the end of the procedure and external pads are required in case the pacemaker fails to terminate the arrhythmia.

At the end of the procedure, emergence from anaesthesia should be conducted as smoothly as possible, avoiding coughing to prevent bleeding from the catheter access point in the femoral vessels. Post-procedure nausea and vomiting should be avoided for the same reason. Cardiac catheter procedures are not especially painful and if required simple analgesics such as paracetamol can be used.

Anaesthetic Drugs and EP Procedures

There is some controversy surrounding the use of anaesthetic agent for maintenance. Volatile anaesthetics are said to suppress arrhythmias and therefore interfere with mapping and accurate ablation. Desflurane in particular has been reported to have this problem. Sevoflurane and isoflurane both prolong the cardiac action potential and—experimentally—make it more difficult to induce tachyarrhythmias. Halothane and isoflurane are said to increase automaticity and cause ectopic beats. Despite these claims, no studies have been able to demonstrate a clinical difference or difference in outcome between inhalational agents and total intravenous anaesthesia (TIVA). Indeed, propofol has also been implicated in the suppression of some arrhythmias, although has also been shown not to be clinically significant. Midazolam may cause either reduction in heart rate by anxiolysis or tachycardia due to its vagolytic action. Opiates have anti-arrhythmic effects via the κ opioid receptor, and cause bradycardia via a central mechanism. Although remifentanyl causes bradycardia because of an effect on sino-atrial node automaticity and reduced atrioventricular node conduction, it does not appear to suppress intra-atrial conduction and is used successfully during ablation of both atrial and ventricular arrhythmias.

Possible Complications of EP Procedures

The most common complication of arrhythmia ablation in the cath lab is vascular injury to the vessel used for access followed by cardiac perforation and tamponade (1.3%), which may happen very rapidly and be catastrophic. Other complications include oesophageal rupture, atrio-oesophageal fistula, and those of the anaesthetic such as airway problems, anaphylaxis, hypotension, and nerve injury or

Table 2 Complications of EP procedures under GA

Vascular	Femoral haematoma Pseudoaneurysm Retroperitonal haematoma Arteriovenous fistula Aortic root puncture Coronary thrombosis / puncture (especially circumflex artery)
Neurological	TIA / stroke Peripheral nerve injury due to positioning Phrenic nerve palsy (cryoablation)
Pulmonary	Pulmonary vein thrombosis Pneumothorax Pulmonary oedema
Intracardiac	Atrial perforation / new ASD Cardiac tamponade Valve damage (including PV and resulting pulmonary stenosis) Coronary artery spasm
Oesophageal	Perforation Atrio-oesophageal fistula Injury due to TOE
Anaesthetic	Airway complications / dental damage Anaphylaxis
Miscellaneous	Infection Renal impairment due to contrast nephropathy Skin irritation / burns due to electrodes or defib pads

pressure-related trauma due to poor positioning (see Table 2). Major complications occur in 0.8% (SVT ablation) to 6% (VT ablation in a structurally abnormal heart) with an overall incidence of 3.6%. The mortality rate for AF ablation is 0.1%.

Recommended Readings

1. Ashley EM. 2012. Anaesthesia for electrophysiology procedures in the cardiac catheter laboratory. Continuing Education in Anaesthesia, Critical Care and Pain, 12, 230–236.
2. Bohnen M, Stevenson WG, Tedrow UB, Michaud GF, John RM, Epstein LM, Albert CM and Koplan BA. 2011. Incidence and predictors of major complications from contemporary catheter ablation to treat cardiac arrhythmias. Heart Rhythm, 8, 1661–6.
3. Cappato R, Calkins H, Chen SA, Davies W, Iesaka Y, Kalman J, Kim YH, Klein G, Natale A, Packer D. & Skanes A. 2009. Prevalence and causes of fatal outcome in catheter ablation of atrial fibrillation. J Am Coll Cardiol, 53, 1798–803.
4. Cleland JG, Daubert JC, Erdmann E, Freemantle N, Gras D, Kappenberger L, Tavazzi L. & Cardiac Resynchronization-Heart Failure Study, I. 2005. The effect of cardiac resynchronization on morbidity and mortality in heart failure. N Engl J Med, 352, 1539–49.
5. Schwarzwald SN, Kersten DJ, Shaikh ZA, Needelman BS, Feldman AM, Germano J, Islam S. & Cohen, T. J. 2018. Mechanisms of Lead Failure by Recall Status and Manufacturer: Results From the Pacemaker and Implantable Defibrillator Leads Survival Study ("PAIDLESS"). J Invasive Cardiol, 30, 147–151.
6. Seiler J, Steven D, Roberts-Thomson KC, Inada K, Tedrow UB, Michaud GF. & Stevenson WG. 2014. The effect of open-irrigated radiofrequency catheter ablation of atrial fibrillation on left atrial pressure and B-type natriuretic peptide. Pacing Clin Electrophysiol, 37, 616–23.

Myocardial Revascularization

Catherine Ashes and Saul Judelman

Coronary Anatomy

The coronary arteries arise from the coronary ostia in the sinuses of Valsalva. The left main coronary artery bifurcates shortly after its origin into the left anterior descending (LAD) and circumflex arteries. The LAD supplies the anterior and anteroseptal walls. The circumflex supplies the lateral and posterior walls. The LAD gives rise to the diagonal branches, and the circumflex gives rise to the obtuse marginal branches.

The right coronary artery (RCA) supplies the right ventricle, inferior and septal walls, and gives rise to the posterolateral branch. Coronary dominance refers to which artery (RCA or circumflex) gives rise to the posterior descending artery (PDA), the artery that supplies the posterior 2/3 of the interventricular septum and the AV node (Fig. 1).

Physiology of Coronary Blood Flow

The coronary circulation receives approximately 5% of the total cardiac output or approximately 250 mL/min. The myocardium has very high oxygen extraction (70–80%) compared with 25% for the rest of the body, therefore increases in oxygen demand must be met by increasing oxygen supply via increased coronary blood flow.

C. Ashes (✉)
St Vincent's Hospital, Sydney, Australia
e-mail: catherine.ashes@svha.org.au

S. Judelman
Royal North Shore Hospital, Sydney, Australia
e-mail: saul.judelman@health.nsw.gov.au

M. Vives and A. Hernandez (eds.), *Cardiac Anesthesia and Postoperative Care in the 21st Century*, https://doi.org/10.1007/978-3-030-79721-8_15

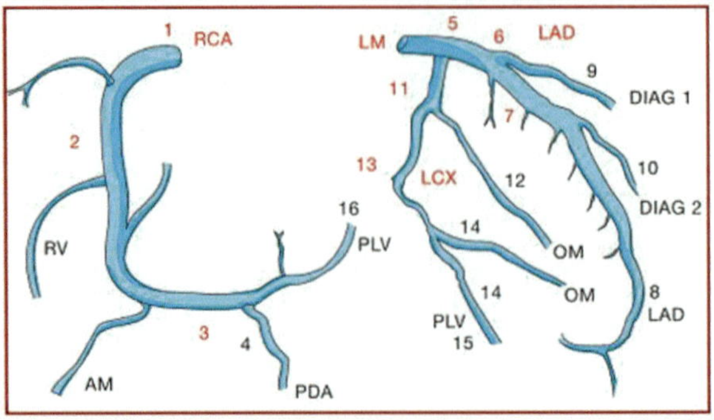

Classification of the American Heart Association. *RC* right coronary artery, *RV* right ventricular branch, *AM* acute marginal branch, *PLV* posterolateral ventricular branch, *PDA* posterior descending artery, *LCA* left coronary artery, *LM* left main artery, *LAD* left anterior descending artery, *DIAG 1* first diagonal branch, *DIAG 2* second diagonal branch, *LCx* left circumflex artery, *OM* obtuse marginal branches

Fig. 1 Coronary anatomy. Reproduced with permission from Fioranelli M, Gonnella C, Tonioni S et al. Clinical anatomy of the coronary circulation. Imaging coronary arteries pp 1–11. Ed Dowe D, Fioranelli M, Pavone P

Coronary blood flow is phasic. In the left ventricle, during systole, the coronary vasculature is compressed by the forceful contraction of ventricular myocardium. In diastole, as the ventricle relaxes, the extrinsic compression of the vessels is released and antegrade flow resumes. Right ventricular perfusion is less phasic due to lesser force of contraction.

Therefore, coronary blood flow is determined by:

1. **Coronary perfusion pressure.** In the left ventricle this is determined by the difference between the aortic root diastolic pressure and the left ventricular end diastolic pressure.
2. **Diastolic filling time.** Any increase in heart rate shortens the duration of diastole and the time for myocardial perfusion.
3. **Vessel wall diameter.** Dynamic changes in coronary vascular tone are influenced by both systemic neurohumoral factors and local conditions in the coronary vascular bed, which generally favour vasodilation. Fixed coronary lesions such as atherosclerotic plaque or coronary thrombosis may render these compensatory mechanisms redundant, and lead to myocardial ischaemia in the presence of reduced perfusion pressure, reduced diastolic filling time or increased myocardial demand.

Myocardial oxygen demand is predominately determined by the factors that influence myocardial work, namely myocardial wall tension (or afterload), contractility and heart rate. Unless an increase in myocardial work is able to be met with an increase in myocardial oxygen supply, ischaemia will ensue. In many patients with fixed coronary lesions, although myocardial oxygen supply will be sufficient at rest, when oxygen demand is increased (such as during sympathetic stimulation with tachycardia and increased myocardial contractility) the normal compensatory vasodilation may be unable to increase.

Anaesthetic Technique

With the pathophysiological considerations of coronary vascular disease in mind, anaesthesia for coronary artery bypass graft (CABG) surgery must facilitate the maintenance of haemodynamic goals that maintain the oxygen supply–demand balance.

Monitoring

Standard anaesthetic monitoring should be used. In addition, 5 lead ECG adds monitoring of lead II and V5 to improve detection of myocardial ischaemia. Continuous arterial pressure monitoring is established prior to induction of anaesthesia, taking care to avoid the side of a planned radial harvest. This is essential during CABG to maintain coronary perfusion, detect sudden haemodynamic changes related to the surgery, and guide vasoactive therapy. Arterial access also facilitates point of care (POC) blood testing (e.g. blood gas, ACT and other POC coagulation testing). Central venous cannulation is usually established post induction of anaesthesia, allowing monitoring of central venous pressure and administration of vasoactive medications.

According to current guidelines, transoesophageal echocardiography (TOE) should be considered in CABG surgery to confirm and refine the preoperative diagnosis, detect new or unsuspected pathology, adjust the anaesthetic and surgical plan and assess the results of surgical intervention. Global and segmental left and right ventricular function, and volume status can be monitored in real time. Myocardial ischaemia may be detected earlier by echocardiography (as new regional wall motion abnormalities) than by ECG changes. Newer modalities such as myocardial strain imaging may allow even earlier, subclinical detection of myocardial ischaemia.

Institutions vary in their practice regarding routine placement of pulmonary artery (PA) catheters. Although there appears to be no mortality benefit in routine PA catheterization for cardiac surgery, effect on morbidity is mixed. A PA catheter should be considered in patients with at least moderate pulmonary hypertension, reduced ejection fraction, and complex procedures (such as combined CABG plus valve).

Cerebral oximetry may be used during cardiac surgery to detect cerebral ischaemia, particularly in those with additional risk factors for cerebral ischaemia such as known cerebrovascular disease.

Haemodynamic Goals

It is important throughout all phases of the anaesthetic to maintain a favourable myocardial oxygen supply demand balance.

Specifically:

- **Blood pressure control.** Avoid hypotension which may reduce coronary perfusion pressure, and hypertension which increases wall tension and myocardial oxygen demand.
- **Low normal heart rate.** Tachycardia both increases myocardial oxygen demand and reduces oxygen supply.

Induction of Anaesthesia

With the above goals in mind, an induction technique should be selected that allows a stable blood pressure and avoids tachycardia. A balanced technique involving combinations of benzodiazepines (e.g. midazolam 0.03–0.06 mg/kg), opioids (e.g. fentanyl 2–4 mcg/kg), propofol (e.g. 0.5–1 mg/kg) and a non-depolarizing muscle relaxant may achieve this goal. Ketamine may be included for its favourable effect on blood pressure, however it may result in a mild tachycardia. High dose opioid techniques (e.g. fentanyl 50 mcg/kg) were previously common but may be associated with longer time to extubation and intensive care length of stay. Regardless of induction technique, blood pressure may decrease due to systemic vasodilation and myocardial depression. Hypotension should be corrected with vasopressors (e.g. phenylephrine or metaraminol) to avoid reductions in myocardial oxygen supply.

Maintenance of Anaesthesia

Volatile anaesthesia has been associated with reduced mortality and complications after cardiac surgery. This may be due to anti-inflammatory and cardioprotective properties of these agents.

Different phases of the surgical procedure have different levels of surgical stimulation requiring adjustment of depth of anaesthesia in anticipation of these dynamic changes. For example, following induction, there is a period of relative low stimulation during central venous catheterization, urinary catheterization, patient positioning and skin preparation. This is followed by sternotomy, which requires interruption of ventilation and deepening of anaesthesia, typically with a combination of maintenance agent and opioids. The placement of the sternal retractor signals left internal mammary artery (LIMA) harvest, a period of relative haemodynamic stability. Tidal volume may need to be reduced to improve surgical exposure. Heparin is administered toward the end of mammary harvest.

Initial TOE

A comprehensive TOE examination should be performed following induction of anaesthesia. Important findings which may influence the anaesthetic, surgical or perfusion planning for CABG are outlined in Table 1.

Table 1 Relevant findings on intraoperative TOE for CABG

Structure		
Left ventricle	Global systolic function	Should be graded by qualitative or quantitative (e.g. LVEF) methods as a baseline and to guide inotrope administration
	Regional systolic function	Regional wall motion abnormalities (RWMA) should be diagnosed and documented according to the 17 segment model for comparison with the post-operative study
New RWMA indicate acute coronary ischaemia and warrant immediate evaluation		
	Diastolic function	Associated with adverse outcomes after CABG
	Thrombus	Patients with myocardial infarction may have LV thrombus, particularly if there is severe global LV impairment or apical akinesis
Right ventricle	Global systolic function	Right coronary artery ischaemia may impair right ventricular systolic function. Patients with preoperative impairment of RV function may not tolerate periods of apnoea and hypoventilation during mammary harvest
Aortic valve	Aortic regurgitation (AR)	Significant AR may limit the ability to deliver antegrade cardioplegia into the aortic root, requiring alternative methods (e.g. retrograde cardioplegia administration)
Greater than mild AR is a relative contraindication to IABP placement		
Mitral valve	Mitral regurgitation (MR)	Ischaemic MR is associated with poor prognosis after MI. Moderate or greater MR may be considered for repair or replacement
Thoracic aorta	Atheroma in aorta	Descending aorta atheroma predicts ascending aorta atheroma, stroke and death after CABG
Epiaortic ultrasound may be used to better identify atheromatous disease in the ascending aorta around the sites for potential cannulation, cross clamp, side biter clamp and cardioplegia delivery		

Post Procedure TOE

LV global and regional systolic function should be reassessed. Pre-existing regional wall motion abnormalities (RWMA) may improve if the newly reperfused myocardium was ischaemic or hibernating. Wall motion may also unchange due to stunning. Any worsening or new RWMA should raise suspicion of acute graft failure, kinking or thrombosis, however distal embolization of air can also produce the same clinical picture. Similarly, new or worsened mitral regurgitation should be evaluated for an associated new or worsened RWMA which may indicate an ischaemic aetiology.

High Risk Patients

Patients at elevated risk for perioperative myocardial ischaemia or haemodynamic instability include, but are not limited to, those with critical left main coronary artery lesions, refractory anginal symptoms, reduced cardiac function, cardiogenic shock or uncontrolled arrhythmias. These patients may require additional interventions including:

- Defibrillator pads placed pre-induction
- Central venous access pre-induction
- Intra-aortic balloon counter pulsation pre- or post-induction
- Inducing the patient prepped, draped and catheterized, ready for immediate sternotomy if required.

Surgical Approaches

On Pump CABG

Following the systemic anticoagulation, preparation for cardiopulmonary bypass (CPB) will commence, including cannulation of the ascending aorta and right atrium, cannulation for delivery of cardioplegia to the aortic root and/or coronary sinus, administration of antifibrinolytic therapy (for example tranexamic acid).

The distal coronary anastomosis are generally performed following aortic cross clamping and delivery of cardioplegia on a non-beating heart. The “top ends” or aortic anastomoses may be performed after the aorta has been unclamped with the heart beating, using a “side biter” clamp.

Off Pump CABG

Off pump CABG refers to the performance of coronary artery grafting without the use of CPB. The technique includes other variations such as the absence of any aortic manipulation and the use of total arterial grafts. Off pump CABG is a technically difficult procedure due to the moving heart during grafting. Much of the operation remains the same including sternotomy and conduit harvesting. Grafting is aided by the use of stabilizing devices which reduce cardiac movement, and intra-coronary shunts to allow continued coronary blood flow during the grafting procedure. The positioning required to reach the target arteries and the use of stabilizer devices can cause haemodynamic instability largely due to reduced venous return. This necessitates ongoing and clear communication between the surgeon and anaesthetist.

Off pump CABG entails additional considerations to a standard procedure. These include coronary ischaemia, arrhythmias and haemodynamic instability. There may be a need to institute CPB if stability cannot be achieved. Much of the anaesthetic technique is similar to a standard CABG, however in general larger volumes of intravenous fluids are required to support venous return. Beta blocker medications may be used to decrease the heart rate to aid grafting. Hypothermia is common due to the lack of CPB to assist rewarming. Active warming of IV fluids and surface warming including preoperatively are necessary.

The proposed advantages of off pump surgery are based upon the avoidance of CPB and minimising aortic manipulation. Benefits include lower transfusion rates, lower reoperation for bleeding and better renal outcomes. Lower stroke rates have been purported as a major benefit, which have been demonstrated in single-centre trials and observational studies. There remains a lack of robust evidence showing reduced mortality in large randomized trials supporting the wide spread use of off pump techniques.

Minimally Invasive Cardiac Surgery

Minimally invasive coronary artery surgery includes a range of techniques that avoid a midline sternotomy. Access is achieved via a left anterior thoracotomy or endoscopically with the use of a surgical robot. The anaesthetic technique may vary due to fast track recovery pathways which involve extubating the patient in the operating theatre or shortly thereafter. Lung isolation with a double lumen endotracheal tube allows access through the left hemithorax. Mammary artery harvest can be performed through the thoracotomy or with the use of a surgical robot. The distal anastomosis is most commonly performed directly but can be performed robotically if a robotic stabilizing device is available. CPB if needed can be instituted peripherally via the femoral vessels.

The major concern with a minimally invasive approach is uncontrolled bleeding or instability with limited direct access to the heart. Cardiac arrhythmias can only be treated with external defibrillation pads. Bleeding which cannot be controlled or other surgical complications may necessitate conversion to sternotomy in order to achieve control.

In general, minimally invasive coronary surgery is performed on patients with fewer coronary lesions and mainly in the LAD or circumflex territory. Access to the right coronary artery is very difficult but has been performed with the use of surgical robots. A hybrid approach with surgical revascularization of the LAD and percutaneous intervention to other territories can also be performed.

Coronary Angiography, Angioplasty and Stenting

Many coronary lesions are amenable to percutaneous angioplasty and stenting. These procedures are usually performed under conscious sedation without involvement of an anaesthetist. A minority of patients require the anaesthetic input. Typically these are haemodynamically unstable patients at high risk of periprocedural complications.

The care of the patient for urgent coronary angioplasty and stenting is challenging. The anaesthetizing location is remote and often unfamiliar to the anaesthetist. The patient is potentially unstable with symptomatic coronary ischaemia and haemodynamic instability. The same haemodynamic considerations should be observed as for patients with ischaemic heart disease presenting for surgical intervention. As these patients are at high risk of haemodynamic compromise, securing adequate intravenous access and monitoring is essential. This must occur without undue delay to the procedure to allow prompt revascularization. Arterial monitoring can be achieved using the femoral arterial sheath inserted by the proceduralist. Femoral central venous access may also rapidly be gained at the same time as arterial cannulation. Clear communication is essential to ensure timely provision of safe anaesthetic care.

Recommended Readings

1. Ramanathan T, Skinner H. Coronary blood flow. Contin Educ Anaesth CritAl Care Pain. 2005;5(2):61–4.
2. American Society of Anaesthesiologists and Society of Cardiovascular Anaesthesiologists Task Force on Transesophageal Echocardiography. Practice guidelines for perioperative transesophageal echocardiography. An updated report by the American Socity of Anesthsiologists and the Socity of Carediovascular Anesthesiologists Task Force on Transesophageal Echocardiography. Anesthesiology 2010;112:1084.
3. Barbeito A. Anesthesia for coronary grafting surgery. UpToDate, Post TW, Waltham MA, 2019.

4. Wong W-T, Lai VWK, Chee YE, Lee A. Fast-track cardiac care for adult cardiac surgical patients. Cochrane Database Syst Rev. 2016;12(9):CD003587.
5. Afilalo J, Flynn AW, Shimony A, Rudski LG, Agnihotri AK, Morin JF, Castrillo C, Shahian DM, Picard MH. Incremental value of the preoperative echocardiogram to predict mortality and major morbidity in coronary artery bypass surgery. Circulation. 2013;127 (3):356–64.

Valvular Surgery

Matias Caceres Quinones and Jacobo Moreno Garijo

Valvular Surgery

Valve heart surgery is one of most frequent and challenging procedures for the cardiovascular anesthesiologist. Different types and stages of valvular disease will influence the physiological conditions and the potential hemodynamic changes in the operating room.

During the perioperative period there are constant changes in the physiologic and hemodynamic conditions that are readily influenced by anesthesia, thus requiring a thorough understanding of the natural history and pathophysiology of valve defects.

Aortic Stenosis

History and Clinical Features

Aortic Stenosis (AS) is the most common valve lesion leading to surgery or catheter intervention in Europe and North America. It can be divided in congenital and acquired AS. The former can be classified as valvular, subvalvular and

---

The original version of this chapter was revised: This Chapter title has been changed from "Cardiac Anaesthesia and Postoperative Care in the Twenty-First Century" to "Valvular Surgery". The correction to this chapter can be available at https://doi.org/10.1007/978-3-030-79721-8_33

M. Caceres Quinones · J. Moreno Garijo (✉)
Department of Anesthesia and Pain Medicine, University Health Network, Toronto General Hospital, Toronto, ON, Canada
e-mail: Jacobo.Moreno@uhn.ca

M. Caceres Quinones
e-mail: Matias.CaceresQuinones@one-mail.on.ca

M. Vives and A. Hernandez (eds.), *Cardiac Anesthesia and Postoperative Care in the 21st Century*, https://doi.org/10.1007/978-3-030-79721-8_16

supravalvular AS based on the location. Valvular AS might occur in an unicuspid, bicuspid or tricuspid valve as a consequence of a degenerative process or secondary to rheumatic disease. Bicuspid aortic valve is found in 1–2% of the population, being the most common cause of AS below the age of 70. Clinically significant AS can develop in 2% of patients older than 65 years and this can increase to 5.5% in patients older than 85 years.

A normal aortic valve has an aortic valve area (AVA) that goes between 2.6 to 3.5 cm^2, and 2 cm^2/m^2 indexed with a rate of progression on average of a decrease of 0.1 cm^2/year. Clinical progression may manifest with classical symptoms like angina (initial symptom in two thirds of patients), syncope (first symptom in 15–30% of patients), and congestive heart failure (CHF), all signs of prognostic significance. Life expectancy when angina develops is about 5 years, 3–4 years for syncope, and 1–2 years once signs of left ventricle failure occur.[4]

Pathophysiology

The maintenance of normal stroke volume (SV) is associated with an increasing pressure gradient between the left ventricle (LV) and the aorta. This gradient results in pressure overload that triggers remodeling with compensatory concentric LV hypertrophy (Fig. 1). This induces changes in diastolic compliance with increases in left ventricle diastolic pressure (LVEDP) ultimately altering coronary perfusion pressure (CPP) and deterioration of exposing the LV to a higher risk of ischemia.

Preoperative Assessment

Echocardiography is the standard method for quantifying AS severity. This includes the measurement of AS peak jet velocity, mean transvalvular pressure gradient by Bernoulli equation and AVA by continuity equation as reflected in Table 1. Intraoperatively, transesophageal echocardiography (TEE) is the required method for the assessment of AS surgery as seen in Fig. 2.

Up to 30% of patients with severe AS may have transvalvular gradients and velocities bellow the range for severe stenosis, despite AVA < 1 cm^2. Intervention in these patients carries a higher risk of mortality and worse prognosis. The characteristics of this groups have been summarized in Table 2.

Timing for Intervention

Intervention is based upon the stage of the disease, and the stage of disease takes into account the severity and the presence or absence of symptoms. The four stages of AS as per the American Heart Association (AHA) guidelines recommendation are summarized in Tables 3 and 4. The less invasive nature of transcatheter aortic

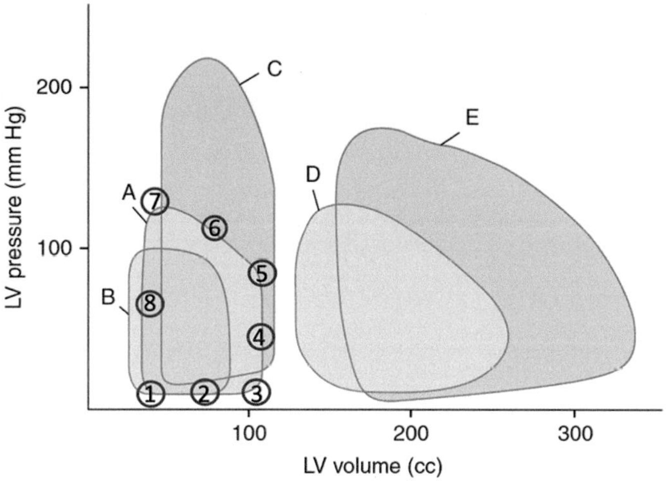

Fig. 1 Typical pressure-volume loop in a patient with AS (**c**). There is a higher peak pressure generated during systole compared to a normal LV (**a**) because of the high transvalvular pressure gradient. There is a preserved systolic function reflected in a normal stroke volume and ejection fraction. The diastolic limb is steeper, which reflects a reduced LV compliance, and thus, impaired diastolic function. Clinically, small changes in diastolic volume produce relatively large increases in ventricular filling pressure. This stiffness makes the contribution of atrial systole to ventricular filling account for up to 40% of the LV end-diastolic volume (LVEDV), rather than the 15–20% on a normal LV. 1. Mitral valve opening; 2. diastolic filling of the left ventricle; 3. mitral valve closure at end diastole; 4. isovolumetric contraction; 5. aortic valve opening; 6. ventricular ejection; 7. aortic valve closure at end systole; 8. isovolumetric relaxation of the LV. Modified from Jackson JM, Thomas SJ, Lowenstein E. Anesthetic management of patients with valvular heart disease. Semin Anesth. 1982;1:240

Table 1 AS grading as per the ASE

Parameters	Mild moderate severe
Peak velocity (m/s)	< 2.6–2.9 to ≥ 4.0
Mean gradient (mmHg)	< 20 to ≥ 40
AVA (cm^2)	> 1.5 to < 1.0
Indexed AVA (cm^2/m^2)	> 0.85 to < 0.6
Velocity ratio	> 0.5 to < 0.25

AS: Aortic Stenosis, ASE: American Society of Echocardiography, AVA: Aortic Valve Area. Modified from Baumgartner et al. *J Am Soc Echocardiogr*. 2017 Apr;30(4):372–392

valve replacement (TAVR), as compared to surgical aortic valve replacement (AVR), has changed the landscape of patients presenting for AVR with symptomatic AS. TAVR has been proven superior to AVR even in low risk patients as per results of the PARTNER-3 and the EVOLUT low risk trial, suggesting that current guidelines might be modified in the future. Current recommendations for intervention in symptomatic AS patients are reflected in Fig. 3.

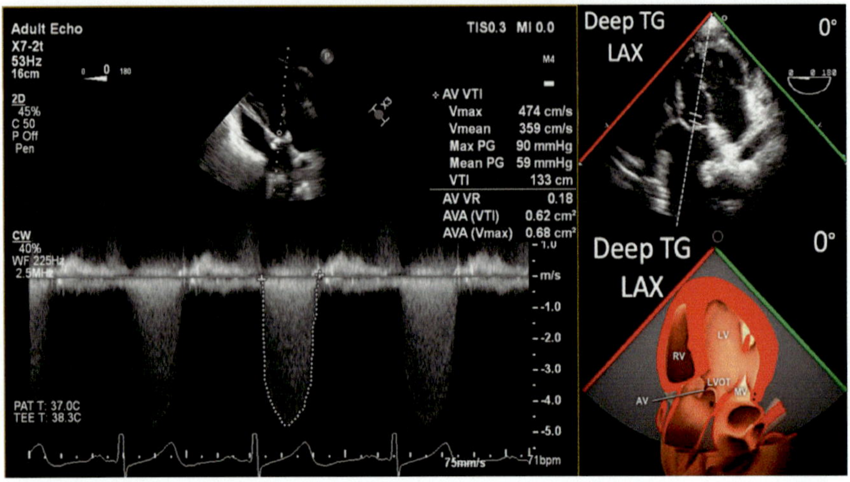

Fig. 2 Severe aortic stenosis with mean transvalvular pressure gradient (Mean PG) determined by Bernoulli equation derived from the aortic valve peak velocity (Vmax) and aortic valve area (AVA) by continuity equation (VTI). Parameters obtained from a long axis (LAX) aortic valve deep transgastric (TG) transesophageal echocardiography (TEE) view. Modified from pie.med.utoronto.ca

Table 2 Low flow, low gradient AS with reduced ejection fraction vs paradoxical low flow, low gradient AS with preserved ejection fraction

Low flow, low gradient AS with reduced ejection fraction	Paradoxical low flow, low gradient AS with preserved ejection fraction
• LV EF < 50% with a low-flow state defined as a stroke volume index (SVi) < 35 mL/m^2 along with mean gradient < 40 mm Hg, peak velocity < 4 m/s, and AVA < 1 cm^2. • Dobutamine stress echocardiography (DSE) should be performed in these cases to help differentiate two clinical situations: • Severe AS causing LV systolic dysfunction (true severe AS) • Moderate AS (pseudosevere AS) with another cause of LV dysfunction (ischemic cardiomyopathy, primary cardiomyopathy, etc.) • If the addition of inotropic support results in a mean gradient > 40 mm Hg and the calculated AVA remains less than 1 cm^2, the diagnosis of true severe AS is confirmed. • If the mean gradient remains less than 40 mm Hg, but the calculated AVA increases to greater than 1 cm^2, then a diagnosis of pseudosevere AS is made.	• The patient has a valve area < 1 cm^2 with a peak velocity <4 m/s and a mean pressure gradient <40 mmHg despite normal LVEF. • This is usually found in the setting of elderly patients with hypertrophied, small ventricles secondary to concentric remodeling and impaired diastolic filling that result in reduced transvalvular flow (SVi < 35 mL/m^2) despite normal EF. • Other more frequent reasons must be first excluded and may be more likely such as technical factors in AVA calculation. DSE is also helpful for diagnosis.

Table 3 Aortic stenosis classification

Stage (clinical)	Definition	
A	At risk of AS	
B	Progressive AS	
C	Asymptomatic severe AS	
	C1	LVEF $\geq 50\%$
	C2	LVEF > 50%
D	Symptomatic severe AS	
	D1	High Gradient AS
	D2	Low flow, Low gradient AS, LVEF < 50%
	D3	Low flow, Low gradient AS, LVEF $\geq 50\%$

Modified from Nishimura et al. *J Am Coll Cardiol*. 2014;63(22):2438–2488

Table 4 Recommendations for timing of AVR in aortic stenosis (AS)

Class I indications
• Symptomatic patients with severe high-gradient AS who have symptoms by history or on exercise testing • Asymptomatic patients with severe AS and LVEF <50% • Severe AS when undergoing other cardiac surgery
Class IIa indications
• Asymptomatic patients with very severe AS (aortic velocity ≥ 5 m/s) and low surgical risk • Asymptomatic patients with severe AS and decreased exercise tolerance or a fall in blood pressure with exercise • Asymptomatic patients with low-flow/low-gradient severe AS with reduced LVEF with low-dose dobutamine stress study showing an aortic velocity ≥ 4 m/s (mean pressure gradient ≥ 40 mm Hg) with a valve area $\leq 1cm^2$ at any dobutamine dose • Symptomatic patients who have low-flow/low-gradient severe AS who are normotensive and have an LVEF $\geq 50\%$ if clinical, hemodynamic, and anatomic data support valve obstruction as the most likely cause of symptoms • Patients with moderate AS (aortic velocity 3–3.9 m/s) who are undergoing other cardiac surgery
Class IIb indication
• Asymptomatic patients with severe AS and rapid disease progression and low surgical risk
AVR, aortic valve replacement; LVEF, left ventricular ejection fraction. Adapted from Nishimura et al. *J Am Coll Cardiol*. 2014;63(22):2438–2488

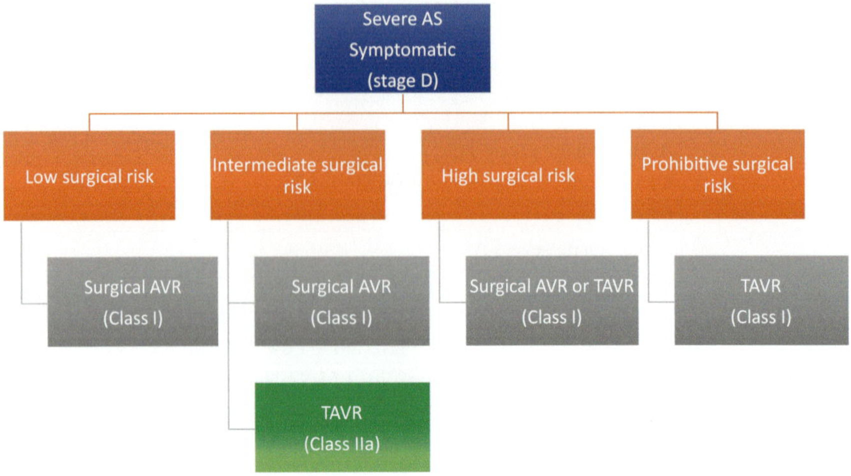

Fig. 3 Choice of TAVR versus surgical AVR in the patient with severe symptomatic AS. AS indicates aortic stenosis; AVR, aortic valve replacement; and TAVR, transcatheter aortic valve replacement. Nishimura, Rick A., et al. *J Am Coll Cardiol*. 2017; 70(2):252–289

Anesthetic Considerations

Regardless of the type of procedure, anesthetic management is based on the avoidance of systemic hypotension, maintenance of sinus rhythm, adequate rate avoiding tachycardia and bradycardia, preserving preload and contractility, and avoidance of potential myocardial ischemia due to impaired CPP and fixed forward flow. Considerations and goals for AS patient's management are summarized in Tables 5 and 6, respectively. Both, TAVR patients who receive general anesthesia and surgical patients can often be extubated shortly after arrival in the intensive care unit, as per fast-track protocols.

Hypertrophic Obstructive Cardiomyopathy (HOCM)

History and Clinical Features

Hypertrophic cardiomyopathy (HCM) is a genetic disorder with autosomal dominant inheritance and variable penetrance that affects around 0.2% of the general population (1:500 births). Around 25% of patients with HCM presents with dynamic obstruction (HOCM) to systolic outflow through the left ventricular outflow tract (LVOT) due to systolic anterior motion (SAM) of the mitral valve. The different types of HCM are summarized in Table 7 and anatomically represented in Fig. 4.

Table 5 Anesthetic considerations in AS

• The surgeon should be present during the induction period and the perfusionist ready to initiate emergency CPB in case of acute deterioration and blood must be readily available. • Premedication to reduce anxiety may be beneficial to prevent preoperative tachycardia and the potential for exacerbating myocardial ischemia due to increased gradient. Careful titration of narcotic-based anesthesia is usually chosen to meet hemodynamic goals, low concentrations of volatile anesthetics for maintenance are usually safe. • Additional to standard monitoring, five-lead ECG system with V5, large bore peripheral venous access, invasive arterial lineon pre-induction, external defibrillator pads and central line are recommended. • Pulmonary artery catheters (PACs) are helpful to assess cardiac output and mixed venous oxygen, capillary wedge pressures (PCWP) are not reliable in a non-compliant left ventricle (LV) and might overestimate LV end diastolic pressure (LVEDP).	• PACs carry the risk of inducing hypotension secondary to arrhythmias. The most conservative approach is leaving the catheter tip in a central venous position until the chest is open. • The post-bypass period is not likely to be marked by myocardial failure or low output states, and therefore PACs should be best reserved for patients with low LVEF preoperatively. • Transesophageal echocardiography (TEE) is useful for LV function, preload, and afterload assessment. Can also predict prosthetic aortic valve size based on the LV outflow tract width and AVA. Is also the method of choice for post-bypass assessment of the prosthetic valve to rule out paravalvular leaks or residual prosthetic valve gradient and assess other complications. • Myocardial function and stroke volume improve fast after the relief of the obstruction, but the hypertrophy will resolve more slowly over time, thus after surgery they still require elevated preload.

Table 6 Aortic stenosis hemodynamic goals

Preload	Increased
Contractility	Normal
Afterload	Increased
Rhythm/ Rate	Sinus rhythm, HR 50 70
Avoid	Hypotension, Tachycardia, Bradycardia and high myocardial oxygen demand situations

Table 7 HCM types

Non obstructive	LVOT peak gradient < 30 mmHg (rest/provocation)
Obstructive (HOCM)	LVOT peak gradient ≥ 30 mmHg
Latent obstructive	LVOT peak gradient > 30 (provocation)

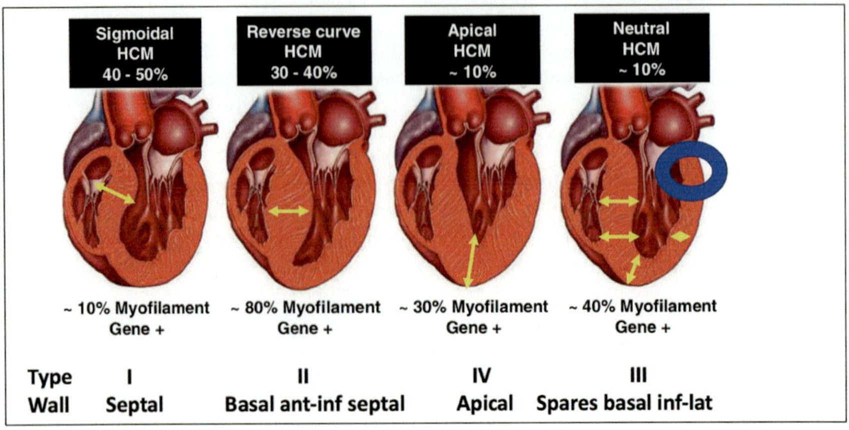

Fig. 4 Septal morphologies in HCM. Adapted from Bos et al. *J Am Coll Cardiol*. 2009;54:201–11

Clinically, it might be asymptomatic or present as dyspnea on exertion and poor exercise tolerance (most common symptom), syncope, chest pain, fatigue, or palpitations. There is no direct relationship between the degree of left ventricle outflow tract (LVOT) obstruction and the occurrence or severity of symptoms. Other symptoms might be secondary to diastolic dysfunction, dysrhythmias, mitral regurgitation (MR), and an imbalance of myocardial oxygen supply and demand. Sudden cardiac death or cardiac arrest may be the first manifestation in more than 50% of patients. The highest-risk group for sudden death include those with a family history of HCM and young patients with high physical demand (i.e., athletes), with an associated mortality of less than 1% a year.

Pathophysiology

HCM is characterized with asymmetrical hypertrophy of the myocardium without any identifiable cause for the hypertrophy, normal or even increased LV systolic function, impaired diastolic function and rarely dilated LV. Abnormal cellular architecture and interstitial fibrosis with patchy myocardial scarring contribute to impaired diastolic filling and relaxation and to derangement in the electrical tissue, putting them at risk of fatal dysrhythmias.

SAM of the anterior mitral valve leaflet (AML) is the underlying cause for dynamic outflow tract obstruction. The LV septum is narrowed by the severe hypertrophy, with further narrowing of the LVOT during systole that leads to an increase in the blood flow velocity and pressure gradient through the LVOT. There is also basal septal hypertrophy that shortens the distance between the AML and the septum, along with hypertrophied anteriorly displaced papillary muscles and elongated mitral valve leaflets that causes a closer coaptation of the posterior mitral leaflet (PML) to the base of the AML and slack tissue extending beyond the coaptation point. Acceleration of flow through the LVOT creates a "Venturi effect" in which the hydraulic forces pulls the AML slack tissue into the LVOT generating a high gradient. Also, a drag force generated by the LV pulls the AML into the LVOT in early systole, currently being this mechanism the predominant cause of SAM. This leads to dynamic obstruction that varies with different loading conditions and contractility. This mid-late systole subaortic obstruction, increases with high contractility, higher rates, and decreases with high preload and afterload conditions. A posteriorly directed jet of MR results as a consequence of SAM, with its severity related to the degree of LVOT obstruction.

Preoperative Assessment

Echocardiography is the method of choice to assess the different types of HCM, severity and location of the obstruction and the presence of SAM. TEE exam at baseline is critical for the surgery providing different measurements to help guiding the extent of myectomy, including maximum basal septum thickness, distance from the AML impact into the septum to the AV annulus and depth of apical extent of the septal bulge as reflected in Fig. 5. SAM can be demonstrated with color flow Doppler showing a high-velocity turbulent flow (aliasing) in the LVOT. Predictor

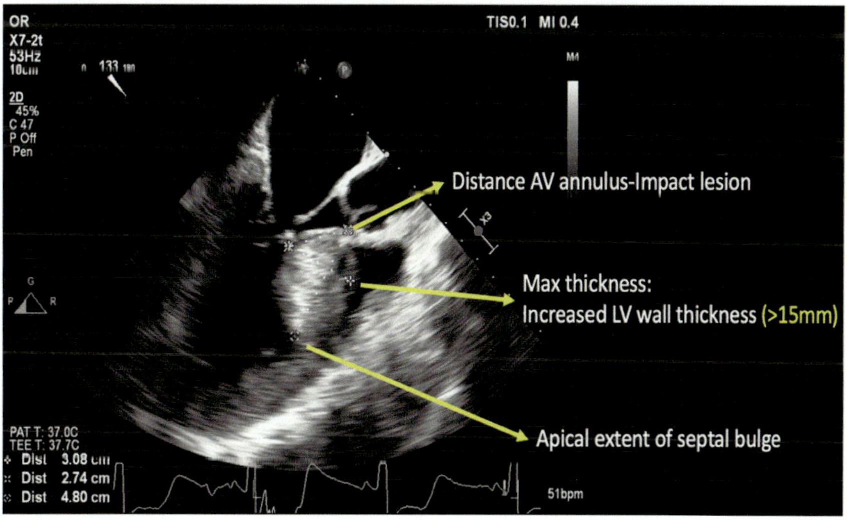

Fig. 5 TEE image of the mid-esophageal AV long axis view with the required measurements before septal myectomy in HOCM patients. AV: Aortic valve, Max thickness: maximum basal septum thickness

Table 8 Echocardiographic predictors of systolic anterior motion (SAM)

Measurement	Echocardiographic view	Time of cardiac cycle
Basal septal thickness >1.5 cm	ME LAX[a]	End diastole
C-sept distance < 2.5 cm[b]	ME LAX or ME 5 Chamber[c]	Onset of systole
PMVL length > 1.5 cm AMVL length > 2.0 cm AMVL:PMVL ratio < 1.3	ME LAX or ME 5 Chamber	Onset of systole
Mitral-aortic angle < 120°	ME LAX or ME 5 Chamber	Onset of systole

PMVL = posterior mitral valve leaflet; AMVL = anterior mitral valve leaflet
[a]Midesophageal long-axis view (ME LAX)
[b]Minimum distance from the coaptation point to the septum
[c]Midesophageal 5-chamber view
Adapted from Hymel et al. *Anesthesia & Analgesia, 118(6),2014:1197–1201.*

of SAM are summarized in Table 8. A characteristic finding of SAM due to dynamic subaortic obstruction of the LVOT is a late peaking, “dagger-shaped” of high-velocity Doppler flow due to the onset of obstruction in mid-to-late systole measured by continuous wave Doppler, as reflected in Fig. 6.

Anesthetic Considerations

The goals of management should be focused in avoiding aggravating the subaortic obstruction. It is critical to maintain an appropriate intravascular volume and prevent increases in contractility or heart rate. The considerations and goals are summarized in Tables 9 and 10.

Aortic Regurgitation

History and Clinical Features

Aortic regurgitation (AR) can be caused by a primary abnormality of the valve cusps and/or from abnormalities of the aortic root and ascending aortic geometry. About two-thirds are degenerative tricuspid and bicuspid AR. There may be also rheumatic or infectious origin, or it may occur in association with any condition producing dilatation of the aortic root and leaflet separation. A practical approach is based in a modification of the Carpentier classification for the mechanism of mitral valve regurgitation by El Khoury et al. reflected in Fig. 7.

Chronic AR remains asymptomatic for a long time during which valvular incompetence and secondary ventricular dilatation become more severe. Symptoms

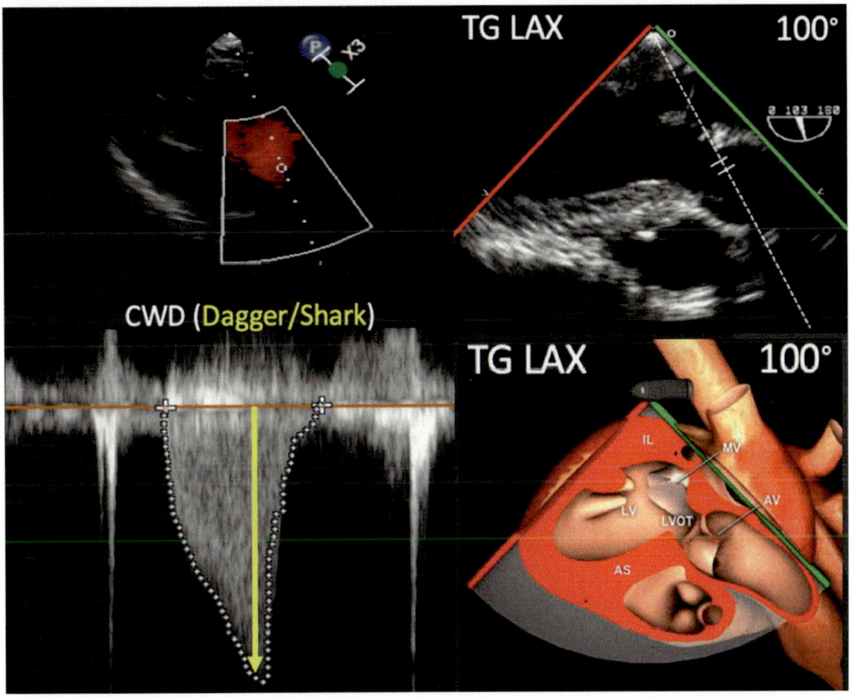

Fig. 6 Transesophageal echocardiography (TEE) long axis (LAX) transgastric view to determine dynamic subaortic obstruction of the left ventricle outflow tract (LVOT) due to systolic anterior motion (SAM) of the anterior mitral valve leaflet, by continuous wave Doppler (CWD). Modified from pie.med.utoronto.ca

Table 9 Anesthetic considerations in HOCM

• Most of patients with HOCM are treated with β-blockers to reduce LVOT obstruction due to their negative inotropic effects and reduction in heart rate and Calcium channel blockers for their effect on diastolic compliance. High risk patients for malignant dysrhythmias have an automated implantable cardioverter–defibrillator (AICD). In the preoperative period is better to keep those therapies and continue them throughout the perioperative period. • Additional to standard monitoring, five-lead ECG system with V5, large bore peripheral venous access, invasive arterial lineon pre-induction and central line are recommended. • AICDs can be deactivated once external defibrillator pads are available.	• Avoid sympathetic stimulation leading to increases in heart rate and contractility and avoid decreases in afterload. Narcotic based anesthesia along with volatile anesthesia might be of benefit due to his negative inotropic effect. • TEE allows to assess the location and extent of hypertrophy, the degree of SAM and LVOT obstruction, and degree of MR. It is also more reliable to accurately assess volume as opposed to CVP and PCWP since they overestimate volume status in the hypertrophied LV. More important, allows to assess the adequacy of surgical repair and possible complications. • Immediate postoperative complications of myectomy that must be ruled out include residual LVOT obstruction, residual SAM, residual MR, complete heart block, and ventricular septal defect.

Table 10 HOCM hemodynamic goals

Preload	Increased
Contractility	Normal or lower
Afterload	Increased
Rhythm/Rate	Sinus rhythm, lower rates 50–60 bpm
Avoid	Tachycardia, hypovolemia, and sympathetic stimulation

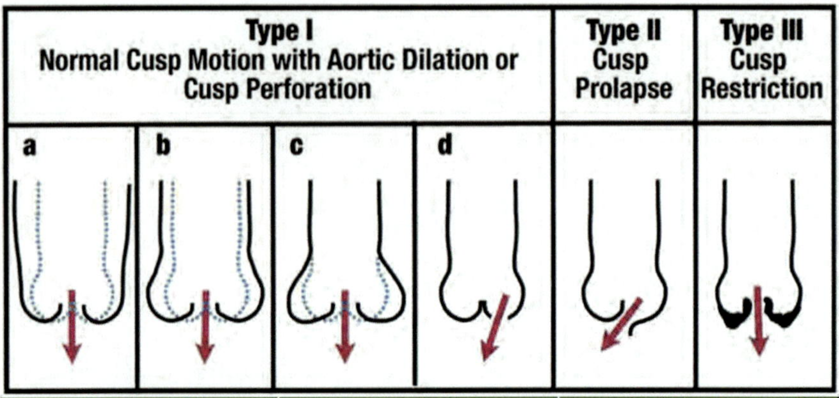

	Valve	Aorta
Acquired	Rheumatic Calcific Endocarditis Traumatic Radiotherapy Toxins	Aneurysm Aortic dissection Autoimmune (SLE, ankylosing spondylitis) Aortitis (Syphilis, Takayasu´s arteritis) Trauma
Congenital	Bicuspid Unicuspid Cuadricuspid	Annulo – aortic ectasia Connective tissue disorders (Marfan´s, Ehlers-Danlos)

Fig. 7 Common Etiologies and Classification of Aortic Regurgitation. Adapted from Zoghbi et al. J Am Soc Echocardiogr. 2017 Apr;30(4):303–371

are usually related to CHF like shortness of breath, palpitations, fatigue, and angina. They usually develop after significant dilatation and dysfunction of the LV. The risk of mortality at 10-years in asymptomatic patient is 5–15%. The prognosis after the onset of symptoms is about 10 years, and the severity and duration of those do not correlate well with the deterioration of contractility. Patients with depressed LV

Table 11 Echocardiographic assessment of aortic regurgitation

Grade	Mild-moderate-severe
Left Ventricular size	Normal to dilated
Jet deceleration rate by Pressure half-time (msec)	Slow (> 500) to Steep (< 200)
Diastolic flow reversal in descending thoracic aorta	Brief to prominent
Vena contracta width (cm)	< 0.3 to > 0.6
Jet width/LVOT width (%)	< 25 to ≥ 65
Jet CSA/LVOT CSA (%)	< 5 to ≥ 60
Regurgitation Volume (ml/beat)	< 30 to ≥ 60
Regurgitation Fraction (%)	< 30 to ≥ 50
EROA (cm^2)	< 0.1 to ≥ 0.3

CSA: cross sectional area, EROA: effective regurgitant orifice Area, LVOT: left ventricle outflow tract. Modified form Zoghbi et al. *J Am Soc Echocardiogr*. 2017;30(4):303–371

function have a higher perioperative mortality rate and higher risk for postoperative heart failure. Acute AR presents with severe symptoms like dyspnea, pulmonary edema and heart failure. Due to the lack of longstanding compensation as in chronic AR, they are not capable of maintaining sufficient forward stroke volume putting the patient at high risk of cardiovascular collapse. The assessment and grading of AR are performed by echocardiography. The parameters used are summarized in Table 11.

Pathophysiology

Left ventricular volume overload is the primary characteristic of aortic regurgitation. The degree of volume overload is determined by the magnitude of the regurgitant flow, which is related to the size of the regurgitant orifice, the aorto-ventricular pressure gradient, and the diastolic time.

Acute AR

There is a sudden major volume overload on the LV. To compensate and keep an adequate forward flow, there is an increased sympathetic tone that leads to tachycardia, an increased contractile state and fluid retention. However, this may not be sufficient to maintain a normal cardiac output and rapid deterioration of LV function can occur, emergency surgical intervention.

Chronic AR

In Chronic AR, there is gradual volume overload that leads to increased LEDV and compensatory eccentric hypertrophy that increases wall tension. The LVEDV increases slowly and the LVEDP remains relatively normal. Cardiac output and CPP is maintained at expenses of high LVEDV, peripheral vasodilation and large SV. As the dilatation progresses, coronary perfusion finally decreases leading to LV dysfunction followed by an increase in PA pressure that leads to CHF symptoms. As a compensatory mechanism for the poor cardiac output and poor coronary perfusion, sympathetic constriction of the periphery occurs to maintain blood pressure, which in turn leads to further decreases in cardiac output. These changes are summarized in Fig. 8.

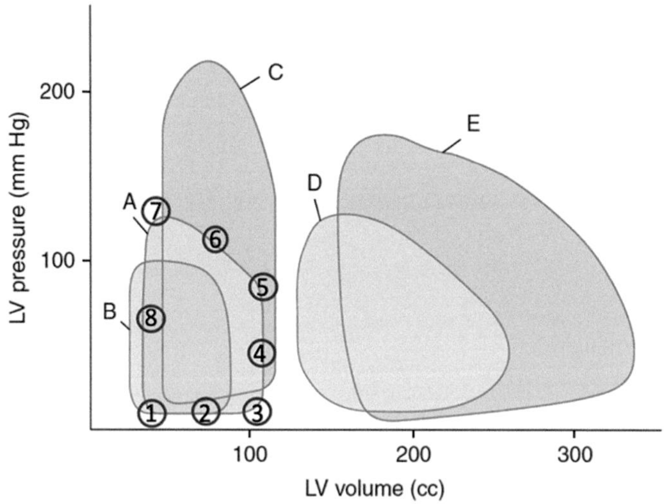

Fig. 8 Figure shows the pressure-volume loops for acute (D) and chronic (E) aortic regurgitation. In chronic AR, the pressure-volume curve is shifted far to the right. There is high diastolic compliance that allows an increase in LVEDV with minimal change in filling pressures. The increase in preload is compensated by ventricular hypertrophy and cardiac output is maintained by the Frank-Starling mechanism. Despite normal cardiac output, contractility is decreased. There is virtually no isovolumic diastolic phase and a brief isovolumic systolic phase. Eventually, with progressive increases in LVEDV, hypertrophy is no longer sufficient to compensate, and a decline in systolic function occurs. In acute AR LVEDV are also increased; however, the ventricle is not adapted to accommodate increased volumes and thus, elevation of filling pressures occurs. 1. Mitral valve opening; 2. diastolic filling of the left ventricle; 3. mitral valve closure at end diastole; 4. isovolumetric contraction; 5. aortic valve opening; 6. ventricular ejection; 7. aortic valve closure at end systole; 8. isovolumetric relaxation of the LV. Modified from Jackson JM, Thomas SJ, Lowenstein E. Anesthetic management of patients with valvular heart disease. Semin Anesth. 1982;1:240

Timing for Intervention

Acute AR is always an emergency and requires prompt surgical intervention. For chronic AR, surgical intervention is recommended in symptomatic patients with severe AR, regardless of LV systolic function. In asymptomatic patients with severe AR and LV systolic function (EF < 50%) should also undergo AVR. The asymptomatic patient with normal LV function should be closely followed clinically and with echocardiography. Surgical intervention is indicated with any sign of LV dysfunction and/or evidence of ventricular dilatation (LVEDD > 65 mm; LVESD > 50 mm). AR classification is summarized in Table 12.

Anesthetic Considerations

Patients with AR may differ widely in their degree of myocardial dysfunction and anesthetic management must be individualized. The general hemodynamic goals are a mild tachycardia, a positive inotropic state, and a controlled reduction in SVR. For the patient with acute AR, the goals are the same but in an "emergency setting" and thus, interventions should be prompt and aggressive. Anesthetic considerations and hemodynamic goals for AR are summarized in Tables 13 and 14 respectively.

Table 12 Aortic regurgitation classification

Stage (clinical)	Definition	
A	At risk of AR	
B	Progressive AR	
C	Asymptomatic severe AR	
	C1	Normal LVEF ($\geq$ 50%) and mild-to-moderate LV dilation (LVESD $\geq$ 50 mm)
	C2	Abnormal LVEF (< 50%) or severe LV dilatation (LVESD > 50 mm or indexed LVESD > 25 mm/m^2)
D	Symptomatic severe AR	

AR: aortic regurgitation, LVEF: left ventricle ejection fraction, LVESD: left ventricle end systolic diameter. Modified from Nishimura et al. *J Am Coll Cardiol*. 2014;63(22):2438–2488

Table 13 Anesthetic considerations in AR

• Light pre-medication is recommended, hemodynamic instability is less frequent during induction since most of the drugs will decrease in some degree the afterload, careful titration must be taken specially in the acute AR setting, since hemodynamic collapse is more likely to happen. • Patients with chronic AR are at risk for acute ischemia with bradycardia since it prolongs diastolic time, increases regurgitant flow, LV diastolic pressure and wall tension. • The CPP is decreased and myocardial perfusion pressure may be insufficient. All this can lead to rapid onset of heart failure and collapse. Inotropes and vasodilators should be promptly used to keep SV and CPP adequate. Pacing might also be considered to increase heart rate to above 70. • Additional to standard monitoring, five-lead ECG system with V5, large bore peripheral venous access, invasive arterial lineon pre-induction and central line are recommended.	• Pulmonary artery catheter (PAC) provides useful information since allows determination filling pressures, cardiac output and response to pharmacologic interventions. In acute AR, PCWP might underestimate LV filling pressures due to premature closing of the mitral valve caused by the regurgitant jet. • TEE is very helpful since it allows for assessment of the AR severity, LV function, preload and response to inotrope/vasodilator therapy both during pre and post- bypass period. It is also critical to assess adequacy of surgical repair and the presence of valvular leaks and/or gradients after replacement of the valve. • Immediately after surgery there is a decrease in LVEDP and LVEDV but there might be a decline in LV function since the eccentric hypertrophy and LV dilatation takes time to improve. Inotropic or intra-aortic balloon pump support might be needed, especially in cases where surgery was not performed early enough.

Table 14 AR hemodynamic goals

Preload	Increased
Contractility	Maintain
Afterload	Decreased
Rhythm/Rate	Sinus rhythm, 70–90 bpm
Avoid	Bradycardia

Mitral Stenosis

History and Clinical Features

Clinically significant mitral stenosis (MS), more common in women than in men (2:1), can be acquired or congenital. Rheumatic disease accounts for up 10% of cases in Europe, being responsible for 99% of all MS surgeries. Congenital MS is a rare cause occurring in younger patients. Without surgery, 20% of all patients are likely to die within 1 year, and 50% die at 10 years of diagnosis.

The normal mitral valve area (MVA) is 4.0 to 6.0 cm^2 and valve index of 4 to 4.5 cm^2/m^2. Symptoms manifest with progressive decreases in valve area, of about

0.1 cm^2 annually. Usually asymptomatic until the valve area reaches 2.5 cm^2 or less. When it goes between 1.5 to 2.5 cm^2, symptoms occur in association with exercise or hyperdynamic states (fever, pregnancy, or tachyarrhythmias). When it becomes 1.5 cm^2 or less, symptoms develop at rest. Dyspnea is usually the first symptom that reflects elevated left atrial (LA) pressure, pulmonary congestion and elevation in pulmonary artery pressures, predisposing to atrial fibrillation, with thromboembolism in 10% to 20% of the cases. Chest pain can also be present in around 10% of patients but does not predict CAD and is more related to right ventricle (RV) enlargement. Severe pulmonary hypertension is a marker of prognosis of MS and is associated with a mean survival of < 3 years. The smallest MVA compatible with life is 0.3 to 0.4 cm^2.

Pathophysiology

The characteristic of MS is a reduced left ventricle end diastolic volume (LVEDV) and pressure (LVEDP) secondary to a restricted flow from the LA to the LV. This restriction reduces the LV filling and decreases the stroke volume. Contractility may also decrease due to LV deconditioning resulting in diminished LV preload reserve. Other mechanism to explain why low contractility persists even after surgery, might be secondary to rheumatic myocarditis, but the true contribution to the LV impairment is uncertain. The contribution of atrial kick to stroke volume might be as high as 30%. The physiology of MS is summarized in Fig. 9.

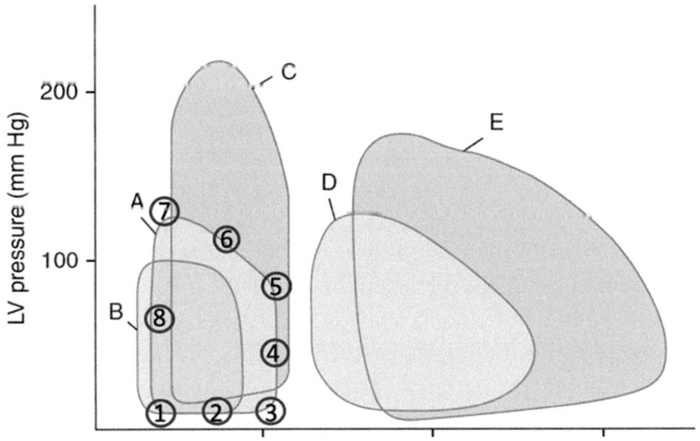

Fig. 9 Pressure volume loop of a normal LV (A) and Mitral stenosis (B). In mitral stenosis the loop is displaced to the left, LVEDV and LVEDP are reduced with decline in SV. LVEDP: left ventricle end diastolic pressure. LVEDV: left ventricle end diastolic volume (LVEDV). Modified from Jackson JM, Thomas SJ, Lowenstein E. Anesthetic management of patients with valvular heart disease. Semin Anesth. 1982;1:240

Timing for Intervention

Early surgery intervention is recommended for symptomatic patients with severe MS. Patients with asymptomatic severe MS and mild to moderate MS should be followed with echocardiography. Hemodynamic severity is best characterized by mitral valve area by planimetry and by pressure half-time. The definition of "severe" MS is based on the severity at which symptoms occur as well as the severity at which intervention will improve symptoms. Thus, a mitral valve area 1.5 cm^2 is considered severe. Usually this means a mean gradient of >5 mm Hg to 10 mm Hg but is highly dependent of loading conditions and heart rate. Once systolic pulmonary artery pressure (sPAP) gets more than 30 mm Hg, surgical intervention will likely be needed.

Anesthetic Considerations

The main goal in severe MS is to prevent and treat promptly tachycardia, keep preload normal without exacerbation of pulmonary vascular congestion and avoid factors that might aggravate pulmonary hypertension and impair RV function. During the postoperative period there is an improve in cardiac output with a dramatic decrease in PA and LA pressures and a significant reduction in PVR. If sPAP do not decrease, is a sign of poor prognosis due to irreversible pulmonary hypertension and/or irreversible LV dysfunction. The anesthetic considerations and hemodynamic goals of MS are summarized in Tables 15 and 16.

Mitral Regurgitation

History and Clinical Features

Mitral regurgitation (MR) can present in acute and chronic forms. Acute MR is an emergency presenting with severe symptoms of heart failure usually secondary to papillary muscle dysfunction due to myocardial ischemia or rupture of the papillary muscle as a complication of infarct or trauma. This can also occur secondary to myxomatous disease of the mitral valve or acute rheumatic fever. The leaflet can acutely deteriorate as a result of infective endocarditis, balloon valvuloplasty and trauma. In Chronic MR, there is a slow progression of symptoms and deterioration of LV function. This can result secondary to mitral valve leaflet abnormalities, mitral annulus dilation, chordae rupture, papillary muscle disorder, global LV dysfunction, or disproportionate LV dilatation.

MR can be classified as organic or functional. Organic MR is due to distortion, disruption, or destruction of the mitral leaflets or mitral apparatus, being the most

Table 15 Anesthetic considerations in MS

• Premedication for anxiety to prevent tachycardia is recommended. Small doses of narcotics or benzodiazepines can be used but carefully titrated, since excessive sedation can produce hypoventilation with hypercarbia, hypoxemia and aggravate pulmonary hypertension. They can also decrease left ventricle (LV) preload limiting stroke volume (SV). • Heart rate control should be continued in the perioperative period. The use of β-blockers and calcium-receptor antagonists may be required to control the ventricular rate in patients with atrial fibrillation (AF), which is the primary goal in managing these patients. Cardioversion should be use if the patient becomes hemodynamically unstable. • Additional to standard monitoring, five-lead ECG system with V5, large bore peripheral venous access, invasivearterial line on pre-induction and central line are recommended. Pulmonary Artery Catheter (PAC) can be of use to monitor cardiac output and pulmonary artery pressures (PAP), but the wedge pressure (PCWP) will overestimate the left ventricle end diastolic pressure (LVEDP).	• Careful must be taken when floating the PAC in patients with severe pulmonary hypertension (PHT) since there is a risk of pulmonary dissection. • TEE is the ideal modality used to monitor volume status intraoperatively and is preferred over more invasive techniques such as pulmonary artery catheters. • Anesthetic technique should aim to avoid increases in pulmonary vascular resistances (PVR) to prevent additional RV dysfunction. It is important to avoid hypoxia, hypercarbia, acidosis and hypothermia. Vasodilators are not useful to reduce PVR and might limit LV filling.

Table 16 MS hemodynamic goals

Preload	Normal or increased
Contractility	Normal
Afterload	Normal
Rhythm/Rate	Sinus rhythm, 50–60 bpm
Avoid	Tachycardia, increase in pulmonary vascular resistance (PVR)

common cause of MR in Western countries. Functional MR occurs in the setting of normal leaflets and chordal structures. Most likely this is the result of global LV dysfunction with disruption of the normal geometric relationship of the mitral valve leaflets, papillary muscles, and LV. MR has been traditionally classified based on the mitral valve motion as per the Carpentier's classification, summarized in Table 17. There prognosis of MR with 5-year survival rates goes from 27 to 97%.

Table 17 Mitral regurgitation Carpentier classification

Types	I	II	IIIa	IIIb
Mitral valve motion	Normal	Excessive	Restricted during diastole/systole	Restricted during systole
Frequent causes	Annulus dilatation Leaflet perforation Cleft	Prolapse flail	Rheumatic	Functional ischemic

Pathophysiology

- **Acute MR**
  Acute MR often presents as biventricular failure with rapid rises in LA and PAP that lead to pulmonary congestion, pulmonary edema, and RV failure. As heart rate increases to compensate the cardiac output, the LV volume and end-diastolic pressure starts rising causing ischemia and more LV dysfunction that leads to collapse development of atrial fibrillation.
- **Chronic MR**
  As a compensatory mechanism of progressive volume overload, eccentric hypertrophy is developed. This keeps LVEDP low despite increased volume and preserves cardiac output by increasing the stroke volume (SV). Once this mechanism can no longer meet the necessary SV to maintain cardiac output, symptoms of CHF appear. LA dilatation occurs secondary to LV dilatation, this also causes widening of the mitral annulus that worsens regurgitation and increases pulmonary congestions, and thus elevated PAPs and ultimately RV dysfunction. There is also high risk of development of atrial fibrillation. The difference in MR physiology between acute and chronic are represented in Fig. 10.

Timing for Intervention

Repair of the valve is the recommended surgical intervention for MR instead of valve replacement whenever is suitable. Repair of the valve avoids chronic anti-coagulation and LV function is better preserved. Symptomatic patients with CHF symptoms and/or chronic or recurrent atrial fibrillation resulting from MR, surgical intervention is strongly endorsed. In asymptomatic patients, the decision to wait or go ahead for surgery depends on the presence of LV enlargement, dysfunction, and pulmonary hypertension, with the onset of LV dysfunction being the most

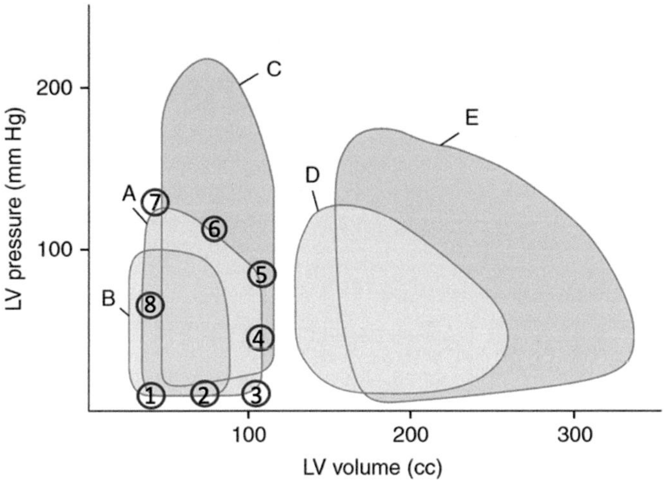

Fig. 10 Pressure volume loop of normal LV (**a**), acute MR (**d**) and chronic MR (**e**). There is a rightward shift in both acute and chronic MR. In acute MR, maintaining the stroke volume requires dilation of the LA. This is accomplished by an increase in the Left ventricle end diastolic pressure (LVEDP). In contrast, in chronic MR, the LVEDP remains normal until the MR has progressed to a severe stage. Modified from Jackson JM, Thomas SJ, Lowenstein E. Anesthetic management of patients with valvular heart disease. Semin Anesth. 1982;1:240

important indicator for surgery. If coronary artery by-pass graft (CABG) is indicated and at least moderate ischemic MR is present, mitral valve repair/replacement at the same time as CABG is recommended. Classification of mitral regurgitation based on echocardiography as per the ASE is summarized in Table 18.

Table 18 Echocardiographic assessment of MR

Grade	Mild-moderate-severe
Morphology	None-mild to severe valve lesions (Flail)
Left atrium/Left ventricle size	Normal to dilated
Left atrium color flow Jet area	Small to large (> 50% or wall-impinging)
PISA	Small to large
Vena contracta (cm)	< 0.3 to ≥ 0.7
Pulmonary vein flow	Systolic dominance to systolic flow reversal
Mitral inflow	A-wave to E-wave dominant (> 1.2 m/s)
EROA (cm^2)	< 0.2 to ≥ 0.4
Regurgitant volume (ml)	< 30 to ≥ 60
Regurgitant fraction (%)	< 30 to ≥ 50
Velocity time integral (VTI) Mitral valve / VTI LVOT	ratio > 1,4

EROA: Effective Regurgitant Orifice Area. Modified Zoghbi et al. *J Am Soc Echocardiogr.* 2017;30(4):303–371

Table 19 Anesthetic considerations in MR

• Special efforts must be done to optimize RV function, by avoiding increases in pulmonary vascular congestion and pulmonary hypertension. • Additional to standard monitoring, five-lead ECG system with V5, large bore peripheral venous access, invasive arterial lineon pre-induction and central line are recommended. • PA catheters helps to optimize left-sided filling pressures following trends of variables to provide adequate preload avoiding fluid overload. Can also be used to assess the response of inotropes with the determination of cardiac output and mixed venous oxygen saturation. Monitoring trends of CVP to assess RV might also be helpful. • Reversible pulmonary hypertension adequately responds to both nitric oxide as well as hyperventilation. Alternatives include inhaled milrinone and prostaglandin E1.	• Intraoperative TEE is the most valuable tool to assess the adequacy of valvular repair and allows to rule out paravalvular leaks or significant residual regurgitation and the presence of SAM or transvalvular gradient. Successfully repaired mitral valves when should have no more than mild MR immediately after CPB. 3DTEE increases the accuracy of quantitative evaluations and gives evidence for long-term durability of the valve providing information of structural integrity. • TEE can identify the cause of hemodynamic derangements, facilitating proper intervention and response to therapies. It is a reliable tool to assess preload and RV/LV performance. • Some very useful methods to estimate LV contractility in MR by Doppler are dP/dT estimation and LV myocardial performance index (MPI or Tei Index) • If a maze procedure was performed for AF, prophylaxis with amiodarone can be used aiming to keep sinus rhythm.

Anesthetic Considerations

In acute MR, the patient might be in cardiogenic shock and emergency surgery is required or can have preserved LV function depending on the underlying cause of MR. For both situations and in the chronic setting, the same hemodynamic goals apply. Maintaining a heart rate of 90 beats/min, preserving ventricular contractility and avoid increases in systemic vascular resistance. Postoperatively, LV function is compromised more severely after mitral valve replacements due to resection of the subvalvular apparatus. They usually require inotropic support compared to mitral valve repairs. The anesthetic considerations and hemodynamic goals on the management of MR are summarized in Tables 19 and 20.

Table 20 MR hemodynamic goals

Preload	Normal or increased
Contractility	Normal
Afterload	Decreased
Rhythm/Rate	Sinus rhythm, 70–90 bpm
Avoid	Myocardial depression, Increase in pulmonary vascular resistance (PVR)

Recommended Readings

1. Cook DJ, Housmans PR, Rehfeldt KH. Valvular heart disease: replacement and repair. In: Kaplan JA, Reich DL, Savino JS, editors. Kaplan's cardiac anesthesia: the echo Era, vol 2011. 7th ed. Elsevier; 2017. pp. 570–614.
2. Nishimura RA, Otto CM, Bonow RO, et al. 2017 AHA/ACC focused update of the 2014 AHA/ACC guideline for the management of patients with valvular heart disease: a report of the American college of cardiology/American heart association task force on clinical practice guidelines. Circulation. 2017;135:e1159–95.
3. Baumgartner H, Hung J, Bermejo J, et al. Recommendations on the echocardiographic assessment of aortic valve stenosis: a focused update from the european association of cardiovascular imaging and the american society of echocardiography. J Am Soc Echocardiogr. 2017;30:372–92.
4. Mack MJ, Leon MB, Thourani VH, et al. Transcatheter aortic-valve replacement with a balloon-expandable valve in low-risk patients. N Engl J Med. 2019;380:1695–705.
5. Popma JJ, Deeb GM, Yakubov SJ, et al. Transcatheter aortic-valve replacement with a self-expanding valve in low-risk patients. N Engl J Med. 2019;380:1706–15.
6. Nagueh SF, Bierig SM, Budoff MJ, et al. American society of echocardiography clinical recommendations for multimodality cardiovascular imaging of patients with hypertrophic cardiomyopathy: endorsed by the american society of nuclear cardiology, society for cardiovascular magnetic resonance, and society of cardiovascular computed tomography. J Am Soc Echocardiogr. 2011;24:473–98.
7. Baumgartner H, Falk V, Bax JJ, et al. 2017 ESC/EACTS Guidelines for the management of valvular heart disease. Eur Heart J. 2017;38:2739–91.
8. Zoghbi WA, Adams D, Bonow RO, et al. Recommendations for noninvasive evaluation of native valvular regurgitation: a report from the American society of echocardiography developed in collaboration with the society for cardiovascular magnetic resonance. J Am Soc Echocardiogr. 2017;30:303–71.
9. Sanfilippo F, Johnson C, Bellavia D, et al. Mitral regurgitation grading in the operating room: a systematic review and meta-analysis comparing preoperative and intraoperative assessments during cardiac surgery. J Cardiothorac Vasc Anesth. 2017;31:1681–91.

Anaesthesia for Surgery of the Thoracoabdominal Aorta

Carlos Corredor and Anne Campbell

Aneurysms involving the descending thoracic and abdominal aorta are referred to as thoracoabdominal aneurysms (TAAAs). The widely accepted definition of TAAAs is a dilatation of at least 50% the expected size of the aorta at the diaphragmatic hiatus. TAAAs are relatively rare and account for only 3% of all aortic aneurysms. The natural history of TAAAs left untreated is continuous expansion with high probability of rupture and death. Patients managed conservatively have a 5-year survival rate of less than 20%.

Aneurysmal dilatation of the aorta occurs commonly as a result of degeneration of the medial layer due to loss of smooth muscle cells and elastin fibres. Dilatation can also develop following an aortic dissection when the intima tears and the aortic wall weakens.

Congenital collagen vascular diseases such as Marfan's and Loeys-Dietz Syndromes are commonly associated with TAAAs. Acquired degeneration of the wall of the aorta occurs as a result of hypertension and atherosclerosis.

The Crawford classification scheme provides a standard framework for surgical planning in TAAAs procedures and facilitates standardized reporting of outcomes. The Crawford classification divides TAAAs aneurysm repairs according to the extent of aorta that needs replacing (Fig. 1).

- Extent I: From origin of left subclavian artery to above the renal arteries origin
- Extent II: From origin of left subclavian artery to aortic bifurcation distally
- Extent III: Replacement of distal half of the descending aorta. From mid descending aorta to aortic bifurcation
- Extent IV: From the diaphragmatic hiatus involving the abdominal aorta.

C. Corredor (✉) · A. Campbell
Department of Perioperative Medicine, St Bartholomew's Hospital, Barts Health NHS Trust, London, UK
e-mail: carlos.corredorrosero@nhs.net

A. Campbell
e-mail: anne.campbell16@nhs.net

M. Vives and A. Hernandez (eds.), *Cardiac Anesthesia and Postoperative Care in the 21st Century*, https://doi.org/10.1007/978-3-030-79721-8_17

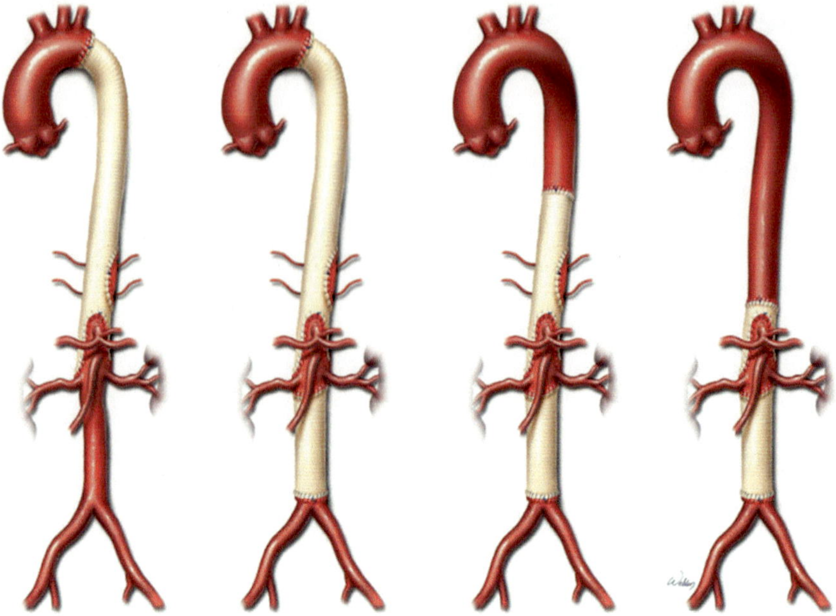

Fig. 1 The Crawford classification scheme for thoraco-abdominal aortic aneurysm repairs

Aortic dissections are classified using the classic Stanford or Debakey classifications covered elsewhere in this book.

Aneurysms of the descending thoracic aorta tend to display exponential growth with a rate of 0.12 cm per year when they exceed a diameter of >5.2 cm. A diameter of 7.0 cm is regarded a critical for risk of rupture in descending aorta aneurysm. When managed conservatively, the survival rate is only 10–20% at 5 years. Indications for surgery include rupture, acute dissection, pain arising from the aneurysm or symptoms related to compression of adjacent structures, enlargement of ≥ 1 cm per year, or absolute size >6.5 cm or >6 cm in patients with connective tissue disorders.

Open surgical repair of TAAAs are lifesaving procedures but are associated with significant perioperative morbidity and mortality. Morbidity such as spinal cord injury, stroke and renal failure requiring dialysis can have a significant impact on long term survival and quality of life for patients. Initial high rates of morbidity and mortality have been significantly reduced by highly specialised multidisciplinary perioperative teams and management strategies that have evolved over the years.

Preoperative Assessment

The pre-anaesthetic assessment evaluates patient specific and surgical procedure related factors that influence the perioperative plan and the conduct of anaesthesia.

Patients presenting for TAAA aneurysm repair often have multiple co-morbidities common to patients with cardiovascular disease that can affect their tolerance to withstanding major aortovascular surgery.

Assessment of cardiovascular fitness includes screening with coronary artery disease with CT coronary angiogram or traditional angiography in patients with risk factors for coronary artery disease. Echocardiography evaluates the function of both ventricles and screens for valvular abnormalities that may affect the conduct of left heart bypass such as aortic insufficiency.

Lung function tests such as dynamic spirometry and transfer factor evaluate tolerance for prolonged one lung ventilation. We believe that functional tests such as the six-minute walk test provide a better indication of cardiovascular reserve and tolerance. Patients with borderline respiratory function are counselled about the possibility of postoperative pulmonary complications and the risk prolonged respiratory wean in the ICU.

Lung isolation with double lumen tubes (DLT) can be challenging as large aneurysms can compress the lower airway with significant deviation of the trachea. This issue can be identified and planed for with careful evaluation of the preoperative CT scan of the Thorax.

Pre-existing renal dysfunction with reduced eGFR is a risk factor for requiring postoperative dialysis in patients undergoing major aortovascular surgery. Preoperative hydration is crucial, and patients are encouraged to drink clear fluids up to 2 hours before surgery.

Anaemia is associated with increased bleeding and transfusion requirements. Whenever possible patients with anaemia (Hb <130 g/l) are screened for true or functional iron deficiency anaemia and optimised with oral or intravenous iron pre-operatively.

The surgical approach or timing may need to be modified according to the patient functional status and comorbidities. For instance, a patient with very limited respiratory reserve may be assessed for suitability of an endovascular approach rather than an open repair.

Surgical Approach and Positioning

Surgical access for TAAA aneurysm repair is usually obtained through a left thoraco-phreno-laparotomy. The patient is positioned in a left semi lateral position with the use of a deflatable vacuum bag. The right side of the torso is placed in a 60° lateral position with the hip and legs in a semi supine position at 30°.

The thoracotomy incision starts below the scapulae laterally and extends medially in to the abdomen often below the umbilicus.

Aortic clamping sites and sequence will depend on the anatomy and extent of the aneurysm. Partial left heart bypass (PLHB) is desirable in terms of bleeding, coagulopathy and inflammatory response when compared with full cardiopulmonary bypass (CPB). However, PLHB requires a safe clamping area to be present at or beyond the level of the left subclavian artery otherwise full CPB is required. Aneurysms involving the distal aortic arch often require a two-stage approach consisting of an elephant trunk procedure first followed by a replacement of the thoracic descending aorta at a different time.

Physiology of Cross Clamping and Left Heart Bypass

The descending thoracic aorta is cross clamped at different stages of the procedure. Sequential cross-clamping helps to protect the spinal cord. Cross-clamping causes marked physiological changes involving different organ and body systems. It is essential for the anaesthesiologist to recognise and pre-empt the effects of cross clamping. The physiological effects of cross clamping are summarized in Table 1.

Left heart bypass is used to ameliorate the changes in cardiac afterload caused by proximal aortic cross-clamping. Left heart bypass also provides distal perfusion, reduces lower body ischaemia–reperfusion injury and decreases the occurrence of spinal cord injury. A common site of cannulation is the left inferior pulmonary vein (LIPV) that drains oxygenated blood from the left atrium. Blood is then reinfused

Table 1 Physiological effects of aortic cross-clamping. MAP, Mean Arterial Pressure; MPAP, Mean Pulmonary Artery Pressure; PVR, Pulmonary Vascular Resistance; CSF, Cerebrospinal fluid; SCPP, Spinal Cord Perfusion Pressure

System	Effects
Cardiovascular	• Increased afterload and MAP • Decrease in Cardiac Output • Increased myocardial oxygen consumption • Supracoeliac clamping increases preload proximal to clamp • Infracoeliac clamping causes changes in preload depending on the splanchnic vascular tone
Respiratory	• Increase in MPAP and PVR • Increase in pulmonary blood flow with supracoeliac clamping
Gastrointestinal	• Ischaemia–reperfusion insult • Bacterial translocation • Release of pro-inflammatory cytokines TN, IL-6, IL-8 and IL-10
Renal	• Decrease in renal blood flow. Suprarenal > infrarenal cross clamp • Increase in renal vascular resistance
Spinal Cord	• Increase in CSF pressure proximal to clamp • Decrease in SCPP distal to clamp

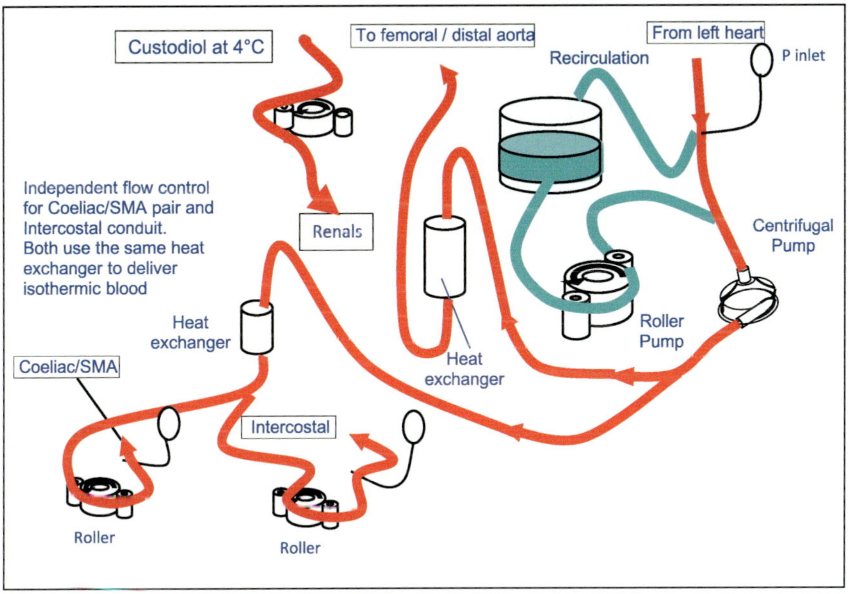

Fig. 2 Left Heart bypass circuit diagram. Drainage from left inferior pulmonary vein and reinfusion by centrifugal pump into the distal aorta/left femoral artery. Balloon-tipped perfusion catheters (10 and 13F) are used for selective perfusion of visceral vessels and the kidneys. A recirculation reservoir (Blue) is used in the rapid transfusion device. SMA, Superior mesenteric artery. (Diagram courtesy of Professor Aung Oo and the Aortovascular Team at St Bartholomew's hospital, London)

using a centrifugal pump into the distal aorta or left femoral artery. LHB circuits typically do not require an oxygenator, therefore only moderate heparinization is required (1 mg/kg) with an ACT target of 250–300 s. Temperature is allowed to drift to 32–34 °C. Mean distal perfusion pressure (MAP) is maintained at 60 mmHg or above with flows usually oscillating between 1.5–2.5 l/min. MAP above the proximal aortic cross clamp needs to be carefully controlled and maintained at 80–90 mmHg. Excessive proximal hypertension increases cardiac afterload and may also result in proximal aortic dissection. On the other hand, excessively low proximal aortic pressures can impair coronary perfusion, lead to spinal cord injury and other organ injury. Balloon-tipped perfusion catheters are used for selective perfusion of visceral vessels using roller pumps from the bypass machine. Isothermic blood is used for visceral vessels and intercostal conduits and Custodiol solution at 4 °C is used for renal perfusion Fig. 2.

Initiation of LHB requires careful coordination and communication between the surgeon, anaesthetist and perfusionist. Proximal hypertension caused by the initial proximal clamp can be mitigated by prompt initiation of LHB. As blood is drained from the LIPV, left ventricle preload is reduced, and proximal aortic pressure reduced. An increase in distal aortic pressure and flow is associated with a decrease in left ventricle preload and proximal aortic pressure.

Once the aorta is opened there can be significant retrograde bleeding from aortic branches. Cell salvage and a rapid infusion devices (Belmont Medical Technologies) capable of fast rates of infusion (up 750–1000 ml/min) are required to return circulation volume to the patient and maintain adequate preload for both the proximal aorta supplied by the left ventricle and the distal aorta supplied by the pump of the LHB machine. Very fast blood loss is returned directly to the Belmont device with slower blood loss being processed through the cell saver devices. Surges in proximal blood pressure may require the use of short acting vasodilatory agents such as glyceryl trinitrate.

Cross clamps need to be repositioned at different stages of the operation which again requires close communication between surgeon, anaesthetists and perfusionists. Removal of the cross clamp can cause precipitous drops in proximal aortic pressure due to the sudden loss of afterload. The fall in pressure can be reduced by gradual release of the cross clamp and use of short acting vasopressor agents may be required i.e. metaraminol or phenylephrine.

Protection of Right Ventricular function is essential during left heart bypass to ensure adequate LV preload. Therefore, situations that cause elevation of pulmonary vascular resistance such as hypoxia or hypercarbia should be avoided. Bradycardia can be problematic as it can interfere with the performance of the right ventricle when faced with rapid infusion of fluids. We use a low dose adrenaline infusion (0.01–0.05 mcg/kg/min) to aid right ventricular performance.

A citrate-dextrose solution (ACD) is used by the cell saver as an anticoagulant exerting its effect by chelating calcium. Therefore, ionised calcium needs to be frequently monitored in arterial blood gas analysis and supplemented during left heart bypass otherwise life-threatening hypocalcaemia may ensue.

LHB is only possible if a safe proximal clamping site distal to the left subclavian artery is identified. Aneurysm involving the aortic arch can preclude safe proximal aortic clamping and surgery needs to be performed using full CPB and Deep Hypothermic Arrest (DHCA) which is associated with significantly higher blood loss and coagulopathy.

Spinal Cord Protection and Neuromonitoring

The spinal cord blood supply depends on an anterior spinal artery that irrigates the motor areas of the spinal cord and originates in the vertebral arteries, and two posterior spinal arteries that originate from the subclavian artery and supply sensory areas of the spinal cord. The anterior spinal artery is crucially supplemented by segmental arteries in the thoracic and lumbar aorta. The artery of Adamkiewicz is a large intercostal artery in the lower thoracic aorta and is a major tributary of the anterior spinal artery. However, recent understanding of the anatomy and physiology of spinal cord supply points to a complex network of segmental intercostal and lumbar arteries rather than a single artery, as responsible for maintaining spinal cord perfusion. These intercostal and lumbar arteries are interconnected both longitudinally and transversely with arterial networks consisting of the anterior spinal artery, epidural arcades, paraspinous muscles and tissues.

Spinal cord deficit (SCD) is a feared complication of open TAAA repairs. Extent II repairs carry the highest risk of SCD with large case series reporting an incidence of 13.6% with 7.7% of the cases being permanent paraplegia.

Spinal cord perfusion is the product of the mean arterial blood pressure (MAP) minus the cerebrospinal fluid pressure (CSFP).

$$SCPP = MAP - CSFP$$

Aortic cross clamping results in reduced arterial blood flow and marked increase in central venous pressure that in turn causes spinal cord oedema and increase in CSFP. If the drop in SCPP is prolonged enough, irreversible damage to neuronal bodies and spinal nerve tracts will occur. Postoperatively, Spinal Cord Injury occurs due to a permanent reduction of blood supply when critical segmental arteries are interrupted by the surgical repair.

Risk factors for spinal cord injury include total extent of the repair with Extent II carrying the highest risk, previous infrarenal aortic repair, compromised left subclavian or internal iliac patency, aortic dissection with visceral malperfusion, emergency repair, prolonged duration of aortic cross clamping, renal disease, type II DM and age > 60 years.

Strategies to prevent Spinal Cord Injury can be divided into pre-operative, Intraoperative and Postoperative Table 2.

Table 2 Perioperative strategies for spinal cord protection in open TAAA repair. CSF, cerebrospinal fluid; MAP, Mean Arterial Pressure; MEP, Motor Evoked Potentials; NIRS, Near Infrared Spectroscopy

Preoperative	• Staged approach to repair if possible, combined endovascular repairs • Segmental artery staged coil embolization
Intraoperative	• CSF drainage pressure <10 mmHg. Max 20 ml/h • MAP >85/90 mmHg SBP >130 mmHg • Hb >100 g/dl • Hypothermia 32–34C • MEP monitoring • Paraspinal NIRS
Postoperative	• CSF pressure <10 mmHg. Max 20 ml/h • MAP >85/90 mmHg SBP >130 mmHg • Early sedation hold and hourly neurological assessment • Hb >100 g/dl

CSF Drainage

CSF drainage and maintenance of CSFP significantly reduces the incidence of paraplegia, especially in the higher risk procedures such as Extent I, II and III repairs. We do not routinely insert CSF drainage for Extent IV repairs. In our institution the drain is inserted following induction of anaesthesia using a midline approach. The patient is placed in a lateral decubitus position with the legs flexed towards the head. The L3–L4 and L4–L5 spaces are the most commonly used to avoid the risk of direct spinal cord injury with higher insertion levels. We use an Integra LifeSciences (Princeton, NJ) lumbar drainage kit containing a Tuohy needle and an 80 cm 5Fr catheter with guidewire. The guidewire is lubricated with saline and pre-loaded into the catheter before insertion. The Tuohy needle is inserted with the bevel facing cephalad and with a 20 degree cephalad angulation. Once free flow of CSF is identified the catheter is inserted to a depth of 8–10 cm past the tip of the Touhy needle. A bloody tap, that does not clear, may lead to postponement of the procedure as there is a risk of intrathecal bleeding or haematoma with heparinisation. Following insertion, the spinal drain is attached to an automated pressure monitoring and drainage system (LiquoGuard; Möller Medical, Fulda, Germany). The LiquoGuard system is capable of volume- or pressure-controlled drainage. We set the system to drain if pressure exceeds 10 mmHg with a maximum drainage of 20 ml/h as excessive drainage may lead to a subdural bleed. Complications of spinal drainage include epidural/subdural haematoma, persistent CSF leak and low CSF pressure headache, subarachnoid haemorrhage, meningitis and puncture site bleeding Fig. 3.

Neurological Monitoring

The integrity of the corticospinal motor pathways can be monitored using motor evoked potentials (MEPs). Measurement of MEPs provides a reliable measure of spinal cord function and can guide interventions to improve spinal cord perfusion such as reimplantation of segmental arteries or augmentation of SCPP. MEP monitoring requires expert staff trained in neurophysiological monitoring and institutional experience. The anaesthesia technique needs to be modified as neuromuscular blockade and inhalational agents affect the amplitude of the MEP signals.

The blood supply to the paraspinous muscles correlates closely with that of the corresponding level of the spinal cord as they are part of a collateral network. This association is utilized by NIRS monitoring of the oxygen saturation in the paraspinal muscles that serve as real-time non-invasive monitoring of spinal cord perfusion. Evidence from small pilot studies suggest that changes in paraspinal NIRS correlates well with MEPs in detecting spinal cord ischaemia.

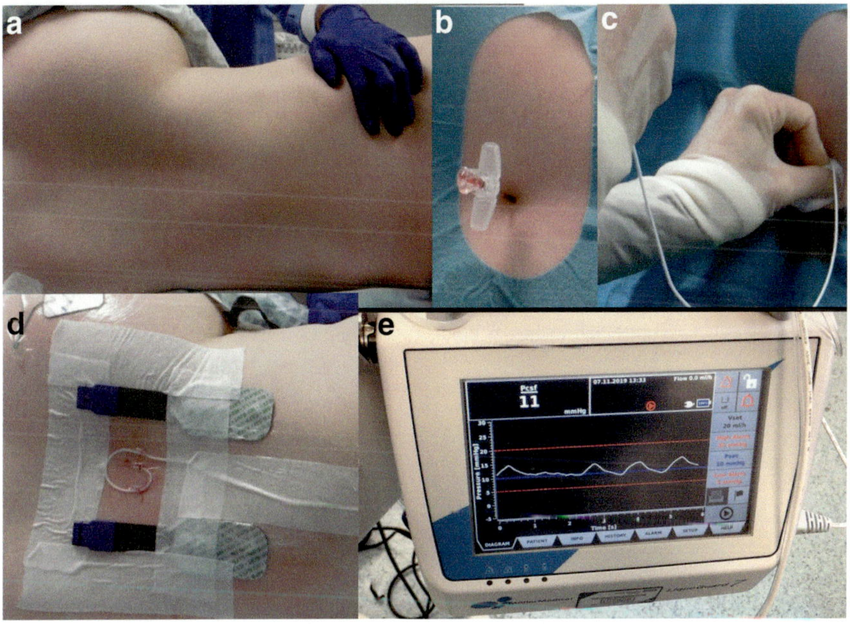

Fig. 3 Insertion of spinal drain catheter for (CSF) drainage. A, Patient is positioned in the right lateral decubitus position with hips and knees flexed. B, L3–L4 or L4–L5 space punctured with a 14 g Tuohy needle and free flowing CSF obtained. C, A 5f silicone lumbar catheter Is inserted into the subarachnoid space. D, Catheter is secured with sutures and adhesive dressings. Near Infrared Spectroscopy (NIRS) sensors are placed at the paraspinal level. E, Drain is connected to automated drainage device (LiquoGuard; Möller Medical, Fulda, Germany) and the system set to drain when pressure exceeds 10 mmHg with a maximum drainage of 20 ml/h. Courtesy of Professor Aung Oo and the Aortovascular Team, St Barthlomew's Hospital, London

Conduct of Anaesthesia

The anaesthesia technique for open TAAA repairs includes very particular considerations that are determined by the anatomical and physiological consequences of the TAAA, complex surgical aspects and the use of specialist neuromonitoring adjuncts. The use of MEP requires significant modification of the anaesthetic plan with avoidance of neuromuscular blockade and use of intravenous agents for maintenance of anaesthesia. The anaesthetist and neurophysiologist need to communicate closely to ensure that anaesthetic agents don't affect the MEP signals. Depth of anaesthesia monitoring is required to avoid deep planes of anaesthesia that may dampen MEP signals.

We administer methylprednisolone 10–15 mg/kg intravenously following induction of anaesthesia and prior to the initiation of left heart bypass. Evidence suggests that steroids lower risk of respiratory failure and reduce length of ICU and hospital stay in patients undergoing complex cardiac surgery.

Particulars of the anaesthesia techniques for TAAA are outlined in Table 3.

Table 3 Considerations for anaesthetic management of open thoracoabdominal aneurysm repair (TAAA). DLT, Double lumen tube; TIVA, Total intravenous anaesthesia; MEP, Motor Evoked Potentials; PAC; Pulmonary artery catheter; CSF, Cerebrospinal fluid; NIRS, Near Infrared Spectroscopy; TEE, Transesophageal echocardiogram; PEEP; Positive End Expiratory Pressure

Airway	• Lung isolation with DLT. Isolation can be challenging when the TAAA causes tracheal deviation or bronchial compression • Bronchoscopic guidance is essential to ensure adequacy of isolation • Exchange to single lumen tube at the end of procedure if safe to do so
Induction	• Avoid surges in blood pressure • Use intermediate acting Neuromuscular blockers i.e. Vecuronium, Rocuronium
Maintenance	• Avoid Neuromuscular blockers • TIVA based technique with Propofol 3–6 mg/kg/h or TCI 3–5 mcg/ml • Use of depth of anaesthesia monitor • Fentanyl 10–15 mcg/kg • Inhaled agents with a MAC not higher than 0.5 as it affect MEPs
Invasive lines	• Right radial artery catheter to monitor proximal aortic 'brain' perfusion pressure • Right Femoral artery catheter to monitor distal aortic pressure • Ultrasound guided insertion of lines as aneurysm can compress mediastinal structures affecting calibre of great veins • Left internal jugular 5 lm central line and 7 French PAC introducer sheath • Right Femoral Vein dialysis catheter (Vascath) attached to rapid infuser
Monitoring	• Nasopharyngeal and bladder temperature monitors • Cerebral and Paraspinal NIRS • TEE • PA catheter If > mild RV or LV dysfunction • MEP • CSF pressure monitoring. Maintain CSF <10 mmHg
Respiratory	• Lung protective ventilation VT <6 ml/kg, patient-specific PEEP • Frequent suctioning and protection of dependant lung (right) from soiling with blood from left lung • CPAP on non-ventilated lung may be required
Circulation	• Prepare infusion and bolus of vasodilator i.e. Glyceryl Trinitrate to lessen hypertensive response to cross clamping • Noradrenaline infusion may be necessary to augment MAP and SCPP • Low dose adrenaline infusion (0.01–0.05 mcg/kg/min) to support RV function and heart rate during LHB • Ionised calcium monitoring and replacement • Rapid infuser (Belmont) capable of high infusion rates (750 ml–1000/min)

Transesophageal Echocardiography

Transoesophageal echocardiography (TEE) is a crucial diagnostic and monitoring tool during open TAAA repairs. A comprehensive and systematic assessment of the thoracic aorta from the aortic root to the distal descending aorta is required using standard imaging planes. The dimensions of the aortic root (i.e. aortic valve

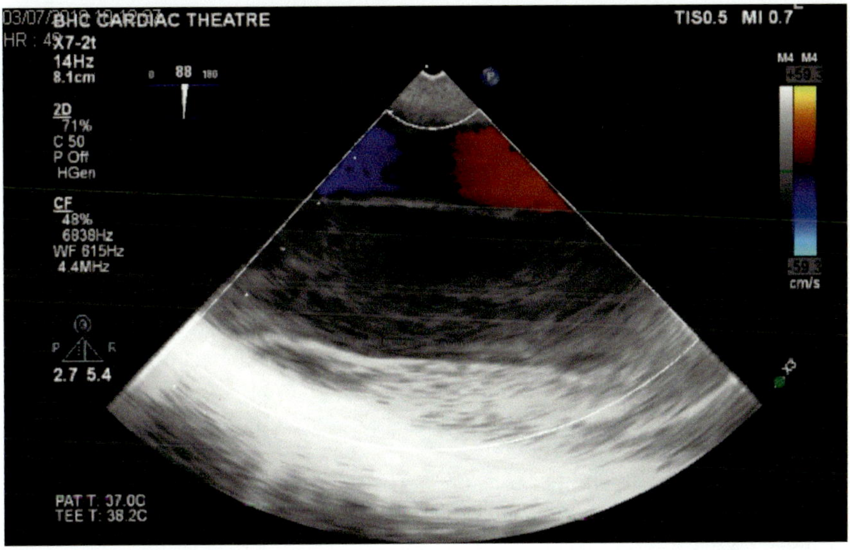

Fig. 4 Descending Thoracic Aorta TOE long axis view demonstrating an aortic aneurysm with chronic type B dissection. Colour doppler examination reveals flow in the smaller true lumen with a larger false lumen with 'smoke' due to stagnant flow

annulus, sinuses of Valsalva, sinotubular junction), ascending aorta, aortic arch and descending aorta should be recorded and taken in diastole from leading edge to leading edge. The maximum diameter and extension of aneurysmal dilatation should also be noted. In the case of dissections, efforts should be made to identify the origin and extension of dissection flap (Fig. 4). Identification of the true lumen is especially important and helps the surgeon to select a safe place for distal cannulation in the descending aorta or femoral artery for LHB. Intraoperative epi-aortic ultrasound can also be used to guide instrumentation of the descending aorta.

Aortic insufficiency should be ruled out and if present, quantified using international guidelines parameters. Anything other than mild aortic insufficiency may lead to left ventricular distension during aortic cross clamping. Ventricular distension can be prevented by initiation of left heart bypass prior to cross clamping and careful management of afterload with intravenous vasodilators. Key aspects of TEE evaluation of TAAA are outlined in Table 4.

Blood Conservation, Coagulation and Haemostasis

Open repair of TAAA causes significant blood loss, coagulopathy and transfusion requirements. Left heart bypass is preferable in terms of coagulopathy and blood loss as lower doses of heparin are required when compared with full cardiopulmonary bypass. However, extensive procedures in LHB can still lead to significant

Table 4 Key points for TEE imaging during open TAAA aneurysm repair. TAPSE, Tricuspid Annular Plane Systolic Excursion; FAC. Fractional Area Change; DTA, Descending Thoracic Aorta

• Right ventricular function: Quantification of Longitudinal (TAPSE) and radial (FAC) function
• Quantification of Left Ventricular function (EF)
• Assessment of volume status
• Aortic valve morphology and presence of regurgitation
• >mild aortic regurgitation
• Size of aortic root, ascending aorta, arch and DTA
• Dissection flaps and differentiation of true versus false lumen

derangements in coagulation homeostasis. The prolonged contact of blood with the extracorporeal circuit leads to activation of coagulation, excessive fibrinolysis, consumption of clotting factors and platelets. Depletion of fibrinogen and platelets can be especially problematic.

We use multiple blood conservation strategies and point of care monitoring to guide management of coagulopathy. The use of cell salvage is routine and essential for open TAAA repairs. We use at least two cell salvage devices.

The use of autologous platelet-rich plasma (PRP) is associated with reduced allogenic blood product utilization and decreased postoperative morbidity in major aortovascular surgery. Our practice is to collect approximately 15 ml/kg of whole blood in a normovolaemic manner following induction of anaesthesia by withdrawing blood from large bore IV access lines inserted for the procedure. The blood is then processed by an autologous transfusion system yielding PRP and red cells. The PRP is given to the patient following administration of Protamine.

Coagulation status is monitored using point of care thromboelastography (TEG 6S global coagulation cartridge, Haemonetics) allowing assessment of all determinants of coagulation. Excessive bleeding associated with coagulation defects may be treated with blood products such as FFP, Cryoprecipitates, platelets or factor concentrates. An algorithm is used to facilitate interpretation and guide therapy according to thromboelastography parameters. Factor concentrates such as prothrombin complex concentrate and fibrinogen may have some advantages when compared with blood products e.g. lower volume of administration, no requirement for thawing and more rapid correction of coagulation abnormalities.

Antifibrinolytics are routinely used with Aprotinin being commonly used in our centre. Tranexamic Acid and aminocaproic acid are also effective at reducing blood loss. The use of cell salvage is essential for blood conservation.

Pain Management

Patients encounter significant acute and chronic pain issues due to the extensive nature of the thoracolaparotomy incision. Gabapentinoids are administered as premedication on the morning of surgery (Pregabalin 150 mg) and continued postoperatively (Pregabalin 75 mg bd) until patients are reviewed in a clinic following discharge. Gabapentinoids have opiate sparing effects and reduce acute and chronic pain after cardiac surgery.

The ideal pain management strategy would facilitate adequate respiratory effort, good cough and secretion clearance with minimal sedation. Acute postoperative pain requires a multimodal analgesia approach with intrathecal diamorphine supplemented by fentanyl administered using a patient-controlled analgesia (PCA) device, dexmedetomidine infusion and intravenous paracetamol. Epidural analgesia may cause significant motor or sensory blocks that will cloud neurological monitoring of the spinal cord. Therefore, we do not use it in our centre. Emerging pain management strategies include novel regional anaesthesia techniques such as the Erector Spine Plane block (ESP) and the use of cryoablation of intercostal nerves.

Early input from a specialist pain team is essential not only for early acute pain management but for follow up of chronic pain issues that are very frequent in this patient population.

Post-operative Management

The composite reported incidence of common complications following open TAAA repairs including paraplegia, paraparesis and renal failure requiring dialysis is 14.4% with Extent 2 TAAA repairs carrying the highest rate of complications. Perioperative mortality ranges between 8–10%. The last two decades have seen major advances in the prevention and treatment of complications arising from open thoracoabdominal aneurysm repair. Crucial to reduction of complications is the seamless continuation of multidisciplinary team treatment and monitoring from the operating theatre into the critical care unit.

Permanent paraplegia is a devastating consequence hence prevention of spinal cord injury is a critical aspect of postoperative care. Therapy is tailored to ensure adequate perfusion and oxygen delivery to the spinal cord. Frequent neurological assessment (hourly whilst CSF drain is in situ) of power and sensation in lower limbs is essential and requires early weaning of sedation postoperatively. If sedation weaning is not possible, monitoring of MEPs is continued in the ICU. Spinal cord deficit can occur intraoperatively, in the immediate postoperative period or be delayed for several days after the procedure. Delayed spinal cord injury has a better prognosis but depends on early detection and intervention.

Detection of neurological impairment triggers the initiation of the COPS protocol. Elements of the COPS protocol include:

- **C: cerebrospinal fluid management**: ensure patency of drain or insert one if not in situ, set CSF pressure ≤ 10 mmHg, drain in place for at least 7 days
- **O: adequate oxygen delivery**: O_2 saturations >92%, Haemoglobin >100 g/l, ensure adequate cardiac index >2.5 l/min/body surface area

- **P: pressure management for perfusion of spinal cord**: MAP >90 mmHg, SCPP >80 mmHg, adequate right sided pressures
- **S: patient monitoring status**: half hourly neurological observations, CT head and spine, MRI spine if feasible.

The extensive nature of the open TAAA repair impacts the homeostasis of practically all of the body's organ systems. Postoperative pulmonary complications are very common following major aortovascular surgery. Mechanisms for lung injury include direct trauma to the lung due to surgical retraction, ischaemia/reperfusion injury, circulatory overload and massive transfusion. Other body systems, potential postoperative issues and suggested interventions are summarised in Table 5.

Table 5 Potential postoperative issues and complications following TAAA repair classified according to body systems, targets and interventions. DLT, Double Lumen Tube; RASS, Richmond Agitation-Sedation scale; CAM-ICU, Confusion Assessment Method ICU; MAP, Mean Arterial Pressure; CSF, Cerebrospinal Fluid; ARDS, Adult Respiratory Distress Syndrome; POC, Point of Care

System	Potential issues	Targets and interventions
Airway	• Airway oedema precluding exchange of DLT • Vocal cord palsy due to recurrent laryngeal nerve injury	• Head elevation to reduce oedema • Speech and Language therapy screening and follow up
CNS	• Stroke (incidence 2%) • Delirium • Subdural Haematoma	• Early sedation holds postoperatively • Target RASS score 0 to −1. We use dexmedetomidine 0.4–1.4 μg/kg/h • CAM ICU screening
Spinal cord	• Prevention of spinal cord injury	• Target MAP >85/90 mmHg. Volume resuscitation and vasopressors i.e. Noradrenaline ± Vasopressin usually required • CSF pressure ≤ 10 mmHg • CSF drainage for 72 hours • Hourly neurological observations
Cardiovascular	• Haemodynamic instability • Right Ventricular dysfunction • Atrial fibrillation	• Adequate filling pressures CVP 8–12 mmHg requiring fluid resuscitation • Positive fluid balance often >5 L in the first 48 hours • Cardiac Index ≥ 2.2 L/min. Inotropes (Adrenaline or Milrinone) may be required. Caution with excessive vasodilatation with Milrinone • Restoration of sinus rhythm (Amiodarone or cardioversion)

(continued)

Table 5 (continued)

System	Potential issues	Targets and interventions
Respiratory	• ARDS • Lung contusion • Pulmonary Haemorrhage • Protracted Weaning	• Lung Protective Ventilation • Ventilator care bundle • Early Respiratory Therapy involvement • Non-Invasive ventilation/High flow oxygen therapy post-extubation • Tracheostomy
Renal	• Acute Kidney Injury • Requirement for Renal replacement therapy	• Monitor urinary output, fluid and acid base balance • Avoid nephrotoxic medications • Renal replacement therapy for hyperkalaemia, severe metabolic acidosis, uraemia or overt fluid overload
Gastrointestinal/ Nutritional	• Postoperative Ileus • Increased catabolism	• Cautious initiation of oral intake • Enteral feeding • Laxatives • Early dietitian input
Haematological	• Postoperative coagulopathy • Thrombocytopenia • Excessive chest drain output • Prevention of thromboembolism	• Haemoglobin >100 g/l • POC thromboelastography guided management of coagulopathy • Blood products ± factor concentrates • Heparin prophylaxis 5000 units subcutaneous tds

Successful recovery and discharge from hospital requires the support of a highly specialised rehabilitation team comprised of physiotherapist, occupational therapists and specialist nurses.

Recommended Readings

1. Lopez-Marco A, Adams B, Oo AY. Thoracoabdominal aneurysmectomy: operative steps for Crawford extent II repair. JTCVS Techniques. 2020.
2. Coselli JS, Green SY, Price MD, et al. Spinal cord deficit after 1114 extent II open thoracoabdominal aortic aneurysm repairs. J Thorac Cardiovasc Surg. 2019.
3. Parotto M, Ouzounian M, Djaiani G. Spinal cord protection in elective thoracoabdominal aortic procedures. J Cardiothorac Vasc Anesth. 2019;33(1):200–8.
4. Rong LQ, Kamel MK, Rahouma M, et al. Cerebrospinal-fluid drain-related complications in patients undergoing open and endovascular repairs of thoracic and thoraco-abdominal aortic pathologies: a systematic review and meta-analysis. Br J Anaesth. 2018;120(5):904–13.
5. Luehr M, Salameh A, Haunschild J, et al. Minimally invasive segmental artery coil embolization for preconditioning of the spinal cord collateral network before one-stage descending and thoracoabdominal aneurysm repair. Innovations (Phila). 2014;9(1):60–5.
6. Whitlock RP, Dieleman JM, Belley-Cote E, et al. The effect of steroids in patients undergoing cardiopulmonary bypass: an individual patient meta-analysis of two randomized trials. J Cardiothorac Vasc Anesth. 2020;34(1):99–105.

Anaesthesia and Intensive Care for Adult Patients Undergoing Aortic Arch Surgery

K. Valchanov, G. Martinez, and A. Valchanova

Introduction

Pathology of the aorta and major vessels is easily diagnosed in the 21 century. Symptoms are now better diagnosed by most healthcare professionals, and imaging is readily available. With the advent of good quality ultrasound devices enlarged and dissected vessels can be diagnosed at bedside, and computerised tomography and magnetic resonance imaging are available in most institutions, as well as the quality of the images is constantly improving. Patients need aortic arch surgery in all its permutations due to 3 reasons: Acute or chronically dissected wall; Enlarged aorta and its branches at a risk of dissection in the future; Re-operation to corrected earlier aortic surgical complications. Surgery for these conditions has evolved since its first description in 1956. However, it still involves cardiopulmonary bypass (CPB) with all its problems.

Despite many minimally invasive techniques (mostly stenting) having been developed as alternative to major, and undisputedly, very high-risk surgery (mortality 16–20%), replacement of the diseased vessels is still the main stay of treatment in 2019. The majority of the operations involve the replacement of the arch and branches with a multi-chimneys vascular graft, in which the distal portion seats in the descending aorta (elephant trunk); or to replace the arch with a multi-branch hybrid prosthesis, where the arch segment is a multi-chimneys conventional graft, but the distal segment is a stent graft (FET-frozen elephant trunk).

Discussions about aortic vessel disease mechanisms and its prognostication are beyond the scope of this chapter. However, when surgery is indicated the team

K. Valchanov (✉) · G. Martinez · A. Valchanova
Department of Anesthesiology & Critical Care Medicine, Papworth Hospital, Cardiac anaesthetist, Cambridge, UK
e-mail: kamen.valchanov@nhs.net

G. Martinez
e-mail: guillermo.martinez@nhs.net

M. Vives and A. Hernandez (eds.), *Cardiac Anesthesia and Postoperative Care in the 21st Century*, https://doi.org/10.1007/978-3-030-79721-8_18

needs to have detailed understanding of the procedure in all its phases. No other type of surgery requires closer team-working than this. Team-work in these cases defines survival, and more importantly the morbidity associated with it. Anaesthetists in these teams need to be involved in the decision- making and planning for surgery, intra-operative monitoring and bypass, coagulation management, and postoperative monitoring and care. Understanding of the exact pathology, and pre-morbid blood flow distribution are essential for the anaesthetist.

Pre-anaesthetic Assessment

In the case of *acute aortic syndromes* (type A dissection (Fig. 1) and aortic ulcers/ ruptures) the pre-assessment is very easy. The patient needs an operation as a matter of urgency. The mortality is increased every hour of delay. If the patient is deemed suitable for surgery (absence of incurable malignancy, advanced frailty), then expediting surgery and haemodynamic monitoring and management take priority over details of pre-operative fasting, family history, etc. It is important that the patients and family have appropriate consent. The focus in such cases is on safe transfer to a cardiac centre; minimal safe blood pressure; management of pericardial collections; extent of dissection; blood transfusion requirements; plan for which vessels would be cannulated. Any pre-existing neurological deficit must be documented. The cerebral perfusion may have been impaired for a period of time, leading to increased risk of neurological deficit.

Elective aortic arch surgery patients have time for thorough assessment. This involves multidisciplinary approach with physicians, imaging specialists, surgeons, anaesthesiologists, perfusionists, and intensive care specialists. Individualised patient anatomy mandates individualised surgical plan. Choice of an aortic graft is

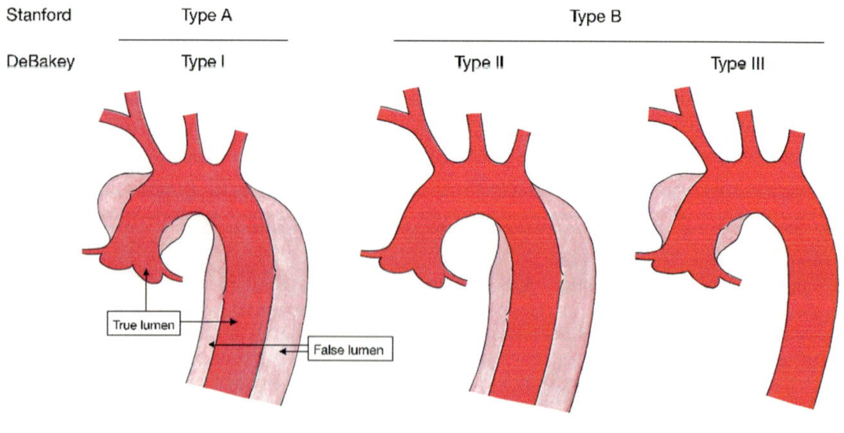

Fig. 1 Dissection types

important and the benefits weighed carefully. As part of the surgery includes cooling to reduce oxygen demand of different organs in times of diminished circulation the temperature planning and monitoring is important. Blood conservations strategies are discussed and the laboratory support enlisted. Cerebral and spinal cord protection is planned. Detailed anaesthetic assessment has to address any airway problems, cannulation of venous and arterial tree, drug and related medical history, and allergies. Finally, after a decision for surgery the patient needs to be presented with the potential benefits of surgery, vs potential complications.

Intraoperative Anaesthetic Management

Full understanding of the surgical plan is paramount to establish the appropriate invasive monitoring and plan for the best possible organ protection. As the nature of replacing the arch is associated with a high risk of brain, spinal cord and heart injury, the anaesthetic and perfusion strategy has to be tailored to prevent organ damage.

Anaesthetic induction: Although it is good practice to have an invasive arterial line monitoring before anaesthetic induction, these vascular patients are overall low risk from the heart performance point of view. The majority have good left ventricular function with some degree of aortic regurgitation that is frequently well tolerated. The 'Re-do' cases, previous Type A repair patients (about 3–11% of arch replacement) could be considered the high-risk group, as they may suffer biventricular dysfunction as a result of compromised coronary perfusion during the first emergency surgery. The selection of volatile or intravenous agent for induction and maintenance has no influence in outcomes; however, the use of high dose of opioids may be associated with higher risk of spinal cord injury. Airway can be secured with a single lumen endotracheal tube. Vascular and tracheobronchial compression as a result of a large aneurysm is rare but it can cause airway obstruction, bleeding and trachea-bronchomalacia.

Monitoring

A central venous catheter is useful for preload monitoring and inotropic support, and it can also be guidance on cerebral drainage, which can be mechanically compromised with clamps and tissue displacement. The innominate vein may need to be divided to dissect a large arch aneurysm or accidentally injured during dissection in re-do cases. Preference is therefore given to the central venous catheter in the right internal jugular, as well as the large-bore cannula for volume resuscitation. Pulmonary artery catheter may be necessary for Re-do cases, where up to 39% of patients have some degree of ventricular dilation or left ventricle dysfunction. Cardiac output monitoring and inotropic support becomes more relevant after the operation, to improve cardiac performance and ensure distal organ perfusion, which can be compromised once the false lumen in the descending aorta becomes excluded (thrombosed) and the remaining rudimentary vascular bed takes over. Echocardiography is essential in the operating theatres for assessment of ventricular function.

Since the ascending aorta and aortic arch are diseased, and they have to be resected for the operation, the CPB arterial cannulation is often peripheral (right axillary, carotid or femoral artery (Fig. 2)), which makes the brain, heart and other organs perfusion retrograde to the arch and ascending aorta. These patients often

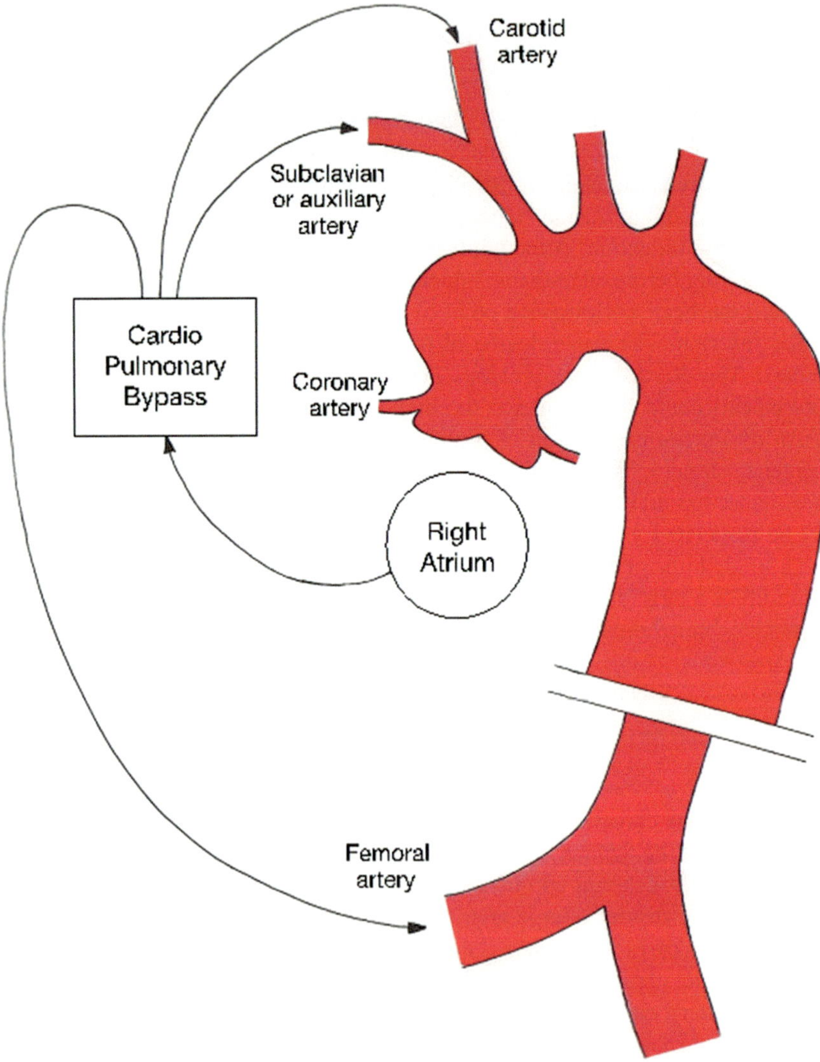

Fig. 2 Bypass cannulation options

have dissected peripheral vessels with flaps or thrombosis at different levels such as innominate artery (10–15% of cases), carotid, or femoral artery, particularly patients who underwent previous type A dissection repair. To ensure effective CPB flow to the arch and descending aorta, the invasive arterial monitoring can be placed in two distant points from the arch such right radial and a femoral artery.

Near infrared spectroscopy (NIRS) can be used to assess cerebral haemoglobin oxygenation. In general terms, cerebral oxymetry values that remain in line with pre-bypass readings, could be considered a good marker of adequate carotid perfusion but the evidence to support this statement is still lacking. Since the NIRS sensors are placed on the forehead, their trends are a good reflection of frontal lobes perfusion. However, it is not clear that using NIRS can influence neurological outcomes after aortic arch replacement. Considering that some patients have an anatomical variance of the circle of Willis, and a posterior communicating vessel is absent in 35% of patients, cerebral NIRS neither guarantee blood supply to the posterior part of the brain, nor offers a reliable guidance on global cerebral perfusion. Despite its limitations, an acute drop in the near-infrared spectroscopy value is highly sensitive to detect mechanical impairment to blood flow, such as cannula malposition, vessel dissection or flow steel into an open vessel.

Perioperative Transoesophageal echo (TEE) is a useful tool for multiple key points during surgery: Assess baseline cardiac function; Grade the aortic regurgitation; Confirm that the aortic arch prosthesis is well-expanded in the descending aorta; Assess cardiac function after the operation. In patients who undergo root replacement, problems with the coronary re-implantation may trigger regional wall motion abnormalities that can be identified and located with TEE guidance. The use of retrograde femoral perfusion can lead to descending aortic rupture or false lumen expansion, and it could be identified with TEE during the operation. When the surgical technique involves continuous antegrade coronary perfusion (400–700 mL warm blood given to the heart through a cardioplegia cannula) the use of TEE is essential to detect LV distension due to poor ventricular venting or aortic regurgitation (i.e. mild aortic regurgitation or washing jet of mechanical valves in previous type A).

Temperature monitoring in at least two territories is important to ensure that the target temperature has been achieved. If the arterial CPB cannulation is close to cerebral vessels (i.e. right axillary), the use of a nasopharyngeal probe as a sole source of temperature can lead to overestimation of hypothermia. Distal organs such as kidneys and spinal cord can remain warm and at risk of ischemic injury during the circulatory arrest. The use of selective cerebral perfusion (SCP) during circulatory arrest can only contribute to the upper spinal cord perfusion up to T3–T5, but not in segments below that level. Therefore, ensuring that the target temperature has been achieved in the lower body is a corner stone in minimising the risk of spinal cord injury. The use of bladder or rectal temperature probe appears to be a good surrogate of spinal cord temperature. In contrast, when return cannulation is placed in the femoral artery, the temperature measured in the upper body (such as esophagus) tends to be higher than that measured in the lower body. A ten degrees gap between blood and nasopharyngeal temperature favours a slow cooling to ensure all regions are cold before circulatory arrest. Rewarming should be preceded by a 5-min interval of cold reperfusion, which has been associated with improved cognitive recovery in experimental studies.

Perfusion

For cases undergoing circulatory arrest with selective cerebral perfusion, more than two or three isolated regional perfusion circuits are running at one particular time to deliver regional blood supply to the brain, the heart and the lower body. Perfusion for deep hypothermic (18–20°) circulatory arrest requires discontinuing circulation for an interval to facilitate the distal anastomosis completion. In that scenario a dynamic and close collaboration between perfusionist, anaesthetist and surgeon is essential.

During the lower body hypothermic circulatory arrest, the two circuits running may include: a cold SCP that is diverted from the arterial line (clamp on the innominate artery) and a second warm circuit to the heart (regional heart perfusion). It is good practice to split the lines at a pump level, rather than on the field, to be able to measure accurately the resistance and amount of flow to any particular area. Once the HCA is finished, a third cold circuit will be added to perfuse the lower body through the graft into the descending aorta.

Spinal Cord Protection

Patients undergoing elective aortic arch replacement may present with a large aneurysm and an intact descending aorta; A previous Type A repair with a chronically dissected descending aorta; or A type B dissection that requires arch replacement to stent the descending aorta in a later stage. The last two types are at higher risk of spinal cord injury. The collateral network of the spinal cord is very complex, and its vascular interconnection between the thoracic, the lumbar spinal plexus and the vertebral circulation play a major role in prevention and treatment of perioperative paraplegia. Although the lower body hypothermic arrest is inevitable, and usually short enough to preserve the spinal cord, it does inflict a degree of sub-lethal ischemia that leaves the spinal cord vulnerable after surgery. The duration of the arrest, the temperature, and the number of segments of thoracic aorta occluded with the stent will impact in neurological outcomes. Delayed perioperative paraplegia is the commonest presentation. In addition to intraoperative sub-lethal ischemia in theatres, the spinal cord swelling, lack of collateral network (i.e. occluded left subclavian), or systemic hypotension can precipitate a delayed spinal shock that if not treated promptly can be permanent. Maintaining high perfusion pressure after the haemostasis has been achieved is paramount. The use of inotropes and vasoconstrictors to achieve mean arterial pressure of 100–120 mm

Hg is often required in symptomatic patients. The insertion of a spinal catheter for cerebrospinal fluid drainage can be beneficial to augment spinal perfusion. High perfusion pressure and spinal drainage will be required for a period of time post-operatively. It appears that between 48 and 96 h after segmental arteries occlusion, a neo-vascular genesis can restore the flow through a dramatic increase in the paraspinal vascular bed, thus the risk of delayed paraplegia is progressively reduced.

Surgical Techniques: (Fig. 3)

Type of surgery is determined by the site of pathology. Surgery for type A aortic dissection aims to restore stability of the integrity of the ascending aortic wall. If the aorta is dissected there must be an intimal tear. The tear has a propensity to expand and the danger is that it may compromise coronary circulation, produce overwhelming aortic valve regurgitation, or tear into the pericardium producing tamponade and death. To avoid these rapid and life threatening complications the ascending aorta needs to be replaced as a matter of urgency.

The aims arch surgery are to resect the primary intimal tear and seal tears extending beyond the transverse aortic arch, as well as to cause false lumen obliteration of the descending thoracic aorta.

Arch replacement: Historically, the classic elephant trunk technique was developed by Borst in 1983. It involves replacement of the ascending aorta and aortic arch with the 3 major branches, not extending to the descending aorta.

Hemiarch: Hemiarch surgery is usually performed in patients who undergo aortic root replacement and present with a distal aorta or proximal arch aneurysm.

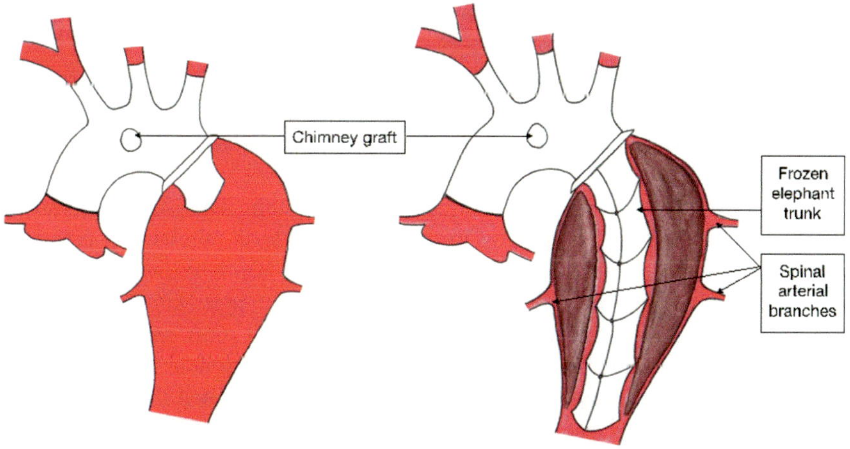

Fig. 3 Conventional elephant trunk (Left) and Frozen Elephant Trunk (Right)

This procedure is similar to interposition graft where ascending aorta is replaced as well as the inferior part of the aortic arch. However, the superior part of the arch where the head vessels are is left uninterrupted. There is a trend to perform hemiarch surgery for type A dissection or elective aortic root replacement when the arch is only mildly dilated, however, it is not clear if that would prevent patients from developing further arch aneurysm. There is controversy around the benefits outweighing the extra risk associated to deep hypothermic arrest and perioperative complications such as stroke, spinal cord injury and bleeding. However, numerous series publications have shown that the mortality and morbidity doesn't differ from isolated aortic root replacement.

Frozen elephant trunk: To overcome the limitations of conventional elephant trunk, a concomitant stented graft was developed and incorporated as an adjunct in the descending aorta, the frozen elephant trunk (FET) procedure. The FET technique has involves antegrade deployment of the descending aortic stent graft through the open arch during hypothermic circulatory arrest. The concerns with this procedure are that the descending aortic graft produces thrombosis of the highest part and can occlude flow in branches, which feed superior part of the spinal cord. The largest international registry including more than 11,000 patients did not show the outcomes of this procedure for Type A dissections to be worse than conventional elephant trunk.

Risks

Bleeding: Bleeding is the commonest complication of aortic surgery. As with any cardiac surgical bleeding the magnitude it is mostly dependent on extravasation from suture lines. The surgical technique and quality of tissues are the most important factor. The anaesthetist in these cases has also major role. Good teamwork with surgeon, perfusionist and blood bank cannot be overestimated. The blood loss in these cases can be very rapid and preparation and experience is very useful.

Correcting coagulopathy associated with long bypass and hypothermia are paramount. It has to be born in mind that prompt correction of coagulopathy with protamine and blood product allows the surgeon to see the bleeding spots that need suturing and allows for prompt haemostasis.

Hypertension during initial haemostasis is undesirable. The role of the anaesthetist is to control the blood pressure to lowest safe level, allowing haemostasis while maintaining perfusion to vital organs. While it is not known what is safe lowest blood pressure, and it varies from patient to patient, mean arterial pressure as low as 50 mm Hg can be tolerated by most patients for a short period of time.

Use of anti-fibrinolytics has been debated over time. High dose tranexamic acid and aprotinin have both been advocated. It has to be appreciated that although the use of aprotinin is associated with acute renal failure, these are high-risk operations and sometimes the risk of this complication is justified by the benefit of avoiding severe coagulopathy.

Myocardial dysfunction: Meticulous intraoperative myocardial protection by the surgeon is paramount for all major cases. The role of anaesthesia in this setting is no other than ensuring that myocardium has been perfused where appropriate, as indicated by ECG changes. In cases when myocardial injury has occurred the choice of post-operative inotropic agents as guided by invasive monitoring, TEE, and cardiac output is important.

Stroke: The second most devastating complication after paraplegia in aortic arch surgery is stroke. While in the general cardiac surgical population the common reason for stroke is embolic, in the aortic surgical patients this is ischaemia related to malperfusion of a carotid artery for a length of time. The incidence of 10% makes this a very frequent complication, and the patient must be warned about it. Ensuring intraoperative perfusion of all of the brain is essential, and use of cerebral oxymetry has been recommended, yet of no proven benefit.

Respiratory failure: It is difficult to define isolated respiratory failure in the post-operative setting in these patients. Hypoxia and hypercarbia are not frequent problems in uncomplicated cases. However, the risk factors are: poor premorbid condition, emergency surgery, prolonged bypass, blood products administration. If this occurs, it has a major impact on the weaning form mechanical ventilation and assessment of neurology. In cases where prolonged mechanical ventilation is required the use of alpha-1 agonists like dexmedetomidine to allow arousal and neurological assessment have been recommended.

Renal failure: It is important to remember that incidence of pre-existing renal impairment in this category of patients is common, and also the duration of cardiopulmonary bypass longer than other operations. It is therefore not surprising that the incidence of acute post-operative renal failure is as high as 21%. No renal protection strategy has been of proven benefit for cardiac surgical patients, and optimal renal perfusion intraoperatively is the best strategy. If the acute renal injury is diagnosed post-operatively the treatment is supportive, via renal replacement therapy. If sure to a dissected segment of the aorta both renal arteries have impaired perfusion then permanent renal failure is likely. The influence of hypothermia on renal protection has also been questioned, and it seems that deep or moderate hypothermia offer the same protection

Complication rate in this group of patients is not inconsiderable. Many studies have presented data, and probably the most consistent is from the Martens publication in 2016: stroke 10%, dialysis 21%, spinal cord injury 5%.

ICU Management

Wake up versus asleep: All patients undergoing aortic arch surgery are postoperatively cared for in an intensive care environment. Once surgery is completed the patient is transferred sedated and mechanically ventilated to the intensive care unit. Immediate or earliest arousal for assessment of neurological function is always the best approach. Early awakening may not be practical for the following reasons:

need for meticulous blood pressure control; bleeding and need for chest re-exploration; and respiratory failure. It has to be remembered that despite advanced monitoring of brain and spinal cord perfusion, the best way to assess these functions is to wake up the patient and ensure arousal and adequate motor function. If sedation has to be continued there is a risk of delayed diagnosis of spinal malperfusion, delayed treatment, and permanent neurological deficit.

Bleeding and open chest: Bleeding is not uncommon in aortic surgery. The goal of good intensive care management is tight blood pressure control and correction of coagulopathy. Proactive management of both is essential. In rare cases massive blood loss and technically challenging operations can lead to swelling of the intrathoracic organs. In such cases the chest cannot be closed, and patients may need to be left with unopposed sternum for several days. Infection control in such cases is important as risk of mediastinitis is high.

Spinal cord monitoring: Replacement of descending aorta mandates spinal cord monitoring intraoperatively, and some form of post-operative monitor. Patients undergoing aortic arch surgery seldom have their regional spinal perfusion interrupted. However, on rare occasions when the patient wakes up with signs of paraplegia aggressive optimisation of spinal perfusion is essential to avoid permanent damage. Spinal drainage and optimising spinal perfusion pressure (i.e. high mean arterial pressure) in the post-operative period are the main stay of treatment.

Pain and delirium management: Postoperative Delirium is common in acute aortic dissection patients (34%). The risk factors include cerebrovascular disease history, surgery and cardiopulmonary bypass duration, postoperative hypoxia. Recognising risk factors early and managing delirium could contribute to early recovery, and avoiding complications associated with prolonged ICU stay. Analgesia is seldom a problem for sternotomy patients and simple morphine infusions or boluses are conventionally used. However, patients who need thoracotomy for surgical access (unusual for aortic arch surgery) may need regional analgesia in a form of epidural and paravertebral blocks.

Gold standards of good intensive care management also include careful Infection vigilance; Mobilisation and nutrition; and Early rehabilitation and discharge planning. Finally, all aortic and cardiac surgical centres maintain rigorous analysis of performance via audit and reporting of results. This ensures high healthcare standards, and best results for patients. Litigation for unexpected mortality or neurological injury in this category of patients is not uncommon, and solid medico-legal defensive practice is helpful in such cases.

Recommended Readings

1. Martens A, Beckmann E, Kaufeldt t, et al. Total aortic arch repair: risk factor analysis and follow-up in 199 patients. Eur J Cardiothorac Surg 2016;50:940–948
2. Guo MH, Appoo JJ, Saczkowski R, Smith HN, Ouzounian M, Gregory AJ, Herget EJ, Boodhwani M. Association of Mortality and Acute Aortic Events With

Ascending Aortic Aneurysm: A Systematic Review and Meta-analysis. JAMA Netw Open. 2018;1(4):e181281

3. Leone A, Beckmann E, Aandreas M, Di Marco L, Pantaleo A, Reggiani LB, Haverich A, Di Bartolomeo R, Pacini D, Sherestha M. Total aortic arch replacement with frozen elephant trunk technique: Results from two European institutes. J Thorac Cardiovasc Surg. 2019 May 11. pii: S0022–5223(19)30970-5
4. Minatoya K, Inoue Y, Sasaki H, Tanaka H, Seike Y, Oda T, Omura A, Iba Y, Ogino H, Kobayashi J. Total arch replacement using a 4-branched graft with antegrade cerebral perfusion. J Thorac Cardiovasc Surg. 2019;157:1370–8.
5. Maier, Sven, Kari, Fabian , et al. Selective Heart, Brain and Body Perfusion in Open Aortic Arch Replacement. The journal of extra-corporeal technology 2016; 48: S122–8
6. Poon SS, Tian DH, Yan T, Harrington D, Nawaytou O, Kuduvalli M, Haverich A, Ehrlich M, Ma WG, Sun LZ, Estrera AL, Field M. Frozen elephant trunk does not increase incidence of paraplegia in patients with acute type A aortic dissection. J Thorac Cardiovasc Surg. 2019 Apr 14. pii: S0022–5223(19)30800-1.

Adult Congenital Heart Disease

Emma Lei Lei and Jane Heggie

Introduction

The Adult Congenital Heart Dosease (ACHD) patient may present for a spectrum of needs including routine cardiac investigations, procedures and interventions under anaesthesia, non cardiac and cardiac surgery. Published guidelines for long-term management and anaesthetic considerations are widely available and recently updated. There is a change from the AHA/ACC 2008 guidelines that now accounts for the patient's current physiology in addition to their anatomical diagnosis. A repaired Tetralogy of Fallot patient, asymptomatic with a competent pulmonary valve and normal exercise testing is considered well in comparison to a Tetralogy of Fallot patient with an aneurysmal right ventricular outflow tract (RVOT), free pulmonary regurgitation and diminished exercise tolerance. Non-adherence to these guidelines, being followed in a general cardiology setting and or being lost to follow up results in increased catastrophic and major complications. Simple, moderate, and highly complex ACHD patients were all at increased risk of adverse outcomes when not managed under specialized ACHD cardiology care (P = 0.04, 0.009, and 0.002). A population based study of 71,463 patients with ACHD in Quebec from 1990 to 2005 found an association between lack of specialized ACHD

E. L. Lei · J. Heggie (✉)
Department of Anesthesia, Peter Munk Cardiac Centre, Toronto General Hospital, University of Toronto, Toronto, ON, Canada
e-mail: jane.heggie@uhn.ca

E. L. Lei
Department of Anesthesia, Westmead Hospital Sydney, University of Sydney, Sydney, Australia

M. Vives and A. Hernandez (eds.), *Cardiac Anesthesia and Postoperative Care in the 21st Century*, https://doi.org/10.1007/978-3-030-79721-8_19

care and all-cause mortality. The mortality risk was largely driven by patients with severe forms of ACHD.

Although it is desirable for patients to be followed by ACHD trained cardiologists the demands exceed capacity even in developed nations. A cardiac anaesthesiologist whether in a reference center or regional center will encounter ACHD patients in emergent, urgent and elective settings for both cardiac and non cardiac interventions and procedures. It is important to screen for cardiac diagnosis that will benefit from referral to a reference center as well as for co morbidities that are a consequence of living with ACHD which in themselves mandate a referral to a tertiary care center. As in all cases it is not only about the skills of the anaesthesiologist and surgeon but about the environment around the patient and the facility's ability to care for the patient's cardiac and non-cardiac physiology.

Recently published 30-day and in-hospital surgical mortality rates for ACHD cardiac surgery range from 3.5 to 4.3%, with variation in reporting of major adverse events and long-term morbidity. Predictors of adverse outcome include anatomical diagnosis, functional capacity, co-morbidities because of living with congenital heart disease, adult acquired comorbid conditions like Chronic Obstructive Pulmonary Disease COPD and the surgical procedure planned. Over time there has been a shift to higher acuity cases with proportionately less 'simple' cases such as Atrial Septal Defects (ASDs) as many of these are referred to interventional cardiologists. Regardless of the patient's booked procedure or surgery there are specific considerations for the ACHD population for anaesthesia and ICU.

General Considerations

One can easily become lost in the attempt to understand the anatomy and complexity of the original diagnosis and subsequent surgery and interventions even when it is documented in detail and readily available. An anaesthesiologist may be faced with no documentation and only the patients and family's recollection particularly in urgent situations such as transesophageal echocardiograms to assess the safety of cardioversion of a new onset atrial arrhythmia. Start with a picture of the original anatomy, then consider how shunts and surgical repairs/palliations have altered the anatomy and the physiological consequences. Table 1 is a list of procedures common to many types of ACHD diagnosis and their timing and staging has changed over the decades. It is by no means exhaustive and many are of historical interest and are no longer offered in current practice yet still existing in ACHD patients or their long-term consequences are experienced by the mature ACHD patient. Fuller et al. using the STS-CHSD registry examined risk of in-hospital mortality on 52 procedural groups and this was a simplification of an extensive list of diagnosis that exceeded 150 categories. A quick internet literature

Table 1 Common previous surgical procedures In adults with congenital heart disease

Procedure	Description
Ballock Hanlon procedure	A surgical or balloon atrial septostomy to promote mixing in newborns with cyanotic heart disease, typically D-Transposition of the Great Arteries
Potts shunt	Left pulmonary artery to descending thoracic aorta to augment pulmonary blood flow but often distorted pulmonary artery anatomy and complicated with unilateral pulmonary hypertension
Waterston shunt	Right pulmonary artery to ascending thoracic aorta to augment pulmonary blood flow but often distorted pulmonary artery anatomy and complicated with unilateral pulmonary hypertension
Blalock Taussig shunt (BT Shunt)	Ipsilateral subclavian artery to pulmonary artery anastomosis. Involves dividing the right subclavian and as a result diminished arterial inflow to the arm. No palpable pulse in the limb, possible distorted pulmonary artery anatomy and potential for unilateral pulmonary hypertension
Modified Blalock Taussig shunt (BT shunt)	Interposition graft between ipsilateral subclavian artery to pulmonary artery. The same sequala as the classic BT shunt but with less severe consequences. Smaller arm and lower blood pressure on the side of the shunt
PA banding	A band placed on the pulmonary artery to limit pulmonary blood flow in the context of a large unrestricted left to right shunt. Usually a precursor to a definitive bi-ventricular repair
Mustard/Senning	Atrial baffle for the correction of D-TGA to redirect systemic venous return to the sub-pulmonary (morphological left) ventricle and pulmonary venous return to the Sub aortic (morphological right) ventricle
Rastelli repair	Physiological repair of a D-TGA with pulmonary stenosis and a VSD. A right ventricle to pulmonary artery conduit is placed and a left ventricle to sub aortic intra-cardiac tunnel
Jatene arterial switch	Physiological repair of a D-TGA with transection of the Great Arteries and reimplantation of the coronary arteries. It has superseded the Senning/Mustard repair
Norwood	Staged treatment of Hypoplastic Heart Syndrome (HLHS) The first stage starts with creating an aorta from the pulmonary artery. The right ventricle supplies the aorta whilst pulmonary and systemic blood flows are balanced by a BT shunt or Sano Shunt. An ASD is created
Sano shunt	A right ventricle to pulmonary artery shunt to augment pulmonary blood flow
Classic Glenn shunt	The Superior Vena Cava (SVC) is divided and the proximal portion anastomosed directly to the Right Pulmonary Artery (RPA). The SVC distally is over sewn as is the RPA at its origin. Complicated by Pulmonary arteriovenous malformations, central venous hypertension. Inability to pass an intracardiac wires via the upper limbs and neck

(continued)

Table 1 (continued)

Procedure	Description
Bidirectional Glenn Shunt	The SVC is divided and the proximal portion anastomosed directly to the confluence of the Main Pulmonary Artery. The SVC distally is over sewn as is the main pulmonary artery at its origin
Fontan	First described in 1971 for the treatment for tricuspid atresia, double inlet left ventricle and single ventricle. Initially the right atrial appendage was anastomosed to the Pulmonary artery. These patients experienced severe right atrial dilatation, arrhythmias and thrombus. Later modifications included the lateral tunnel and total cavopulmonary connection TCPC to try an address the issue of arrhythmias

and image search to conceptualize the anatomy is a helpful start. Congenital bicuspid valves and aortopathy overlap considerably with acquired heart surgery practices and their distribution and allocation may differ between institutions.

Pre-operative Considerations and Red Flags

Regardless of the surgery contemplated, cardiac or non cardiac surgery, or ICU admission, there will be unique cardiac physiological and comorbid conditions that are a consequence of the original diagnosis, subsequent repair and end organ dysfunction due to diminished cardiac output or high venous pressures. Each patient's individual case must be carefully reviewed however there are commonalities and hemodynamic considerations in ACHD lesions and below is a list of questions to resolve when reviewing the patient.

- Is the lesion dependant on pulmonary vascular resistance?
- Are there septal shunts or fenestrations?
- Presence of cyanosis?
- Preload and afterload dependant?
- Pulmonary function?
- Liver disease?
- Blood loss anticipated. Massive?
- Cognitive impairment and Syndromes

Pulmonary Vascular Resistance (PVR)

Right sided heart lesions including Ebstein's, Conotruncal lesions such repaired Tetralogy of Fallot with pulmonary regurgitation, Fontan circulation and Glenn shunts are all dependent on a low pulmonary vascular resistance for successful left atrial filling whether it is passive (Glenn and Fontan) or active with a hypokinetic dilated Right ventricle. Spontaneous ventilation is preferable but may not be possible if neuromuscular blockade is required. Mechanical ventilation must be at volumes close to FRC with little PEEP and low airway pressures.

Septal Shunts, Great Vessel Shunts, Fenestrations, Unrestricted Shunts

Intracardiac shunts (ASD, VSD, fenestrations in ASDs and Lateral tunnel Fontans) and Great Vessel shunts (Patent Ductus Arteriosus, Blalock Taussig, Waterston and Potts shunts) will need thoughtful precautions for venous air emboli. Venous in-line filters are problematic in cases using TIVA or blood transfusion as the filters occlude and if the line is 'tucked' you may lose access to the patient. De-airing the lines ahead of time and attention to detail intraoperatively is paramount. Ensuring the patient has appropriate venous lines with filters with education of their need is important with transfer of care.

Lesions with large unrestricted shunts, meaning there is no gradient between the two chambers or vessels, are dependent on a balance between the PVR and SVR (systemic vascular resistance). These patients have found this balance in their ambulatory life and post induction it is wise to target their room air PaO2 and oxygen saturations. A pre-existing left to right shunt can exacerbated by exuberant ventilation and hyperoxygenation. Ironically a pink patient will have a metabolic acidosis and hyper-perfused lungs. Similarly, cyanotic patients as in the case of massive aorto-pulmonary collaterals, may have temporary increases in saturation but at the expense of systemic oxygen delivery.

Pulmonary Hypertension

The most common cause of pulmonary hypertension in ACHD is due to left heart disease such as regurgitant systemic atrioventricular (AV) valve, aortic regurgitation or a failing systemic ventricle. Specific to ACHD is pulmonary hypertension as a result of an unrestricted left to right shunt that may have been reversible initially but if left uncorrected, progress to the Eisenmenger's syndrome where the shunt is reversed to right to left. In this case the right ventricle is robust as it has seen systemic pressures since infancy and although preload dependent, it is much less vulnerable than the adult with acquired primary pulmonary hypertension. The median survival of a patient with Eisenmenger's syndrome is 40 to 60 years. Anesthetic management should focus on maintaining systemic ventricular afterload and avoid exacerbation of pulmonary hypertension by ventilating at tidal volumes close to FRC and maintaining a normal to alkalotic pH.

Preload and Afterload

Preload and afterload considerations are important for both right and left sided heart lesions. Ventricular compliance is another consideration. For example, a patient with repaired Tetralogy of Fallot may have severe pulmonary regurgitation and tricuspid regurgitation as well as a restrictive right ventricle would require adequate preload and low PVR. Patients with small left ventricles will be sensitive to preload particularly if there is left ventricular outflow tract obstruction. These considerations are familiar to adult cardiac anaesthesiologist and ICU physicians.

Liver Disease

Liver dysfunction and cirrhosis are risk factors for all cardiac surgery patients. Short-term mortality is considerably increased in patients with liver cirrhosis as measured with both the Child Pugh and MELD score classification systems in cardiac surgical populations. ACHD patients with right sided heart lesions, Ebstein's Anomaly, Tetralogy of Fallot and Fontan Circulation, have congested livers due to congestive cardiac cirrhosis. Many who had blood transfusion prior to the 1990s contracted hepatitis C through blood transfusions. An elevated MELD score in ACHD patients have increased in-hospital and one year mortality.

Pulmonary Function

Chest wall incisions are associated with restricted lung function from chest wall deformities and in the case of thoracotomies a proxy for cyanosis and diminished pulmonary blood flow augmented with a shunt. Restriction in lung function is common, as are respiratory and skeletal muscle weakness. These can all lead to worse post-operative outcome, especially prolonged ventilation.

Cognitive Impairment and Syndromes

Causes of cognitive dysfunction associated with ACHD include Down's syndrome, 22q11.2 deletion syndrome (Di George syndrome) or global developmental delay from of chronically low cardiac output or collapse in neonatal period and infancy.

The median survival of Down's syndrome in developed nations is ~ 60 years. Extra cardiac comorbidities include cognitive dysfunction, dementia (50–70% at 60 years), hypothyroidism, acquired mitral valve disease, atlanto-axial instability, obstructive sleep apnea, and epilepsy.

Patients with 22q11.2 Deletion Syndrome co-morbidities include palatal abnormalities, autism spectrum and or schizophrenia, developmental delay, trachea-esophageal disorders, renal anomalies, seizures, immunodeficiency and hypocalcemia. Whether the patient is living with their family or in a supervised care there will be an investment required by both the peri-operative team and the care givers of the patient.

Individual Management-Key Points

Simple

Bicuspid Aortic Valve (BAV) and Aortic Root Surgery

Bicuspid aortic valve is a common cardiac anomaly. It causes premature onset of aortic stenosis, regurgitation or mixed disease. BAV is also associated with concomitant aortopathy with dilated aortic aneurysm, aortic dissections, coarctation and coronary anomalies. The valvular issues are as that for acquired aortic valve disease. Common aortic valve procedures for BAV include aortic valve replacement (tissue or mechanical), Ross procedure and Ross Konno.

Common postoperative ICU complications include increased incidence for bleeding, tamponade and relook sternotomy, and permanent pacemaker insertion. However, over ICU mortality and morbidity is low and prolonged ICU stay uncommon.

Aortic Coarctation

Coarctation is a narrowing of the proximal descending aorta, usually close to the site of ductus arteriosus, at junction of distal aortic arch and descending aorta. The narrowing can be localised or extensive. It can occur in isolation or be associated with other lesions e.g. BAV, VSD, Shone's complex (sequential left heart obstructive lesions). The narrowing causes a gradient across the narrowing and hypertension of upper limbs and relative hypoperfusion of lower limbs.

Endovascular repair has transformed coarctation of aorta management and they rarely require open surgery except in complicated lesion or thoracic aortic aneurysm post coarctation repair. Endovascular dilation and stenting can be performed under sedation or general anaesthetic and to a routine ward post operatively. Some chest and back pain is normal post stenting, but severe back pain is concerning for aortic tear or rupture albeit rare.

Open repair is performed via a left thoracotomy with lung isolation and possibly femoral cannulation for partial cardiopulmonary bypass and deep hypothermic circulatory arrest. Spinal cord protection is less of an issue than in the acquired aneurysm population due to well-developed collaterals. Invasive blood pressure pre and post coarctation i.e. radial and femoral arterial lines are useful. Bleeding can be significant in redo surgery or complicated repair.

Atrial Septal Defects and Ventricular Septal Defects

Atrial septal defect (ASD), a defect in the interatrial septum, is a common CHD, and commonly present in adulthood. There are 4 types of ASDs: Secundum ASD (a defect in fossa ovalis) is the most common type followed by Primum ASD (associated with a mitral valve cleft and is a partial atrioventricular septal defect), Sinus Venosus ASD (due to malformation of sinus venosus and is often associated with partial anomalous pulmonary venous drainage; is can be superior and associated with SVC or inferior and associated with IVC) and the rare Unroofed Coronary Sinus (associated with a persistent left sided SVC). ASDs cause right atrial, right ventricular volume overload and dilation and potentially pulmonary hypertension.

Adults with isolated ASD causing impaired functional capacity, right atrial and/or right ventricular enlargement, and net left to-right shunt sufficiently large to cause physiological sequelae (e.g., pulmonary–systemic blood flow ratio [Qp: Qs] $\geq$ 1.5:1) without cyanosis at rest or during exercise, ASD closure is recommended, provided that systolic PA pressure is less than 50% of systolic systemic pressure and pulmonary vascular resistance is less than one third of the systemic vascular resistance.

Large Secundum ASDs (or if it lacks adequate septal rim), and all other types of ASDs are closed surgically. Pre bypass, it is important to maintaining the patient's baseline level of PVR:SVR ratio and usual air precautions. Management pre and post bypass will depend on the degree of PAH. Specific pulmonary vasodilators such as milrinone, inhaled nitric oxide (NO), or inhaled prostacyclin are all useful and likely dictated by institutional preference and availability. Patients having primary repair at a late age have a high incidence of arrhythmias.

Isolated VSD is the most common CHD in children but they're uncommon in adults as most VSDs are small muscular or peri membranous VSDs and usually close spontaneously. A more common scenario is patients who had their defects closed in childhood and then return for a revision of a defect such as a patch leak, which is not hemodynamically significant but is a risk for paradoxical embolism.

Moderately Complex

Atrioventricular Septal Defect (AVSD)

Complete AVSD repair is usually performed in childhood but partial defects may require repair in adulthood. The main consideration is managing pulmonary hypertension related to the left to right shunt and systemic left atrioventricular valve regurgitation. Post operatively, LVOT obstruction may occur due to the elongated 'goose neck' LVOT and need for temporary pacing.

Ebstein's Anomaly

Ebstein's anomaly is a rare ACHD defect, representing less than 1% of all ACHD. It may present in childhood or as an adult with new onset atrial flutter and right heart failure. It is characterized by abnormal apical displacement of the tricuspid septal and posterior leaflets and a large sail like anterior leaflet resulting in severe tricuspid regurgitation, dilated right atrium and "atrialized" thin walled and hypokinetic small right ventricle. Operative repair involves tricuspid repair (cone repair) or replacement, plication of atrialized right ventricle and closure of intracardiac shunts. In the event of failing small right ventricle post cardiopulmonary bypass may necessitate creating an interatrial fenestration or bidirectional Glenn Shunt.

Post operatively in ICU the main challenge is optimise RV function and reduce PVR using standard techniques. Early conversion to spontaneous ventilation is essential in ICU. Filling can be difficult to assess; they need to be adequately filled but RV volume overload is detrimental to tricuspid repair and will impair LV filling and function through interventricular dependence. Significant post-operative RV dysfunction is associated with a high incidence of renal, gastrointestinal and hepatic dysfunction, and a significant requirement for prolonged respiratory support.

Severe tricuspid regurgitation, congestive hepatopathy and prolonged complex surgery also increase bleeding and coagulopathy post operatively. Ebstein's patients also experience a high incidence of atrial arrhythmias, further complicating the post operative course.

Tetralogy of Fallot and Conotruncal Defects

Tetralogy of Fallot, as well as Double Outlet Right Ventricle, results from malalignment of the outlet portion of the ventricular septum resulting in a large, non-restrictive VSD, the aorta 'overrides' the VSD, right ventricular outflow tract obstruction (infundibular RVOTO), right ventricular hypertrophy. Tetralogy of Fallot rarely presents uncorrected in adulthood. The history of the lesion and its repair have changed with each decade. Older adults likely will have had a temporizing systemic artery to pulmonary artery shunt, Blalock Taussig, Potts or Waterston shunt, and a definitive repair as an older child. Younger adults are likely diagnosed in utero and have had a primary correction as a neonate or more recently as an infant 3–6 months.

Repair of Tetralogy of Fallot as an adult is a rare occurrence in developing nations and should be done at reference centres. Considerations for the cyanotic patient, right to left shunting and risk of stroke as well as post-operative management of the patient's pulmonary circulation. The ICU team must take into account that the lungs will see a full cardiac output for the first time and may have the additional burden of residual aorto-pulmonary collaterals contributing to pulmonary (relative) hyper perfusion.

Common re-presentations for adults include, pulmonary regurgitation due to transannular patch in childhood or an obstructed RV to PA conduit. Increasingly, there are interventional options for this population however a substantial number still need surgery. Having a team strategy for sternal re-entry is vital and should include rehearsal of emergent bypass with drop suction, peripheral (femoral) cannulation. Complications and morbidity are usually associated with right ventricular dysfunction especially in pulmonary regurgitation, whereas the RV tends to do well in pulmonary stenosis. LV dysfunction and ectopy will occur if the annulus of the valve impinges on the left main coronary ostia. The pulmonary valve is in close vicinity of left main coronary artery and the sewing ring may impinge on the artery and will be self-evident with a wall motion abnormality on echocardiogram.

Complex

Transposition of the Great Arteries

There are three common presentations of transposition of great arteries (TGA); D-TGA, D-TGA with VSD and pulmonary stenosis and L-TGA or ccTGA. TGA can present as a combination with other complex lesions (Fig. 1).

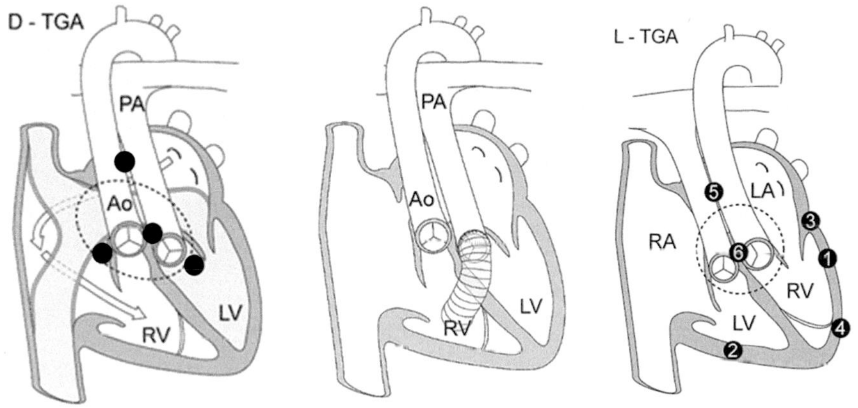

Fig. 1 D-TGA with a Mustard Baffle, Rastelli and L-TGA

D-TGA with Mustard or Senning Baffle Repair

D-TGA have atrial-ventricular concordance and ventricular-great artery discordance and prior to the 1980s had a Mustard or Senning repair. Although rarely performed now there are many adults living with atrial baffles which re-direct atrial blood to the opposite ventricle. The RV remains as the systemic and sub-aortic ventricle. Baffle leaks, sinus atrial arrhythmias, sick sinus syndrome, and systemic ventricular failure occur in midlife. Many will be considered for heart transplant and may be optimized by management of arrhymmia and dual chamber pacing. with an AICD or PPM in-situ. Strategies that optimize function and lower afterload of the systemic ventricle are indicated for operative and ICU management.

D-TGA with Arterial Switch Repair

Early in the 1980s CHD paediatric centers moved from the above repairs to the Jatene or Arterial Switch operation. The aortic and pulmonary arteries are switched with re-implantation of the coronary arteries. The LV is the systemic ventricle and atrioventricular and ventriculoarterial synchrony is restored. Late complications in adulthood include the requirement for aortic or pulmonary valve replacement, and ventricular dysfunction due to coronary disruption. In these patients, post-operative recovery is generally uneventful, and does not significantly differ from standard post-cardiac surgical care. Urgent non-cardiac surgery can be done safely in the community setting with consultation from cardiac anaesthesia and an ACHD cardiologist.

D-TGA with VSD and Pulmonary Stenosis and a Rastelli Repair

Adults living with D-TGA (AV concordance and VA discordance) having a VSD and Pulmonary Stenosis were corrected in childhood with a Rastelli repair. (described in the introduction). Frequently the RV to PA conduit will become obstructed and require balloon dilatation in the interventional lab and a percutaneous pulmonary valve replacement within the RV to PA conduit. Presenting to the operating room are likely associated with right endocarditis with significant sternal entry risks.

L-TGA or cc-TGA

In congenitally corrected TGA (cc-TGA) there is atrioventricular and ventriculoarterial discordance i.e. morphological RV and LV are switched so that subpulmonic ventricle is the morphological LV and systemic ventricle is the morphological RV (see diagram). There may be associated abnormalities of atrial situs, septal defects and/or sub-pulmonary outflow tract obstruction. AV conduction abnormalities are common. Most of these patients have an Ebstein's like malformation of the tricuspid, systemic AV valve, with moderate to severe systemic AV valve regurgitation. Tricuspid valve replacement for regurgitation is the most commonly performed procedure. They are managed like a dilated cardiomyopathy as the morphological RV which is the systemic ventricle is more likely to fail with time. Post operatively in ICU they may experience significant ventricular failure and if medical inotropic support is inadequate, mechanical circulatory may be required to allow the systemic ventricle to recover to recover.

Single Ventricle with Glenn and Fontan Type Connections

Tricuspid Atresia and Pulmonary Atresia

Double Inlet Left Ventricle (DILV)

Hypoplastic Left Heart Syndrome (HLHS)

Adults with single ventricle physiology such as tricuspid atresia, pulmonary atresia, DILV and HLHS will likely have had at least a Glenn shunt followed by a form of the Fontan procedure. This patient population is complex and now living well beyond 18 years and may present to adult centers for cardioversion, diagnostic and interventional procedures as well as non-cardiac surgery. The population of HLHS is disadvantaged with a morphological RV as their single ventricle and is an increasing proportion of the noncyanotic single ventricle population over the age of 18 years.

The Fontan palliation was first described in 1971. The original procedure was anastomosis of the RA to main PA. The original Fontan suffered severe RA dilation overtime leading to arrhythmias and thrombus formation, and these complications led to recent revisions. Subsequent modifications were made to improve the

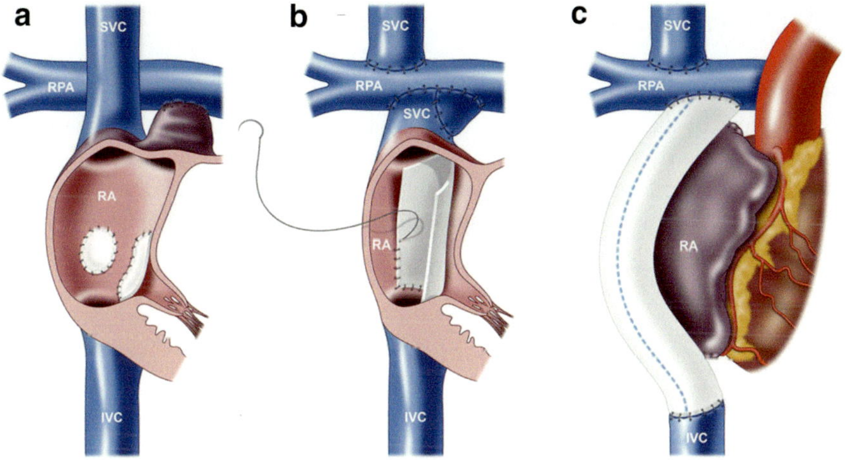

Fig. 2 An illustration of the evolution of the Fontan procedure

efficiency of the circulation, to the current version of either lateral tunnel Fontan or the total Cavopulmonary connection (TCPC). In TCPC, both SVC and IVC are anastomosed end to side to RPA, bypassing the heart completely. In the Fontan circulation, pulmonary blood flow is passive and reliant on central venous pressure – pulmonary pressure gradient, requiring adequate filling pressures, low PVR, unobstructed pulmonary veins, compliant LA, AV synchrony, compliant LV without outflow tract obstruction and a low SVR. Fenestration of in the Fontan circulation acts as a pressure pop off valve during times of raised PVR allowing blood flow from right to left heart to maintain cardiac output but at the expense of desaturation. These fenestrations can be source of paradoxical embolus.

Spontaneous breathing is better than positive pressure ventilation as negative intrathoracic pressure generated during inspiration increased pulmonary flow where as PPV reduces cardiac output. Pleural collections should be drained, avoid pulmonary vasoconstrictors, optimise ventilation settings with short inspiratory time and low PEEP, iNO, nebulised prostaglandins and milrinone. In those with a fenestration, hypoxia can be from excessive right to left shunting in presence of pulmonary hypertension. Post operative ICU stay can be prolonged with multi-system dysfunction and prolonged ventilation (Fig. 2).

Rychik J, et al. Evaluation and Management of the Child and Adult with Fontan Circulation: A Scientific Statement from the American Heart Association. Vol. 140, Circulation. 2019.

Key Points and Summary

Mortality and morbidity increase with complexity of the underlying disease. Management of the post-operative ACHD patient requires a highly trained multidisciplinary approach with in-depth ACHD knowledge. Specific conditions and interventions merit special consideration and expectantly managing common post-operative complications can potentially avoid those complications and improve outcome.

Recommended Readings

1. Aboulhosn JA, Daniels CJ, Van Hare GF, Gurvitz M, Dearani JA, Crumb SR, et al. AHA/ACC guideline for the management of adults with congenital heart disease: executive summary. Circulation. 2018;2018:1–113.
2. Goeddel LA, Jung YH, Patel P, Upchurch P, Fernando RJ, Ramakrishna H. Analysis of the 2018 American Heart Association/American College of Cardiology Guidelines for the Management of Adults With Congenital Heart Disease: Implications for the Cardiovascular Anesthesiologist. J Cardiothorac Vasc Anesth. 2019.
3. Lui GK, Saidi A, Bhatt AB, Burchill LJ, Deen JF, Earing MG, et al. Diagnosis and management of noncardiac complications in adults with congenital heart disease: a scientific statement from the American Heart Association. Circulation. 136;2017.
4. Khan I, Tufail Z, Afridi S, Iqbal M, Khan T, Waheed A. Surgery for tetralogy of fallot in adults: early outcomes. Brazilian J Cardiovasc Surg. 2016;31(4):300–3.
5. D'udekem Y, Iyengar AJ, Galati JC, Forsdick V, Weintraub RG, Wheaton GR, et al. Redefining expectations of long-Term survival after the fontan procedure twenty-five years of follow-up from the entire population of Australia and New Zealand. Circulation. 2014;130(11): S32–8.
6. Rychik J, Atz AM, Celermajer DS, Deal BJ, Gatzoulis MA, Gewillig MH, et al. Evaluation and management of the child and adult with Fontan circulation: a scientific statement from the American Heart Association. Circulation. 140;2019.

Anaesthesia for Heart Transplantation

Andrew Gaunt

Background

Around 5000 heart transplants are carried out annually worldwide, and heart transplantation remains one of the most challenging cases that a cardiothoracic anaesthetist can undertake. Heart transplantation is indicated if there is end-stage heart disease with a life expectancy of 12–18 months, if there is NYHA grade III or IV heart failure, or pathology that is not remediable by medical or surgical means.

The International Society for Heart and Lung Transplantation (ISHLT) registry suggests there is an 8% mortality in the first month after transplantation, with approx. 40% of these deaths related to primary graft failure (PGF), and so heart transplantation is best reserved for those with a significant threat to life. Median survival after heart transplantation is 12.4 years and is improving slightly, although all of the recent improvement in survival is entirely due to a reduced early mortality. The mortality rate in the years following heart transplantation is remarkably consistent and hasn't changed relative to the 1982–1991 cohort.

Recipient Selection

The majority of heart transplant recipients are in the 40–59 age group, although the proportion of organs going to the over 60 s is increasing. Heart transplantation has been successfully carried out on septuagenarians but remains uncommon. Dilated cardiomyopathy remains the most common indication for heart transplantation (Fig. 1).

A. Gaunt (✉)
Department of Anaesthesia & Intensive Care, Royal Brompton and Harefield NHS Foundation Trust, Hillingdon, London, England
e-mail: A.Gaunt@rbht.nhs.uk

M. Vives and A. Hernandez (eds.), *Cardiac Anesthesia and Postoperative Care in the 21st Century*, https://doi.org/10.1007/978-3-030-79721-8_20

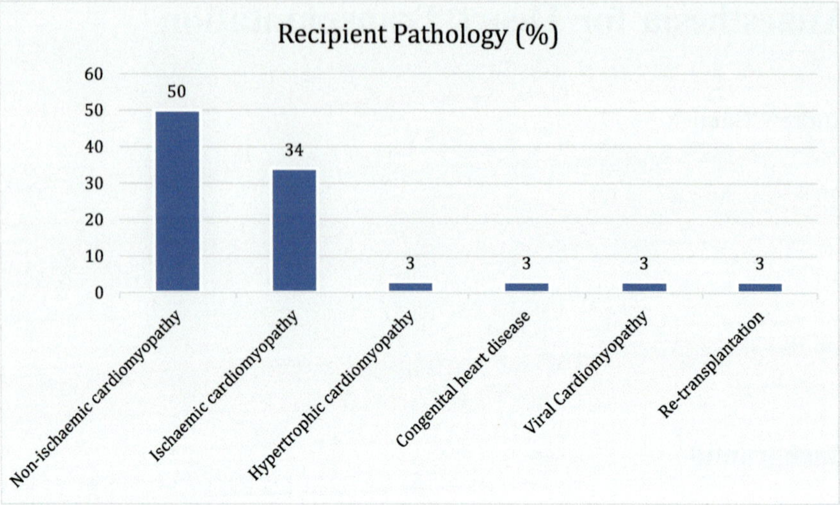

Fig. 1 Recipient pathologies

The increasing complexity of both recipients and available donors represent some of the greatest challenges to the current practice of heart transplantation. An increasing number of heart recipients have undergone previous cardiac surgery. In the 2009–2016 cohort of adult heart recipients, 50.7% of patients were undergoing re-sternotomy for heart transplantation, with an increasing number (42%) of so called "bridge to transplantation" recipients, who have already undergone implantation of mechanical circulatory support. Heart transplantation in these patients is a much more complex and demanding procedure. Performing a re-sternotomy where a VAD outflow graft is adherent to the underside of the sternum, the right ventricle is adherent to the sternum, or there are patent grafts from a previous CABG is hazardous and has led to various approaches to reduce the risk. Implantation of ventricular assist devices via bilateral thoracotomies, which avoids the need for midline sternotomy, is a potential solution to make midline sternotomy safer in VAD recipients subsequently undergoing heart transplantation. Careful routing of the VAD outflow graft can help to reduce the risk of iatrogenic complications at the time of transplant. A CT scan of any patient requiring a re-sternotomy is usually carried out at listing for transplantation, to determine the positions of any structures that may be damaged during re-sternotomy. The contraindication to heart transplantation are listed in Fig. 2, but the situation remains fluid as novel therapies are introduced to manage pre-existing conditions. For example, HIV infection is no longer considered a contraindication to transplantation.

Absolute Contraindications

Other medical condition with risk of death within 5 years

Chronic infection

Malignant disease

Cerebrovascular disease

Smoking or excessive alcohol intake

Relative contraindications

High Pulmonary vascular resistance (> 4 woods units)

Transpulmonary gradient (mPAP – PCWP) > 15 mmHg

Chronic renal impairment

HIV, Hepatitis B, C

Secondary organ damage due to diabetes

Amyloidosis

Fig. 2 Contraindications to heart transplantation

Heart Donation

Donated hearts are matched to recipients based on ABO blood group compatibility and size. The majority of donated hearts are removed from donors with head injuries, strokes or cerebral anoxia. With the increasing demand for hearts, the maximum age of donors is gradually being relaxed, with a steadily increasing number of hearts being donated by the over 60 s. Hearts are assessed by the donation team using echocardiography and visual inspection ± pulmonary artery flotation catheter. Hearts should be structurally normal (a small patent foramen ovale is easily dealt with and not a contraindication to transplantation), with no major valvular abnormalities and good ventricular function. They should be free of significant coronary artery disease and significant wall motion abnormalities.

Donor Organ Preservation

Conventionally, the donated heart was first flushed with cardioplegia solution and then stored on ice whilst being transported to the implanting hospital. This so called "cold ischaemic time" was a risk factor for poor outcomes, with increasing rates of early graft failure and mortality beyond three and a half hours of ischaemic time. A number of organ preservation systems have been introduced to try to address organ preservation issues. The TransMedics Organ Care System (OCS, Andover, MA, USA) maintains a donated heart in a functioning state. The heart is perfused with donated blood and nutrients whilst being is transported to the implanting centre. Ischaemic times are reduced to just the time required to harvest, attach to the machine, remove, and implant. This approach reduces ischaemic times markedly and may represent a significant development in organ preservation.

Supply of Organs

Ordinarily, the source of hearts for transplantation was from donors with confirmed brain stem death (so called DBD, donation after brain death), however it is feasible to collect donated hearts from so called "donation after cardiac death", or DCD donors. Indeed, the first successful heart transplant was from a DCD donation. In this group of non-brain death donors, withdrawal of life supporting treatment is carried out in an operating theatre environment until death occurs. Sometimes potential donors do not meet the criteria for donation, particularly if the donor maintains a degree of stability after life support withdrawal, or if they persist in a low cardial output state for a prolonged period. This is regarded as warm ischaemic time, and collection of the heart is often abandoned after more than an hour of haemodynamic instability. After a standard period of cessation of circulation (usually five minutes), a sternotomy is performed to harvest heart and lungs. There are two preservation techniques described. Normothermic regional perfusion (NRP) involves sternotomy and heparinisation in situ, the cerebral vessels are excluded from the circulation to ensure no recovery of cerebral function, and the heart is perfused to allow recovery. During this time, abdominal organ harvest can begin, and after approx. 45 min of re-perfusion the heart is assessed to ascertain its suitability for harvest and transplantation. Alternatively, it is feasible to perform a sternotomy and administer cardioplegia straight away, and then harvest the heart. In both techniques, the heart is then connected on to the TransMedics OCS system for reperfusion and transport. Using this approach, periods of warm ischaemic time are reduced to around 1 h.

There are alternative methods of organ preservation available which are aimed at ensuring a donated heart is kept cold and submerged under preservation fluid. They include the Sherpa Pack (Paragonix Technologies Inc, Cambridge, Massachusetts, USA) and the Asporto organ preservation device (Hibernicor LLC, Delaware, USA)

Operative Management

Pre-anaesthetic Assessment

Due to the fact that patients are frequently called in from home, patients may arrive not starved adequately, and may occasionally require preparation for rapid sequence induction.

An anaesthetic history should be taken, with attention paid to allergy and medication history, airway assessment and any recent changes in physiology. The conduct of the anaesthetic, invasive lines, pain management, post-operative critical care and insertion of a TOE probe should be discussed briefly. The patients latest blood results and recent investigative findings should be summarised.

Induction

Most patients arrive in the anaesthetic room with a fair degree of trepidation. In most cases pre-operative long acting, sedative premedication is undesirable and best avoided. Reassurance and a patient centred approach can go a long way to reduce anxiety, supplemented by short acting intravenous anxiolysis.

Conventional monitoring with ECG (Leads II and V5) and SpO_2 is usual. Cerebral oximetry should be applied pre-induction if it is to be used.

Arterial line insertion can be difficult, particularly when the radial arteries have been cannulated previously. USS guidance can be invaluable, particularly in axial or centrifugal flow VAD recipients, who may not have a palpable pulse.

Patients may present with central access already sited, if they have required pre-operative inotropic support. It is preferable to site new lines prior to the procedure, and the administration of immunosuppressive medication.

Transoesophageal echocardiography is essential during heart transplantation for assessing haemodynamics, volume management, myocardial function, and to guide de-airing.

Choice of induction drugs for heart transplantation is down to individual preference and familiarity, but induction should be slow and careful, with titration to effect. Historically, a high dose opiate (fentanyl 50–100 mcg/kg) anaesthetic supplemented by midazolam with pancuronium was used. Pancuronium was used in cardiac surgery due to its properties as a ganglion blocker, which induces a relative tachycardia, thereby offsetting hypotension from vasodilatation caused by induction drugs. As cardiac anaesthesia has evolved, so has the anaesthetic management of heart transplantation, with most choosing a balanced technique with lower dose opiates, volatile supplementation and shorter acting paralysis. Arm-brain circulation times can be significantly prolonged in severe heart failure, and allowance should be made to avoid accidental over-dosing. Core temperature monitoring is usually facilitated by a nasopharyngeal, oesophageal or rectal temperature probe. Antibiotic prophylaxis is normally given in the anaesthetic room, along with initial immunosuppression, usually 1 g IV methylprednisolone.

Following intubation, large bore access along with central venous catheters are sited using ultrasound guidance. Patients presenting for heart transplantation may have difficult central access due to prior usage, or the presence of devices such as ICDs or pacemakers. A large bore haemofiltration catheter may be useful, both for intraoperative volume and blood product administration, and to provide post-operative renal support.

The ISHLT currently recommends the reversal of warfarin prior to the start of surgery, by the administration of factor concentrates, Vitamin K, or fresh frozen plasma. This may reduce the need for post-operative blood product administration; newly transplanted hearts do not tolerate significant volumes of blood products well, as they are prone to right heart failure. Also, the vasoactive properties of platelets can precipitate sudden heart failure, and anything that can be done to reduce the requirement for allogenic products is prudent. The use of aprotinin to reduce allogenic blood product usage should be considered in re-do cardiac surgery. Many patients have implanted devices such as pacemakers and defibrillators; these should be switched to fixed modes not affected by diathermy, and the defibrillation therapies deactivated prior to surgery. The wires are normally cut when the native heart is explanted, and the devices are usually removed at the end of the operation.

Surgery and Maintenance

After skin preparation and draping, surgery normally commences with skin incision and sternotomy. In cases of re-sternotomy, surgery may begin with femoral vessel or subclavian access to facilitate emergent cannulation in the event of damage to intrathoracic structures during re-sternotomy. In extremely high-risk cases, where either heart or VAD outflow is adherent to the sternum, the chest may be opened once cardiopulmonary bypass has been established. If there is significant damage to the heart or great vessels during sternotomy, and it is not feasible to open the chest expeditiously, it may be necessary to rapidly cool on bypass and institute deep hypothermic circulatory arrest prior to continuing to open the chest.

Anaesthesia is usually maintained by a balanced technique using vapour / narcotics and intravenous hypnotics. Heparinisation is achieved by the administration of 300–400iu/kg intravenous heparin and titrated to the required activated clotting time (ACT) depending upon hospital policy.

Cardiopulmonary Bypass

Once an adequate ACT is achieved, the patient can be cannulated and bypass stablished. Maintenance of anaesthesia on bypass is usually achieved by TIVA, although vapour administration via the bypass machine is feasible. The heart $\pm$ VAD can then be explanted, and the vessels prepared for anastomosis. The donated heart is usually given cardioplegia and kept cold with pericardial ice slush prior to re-perfusion. The left atrium, pulmonary artery and aorta are anastomosed, and following de-airing, the aortic cross clamp can be removed and the heart re-perfused to reduce ischaemic time prior to right atrial or bi-caval anastomosis. Suturing right atria (donor and native) together is technically easier, but results in a larger, anatomically abnormal right atrium, which is associated with rhythm disturbances. The heart is then re-perfused after insertion of a vent to decompress the heart, and rhythm is established using biventricular pacing if necessary.

Weaning of Cardiopulmonary Bypass

Following completion of the anastomoses, there follows a period of controlled re-perfusion prior to weaning, to allow heart function to recover following cardioplegia and ischaemia. This is typically at least 30 min, and may be up to 1 h.

During this period, there is an opportunity for surgical haemostasis and it represents a good time for the anaesthetists to make all preparations for weaning of cardiopulmonary bypass. All required inotropes should be connected and running, all emergency drugs should be to hand and inhaled vasodilators such as nitric oxide or inhaled prostacyclin, should be commenced to optimise right ventricular afterload.

Inotropic Support and Weaning

There is no correct "recipe" for inotropic support following heart transplantation that is supported by research, but there is significant experience, and most centres have their own protocols for management. It is likely that the secret to successful heart transplantation lies in recognition of evolving problems and early and appropriate management of these complications. The characteristics of commonly used inotropic and chronotropic drugs are discussed below.

Epinephrine

Epinephrine (adrenaline) is a mixed α and β adrenergic agonist. It is used in heart transplantation to augment ventricular function, heart rate and increase cardiac output. As part of its endogenous activity in the so called "fight or fright" response, it also has significant endocrine activity and decreases insulin secretion, increases glucagon secretion, increases ACTH secretion and causes lipolysis. This results in increased availability of glucose and fatty acids for energy production.

Isoprenaline (Isoproterenol)

Isoprenaline, a β-agonist inodilator, is often used to augment ventricular function.

It has β-1 and β-2 agonist properties, but almost no activity at α receptors.

Its effect is to increase heart rate and cardiac output but can reduce arterial blood pressure due to β-2 mediated vasodilatation.

Milrinone

Milrinone is a phosphodiesterase type 3 inhibitor. It acts by inhibiting the breakdown of c-AMP. It is an inotrope and vasodilator. Its vasodilator effects are potent on both the systemic and pulmonary circulation and may complicate so called "vasoplegic" states after cardiac surgery.

Norepinephrine (Noradrenaline)

Norepinephrine is predominantly used as a vasoconstrictor. It is used to maintain afterload at low-normal levels following cardiac surgery. A SIRS-like responses to cardiopulmonary bypass is common, and vasodilation is a physiological effect of many of the inotropic drugs used in cardiac surgery (e.g., milrinone, dobutamine, levosimendan).

Vasopressin

Vasopressin (antidiuretic hormone) is used as a vasoconstrictor in cardiac surgery. Its primary mode of action is to increase water reabsorption in the kidneys, but it also causes arteriolar constriction. It may allow reduction of norepinephrine doses and help reduce its undesirable effects such as peripheral and gut ischaemia.

Dopamine

Dopamine is a dopaminergic agonist, with mixed α and β receptor agonist properties. Its β effects predominate at lower doses, but it causes significant vasoconstriction at higher doses. It also increases urinary sodium excretion but has no role in the treatment of renal dysfunction. Its use has declined significantly due to concerns about its arrhythmogenic properties.

Dobutamine

Dobutamine is a predominant β-1 agonist and therefore increases heart rate and contractility, with lesser effects on β -2 mediated vasodilatation. It has almost no activity on dopaminergic receptor mediated norepinephrine secretion, and so does not increase afterload.

Levosimendan

Levosimendan is a newer class of inotropic agent, a calcium sensitizer. It exerts its inotropic effects by binding to cardiac troponin C in myocytes and increasing the sensitivity to calcium, and it reduces both preload and afterload due to vasodilation. There is little experience of the routine use levosimendan in heart transplantation, however there are some case reports of beneficial effects in low cardiac output states following heart transplantation.

Nitric Oxide

Nitric oxide is administered as an inhaled drug into the ventilator circuit to cause selective pulmonary vasodilation whilst maintaining systemic perfusion pressures, thus reducing right ventricular afterload. It acts via increasing cGMP mediated vasodilatation. Its adverse effects include increased synthesis of nitrogen dioxide, dinitrogen tetroxide (rocket propellant) and peroxynitrite which can all be cytotoxic, although the real world relevance of these by products in un-known. iNO can only be administered via a breathing circuit, so the patient cannot be extubated until NO is successfully weaned. Sildenafil may facilitate the weaning of inhaled nitric oxide.

Prostacyclin

Inhaled prostacyclin can be used to induce pulmonary arteriolar vasodilatation, as an alternative to inhaled nitric oxide.

Weaning from Cardiopulmonary Bypass

Prior to weaning from cardiopulmonary bypass, certain conditions must be met. Many centres have a checklist for such conditions prior to weaning. These are the same conditions as for conventional cardiac surgery.

Checklist for weaning from cardiopulmonary bypass

1. Patient being ventilated.
2. Drugs connected and emergency drugs available
3. Rate and rhythm acceptable
4. Temperature > 36 degrees C.
5. Potassium 4.5–5 mmol/l
6. Haemoglobin > 70 g/l
7. pH > 7.2

Once the heart begins to eject, it may be feasible to float a pulmonary artery flotation catheter to allow measurement of cardiac index, pulmonary artery pressure, PCWP and SvO2, although this may not be possible until the venous cannula is removed from the heart.

Weaning from cardiopulmonary bypass involves sequential step-wise reduction of flow from the bypass machine, along with consequent reduction of venous drainage in to the pump by the perfusionist, so as to facilitate return of heart function and restoration of cardiac output. Weaning is usually carried out in a stepwise fashion (75, 50, 25%, off CPB). The perfusionist maintains the CVP at pre-determined levels (usually around 10 mm Hg) by varying the degree of venous drainage.

During weaning, multimodal surveillance of heart function is carried out by both anaesthetist and surgeon. Attention is paid to both conventional monitors (ABP, CVP, PA, PCWP, SvO2 and CI) and also to the gross appearance of the heart. TOE guidance of volume replacement and assessment of ventricular function is useful. If any signs are adverse, then a stepwise approach allows for institution of restorative measures prior to the next weaning step i.e. increased inotropic support or removal/ addition of volume.

Primary graft failure (PGF) carries a high morbidity and mortality. In severe cases there is a need for early mechanical circulatory support (IABP, ECMO or Ventricular assist device).

Primary Graft Failure

Primary graft failure is defined in different ways but is perhaps best characterised as poor heart function requiring either high dose inotropic support or mechanical circulatory support in the immediate post-operative period. It occurs in up to 23% of cases. It is implicated directly as a cause of death in approximately 40% of the 8% 1-month mortality following heart transplantation and is a risk factor for reduced survival at one year. Reasons for early failure include preservation issues (where cardioplegia has been inadequate, or the organ has not been cooled adequately), surgical complications, iatrogenic overdistention or hyperacute rejection which is thankfully rare. The increasing age of donors has been implicated as a factor in the high rates of PGF.

TOE for Heart Transplantation

The usefulness of transoesophageal echocardiography in heart transplantation cannot be overestimated. Continuous surveillance of left and especially right ventricular function following transplantation, and early intervention seems key to successful outcomes. TOE is used to guide filling, look for hidden air, assess left and right ventricular function (both qualitatively and quantitatively), check the patency of anastomoses and to guide inotropic therapy.

Bleeding and Coagulation Management

Those patients undergoing relatively uncomplicated heart transplantation may not require blood product administration following reversal of heparinisation. This is fortuitous as newly transplanted hearts do not tolerate excessive circulating volume, and high filling pressures are associated with poor outcomes. Additionally, allogenic blood products contain vasoactive substances which can affect the pulmonary circulation adversely, thereby increasing the risk of right heart failure.

Protamine administration may trigger right heart failure due to pulmonary hypertension, anaphylaxis, hypotension or complement activation and cytotoxicity, so should always be given carefully in this fragile group of patients.

Those recipients undergoing transplantation after re-sternotomy, or in complicated or prolonged surgery, may need supplemental blood product administration to reverse coagulopathy and ensure adequate haemostasis. The availability of factor concentrates may reduce the need for large volumes of blood product administration, but their usefulness in this situation is not yet proven.

Use of thromboelastography (TEG), platelet function analysis and lab based formal clotting studies are used to guide blood product administration.

Common Pitfalls and Early Post Op Management Including Mechanical Circulatory Support

Right Ventricular Failure

Once cardiac output is established, qualitative and quantitative assessment of the heart helps guide further management. Immediately after coming off CPB, the pulmonary vascular resistance (PVR) is typically high and may further compromise RV function. PVR typically falls in the minutes after weaning, and there may be a consequent improvement in function as the RV afterload decreases and left ventricular filling improves. Failure of the right ventricle is not uncommon and once established, it can be difficult to manage.

Signs of a failing RV include a rising CVP (particularly in the presence of a falling PCWP), right ventricular distension (direct observation or on TOE), evolving tricuspid regurgitation, falling cardiac output or an underfilled LV. Treatment includes inotropic support together with pre and afterload reduction, and ultimately either a return to cardiopulmonary bypass, or institution of mechanical circulatory support.

Left ventricular failure occurs in the context of primary graft failure but is less common as a discrete entity than right ventricular failure. Air embolization into the coronary arteries can precipitate LV failure, although this usually affects the right coronary artery, thus affecting the right ventricle and ventricular septum preferentially.

In cases where the heart performs well and requires only low dose support, there is often a deterioration in the early post-operative period as myocardial oedema develops in the graft.

Mechanical Circulatory Support

In the setting of persistent poor ventricular function resulting in poor end-organ perfusion, mechanical circulatory support is required. This can be in the form of either ventricular assist devices (VAD) or ECMO. The aim of mechanical circulatory support is to off load the failing heart and allow recovery of ventricular function by reducing wall stress and buying time for healing or therapeutic intervention (such as steroids or anti-thymocyte globulin for rejection), or to allow time to recover from ischaemic reperfusion injury. Temporary VAD implantation can support both left and right ventricles independently. A right atrial cannula for outflow and a pulmonary artery inflow cannula will allow the siting of a VAD to support the right side, and the left ventricle is supported by insertion of a VAD between the left atrial and aortic cannulas. ECMO support would typically be VA ECMO in this setting, but a left ventricular drainage cannula may be required to properly off load the heart.

Rejection

Early hyperacute rejection is extremely rare, but manifests as sudden inflammation of the affected organ, and is often fatal in the case of heart transplant. It is largely avoided by the process of ABO compatibility matching. Acute rejection can occur in the days following transplantation and is usually represented by a deterioration in the level of cardiac function. It is diagnosed by myocardial biopsy, but often treatment is initiated prior to a histologically confirmed diagnosis. Pulsed steroids or rabbit anti-thymocyte globulin are used to suppress immune function and restore graft function. Exchange plasmapheresis can also be useful.

Recommended Readings

1. Khush KK, et al. The international thoracic organ transplant Registry of the International Society for Heart and Lung Transplantation: Thirty-fifth adult heart transplantation report-2018; Focus theme: multiorgan transplantation. J Heart Lung Transplant. 2018;37 (10).1155–68.
2. Gregoric ID, La Francesca S, Myers T, et al. A less invasive approach to axial flow pump insertion. J Heart Lung Transplant. 2008;27:423–42.

3. Hill JD, Avery GJ, Egrie G, Turley K, Reichenbach S. Less invasive Thoratec LVAD insertion: a surgical technique. Heart Surg Forum. 2000;3:218–23.
4. Popov AF, Hosseini MT, Zych B, Simon AR, Bahrami T. HeartWare left ventricular assist device implantation through bilateral anterior thoracotomy. Ann Thorac Surg. 2012;93:674–6.
5. Costanzo MR, et al. The international society of heart and lung transplantation guidelines for the care of heart transplant recipients. J Heart Lung Transplant. 2010;29(8):914–56.
6. Petaja Liisa M. et al. Levosimendan reversing low output syndrome after heart transplantation. Ann Thoracic Surg. 2006; 82(4):1529–31.
7. Mychaskiw G, Sachdev V, Heath BJ. Sildenafil (viagra) facilitates weaning of inhaled nitric oxide following placement of a biventricular-assist device. J Clinic Anesthesia. 2001; 13:218–20.
8. D'Alessandro C, Golmard J-L, Barreda E, et al. Predictive risk factors for primary graft failure requiring temporary extra-corporeal membrane oxygenation support after cardiac transplantation in adults. Eur J Cardiothorac Surg. 2011;40:962–70.
9. Stehlik J, Edwards LB, Kucheryavaya AY et al. The registry of the international society for heart and lung transplantation: twenty-seventh official adult heart transplant report 2010. J Heart and Lung Transplant. 2010; 29:1089–103.

Anesthesia for Transcatheter Cardiac Interventions in Adults

Jose Luis Carrasco Del Castillo and Marina Urena Alcazar

Introduction

The percutaneous cardiac interventions in adults, for diagnostic and therapeutic reasons, are highly heterogeneous (Fig. 1). The complexity of the planned intervention is widely variable too. The presence of anesthesiologists is required in procedures needing a monitored anesthesia care (MAC), sedation or general anesthesia (GA), either in high-risk procedures or patients at high risk for complications. These interventions often required 2 dimensional (2D) or 3 dimensional (3D) transesophageal echocardiography (TEE). Nonetheless, currently the presence of the anesthesia team is necessary in most procedures to improve safety and comfort of both patients and operators.

These interventions require thorough preoperative preparation and a comprehensive understanding of the procedure and its hemodynamic implications. It is crucial to be able to rapidly adapt treatments to the potential hemodynamic changes, which may be sudden and dramatic, and to have an effective communication with operators and other member's HT.

These challenges, which makes this subspecialty unique and a very attractive opportunity for anesthesiologists, are detailed below.

An unusual environment

The same principles of anesthetic care applied for procedures outside the operating room can be applied to the procedures programmed in cardiac catheterization laboratory (CCL) or hybrid operating room (HOR).

J. L. C. Del Castillo (✉)
Department of Anesthesiology and Intensive Care, Bichat – Claude Bernard Hospital, Paris University, Paris, France

M. U. Alcazar
Department of Cardiology, Bichat – Claude Bernard Hospital, Paris University, Paris, France
e-mail: marina.urena-alcazar@aphp.fr

M. Vives and A. Hernandez (eds.), *Cardiac Anesthesia and Postoperative Care in the 21st Century*, https://doi.org/10.1007/978-3-030-79721-8_21

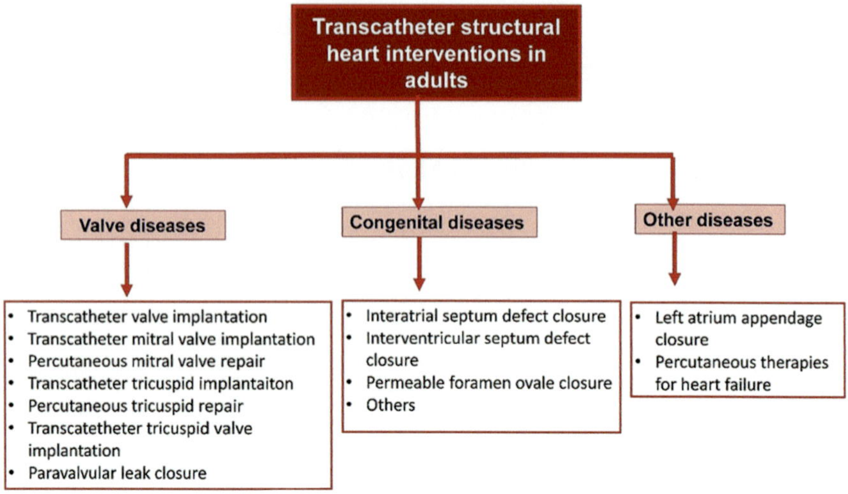

Fig. 1 Transcatheter structural heart interventions in adults

The HORs are configured in an attempt to link the role of all HT's members to get a balanced multidisciplinary approach. Although HORs generally offer a better use of workspace than CCL and significantly improve the work conditions of the anesthesia team, they are still a *friendly* environment that is not designed for the specific requirements of the anesthesia equipment. Thus, the anesthesia's team have to adapt to the environment, learn about the available resources and design a personalized action plan to anticipate potential complications. The lack of familiarity and limitations with the environment can lead to potentially serious safety problems.

The anesthesiologist should meet the following requirements when working integrated into the HT: to perform a thorough preoperative preparation, to understand each procedure's step and their hemodynamic implications, to have the skills and flexibility to a very dynamic critical clinical different scenarios (such as performing an aggressive cardiopulmonary resuscitation, treatment of a massive hemorrhage, performing an emergency endotracheal intubation, an extracorporeal life support indication, etc.), team-working skills, having effective communication and coordination between the members (Fig. 2).

In general, these HORs have the following configuration:

1. **Control room** (Image 1) => it allows continuous communication with the operators and a system for recording the procedure (patient's constants, vascular pressures and radiological images)
2. **Procedure's room** (Image 2) => In general, the configuration including a similar scheme (Fig. 3). These rooms allow the integration of other imaging modalities, such as a biplane system, C-arm CT, integrated ultrasound and electromagnetic navigation systems, fusion image, etc.

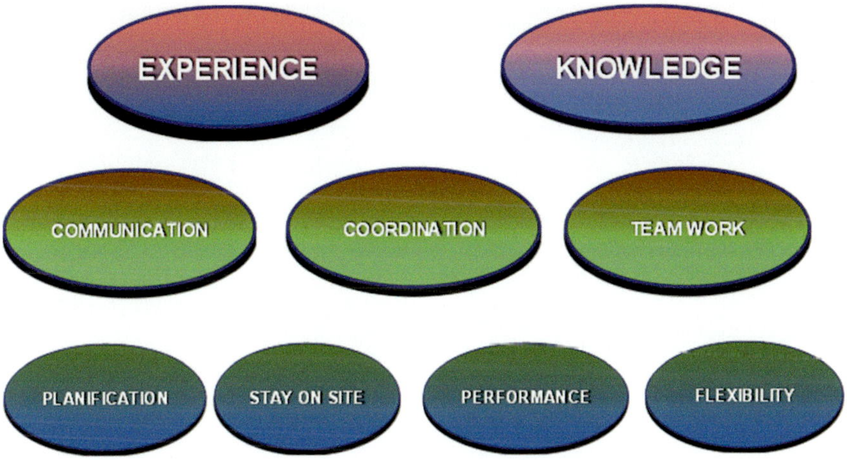

Fig. 2 Anesthesiologist's skills to work in the HOR

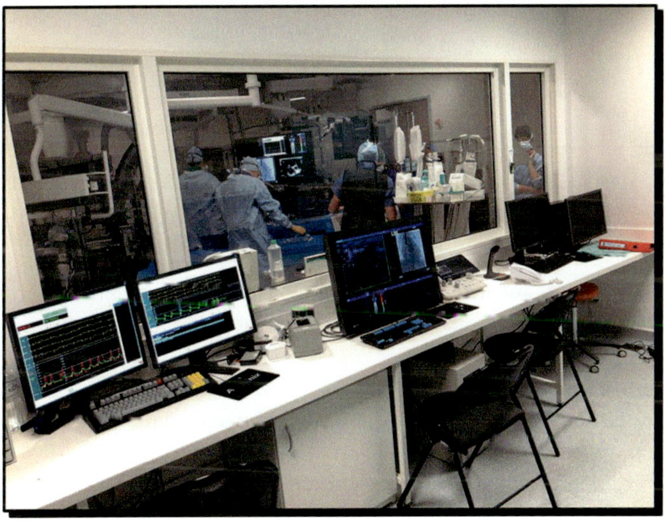

Image 1 Hybrid control room

3. **Radiation safety measures**: doors, glass, mobile lead shields and lead-lined walls
4. System for laminar air flow and positive pressure inside the room.

Some aspects as understanding the pathophysiology of diseases, the environment, the need of a lead apron for radioprotection, have to be kept in mind when working in these rooms (Fig. 4).

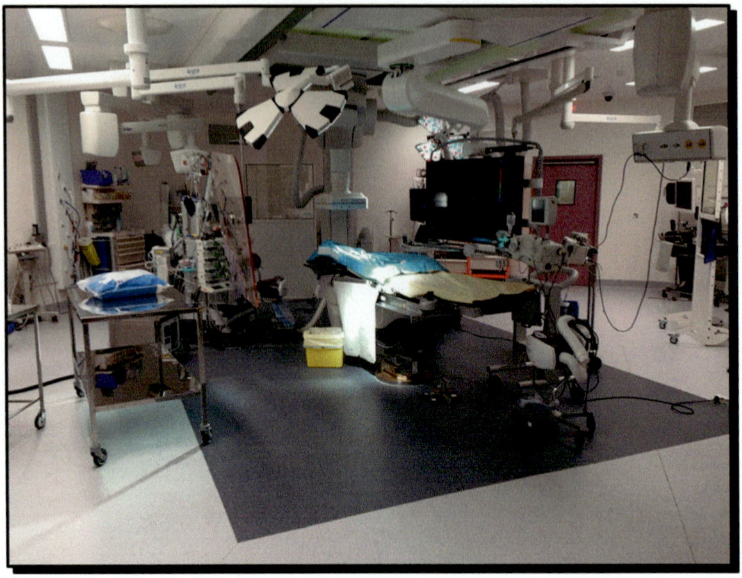

Image 2 Hybrid procedures room

Preparation of patients

In general, the preparation is similar to that used in standards operating rooms (SOR), following the usual anesthetics standards.

However, special attention should be taken to the following:

(A) **Circuits and IV infusion system**: It should be longer than usual, to allow free movement of the table and the C-arm without generating tension or accidental disconnections or extubations.
(B) **Manipulation of the table and of C-arm**: It may cause accidental extubations, clamping or withdrawal of IV infusions and, sometimes, physical injuries to the patient or the HT's members.
(C) **Intubation and central venous catheterization**: It may be difficult, in particular, if the table cannot be placed in the Trendelenburg position.
(D) **Presence of screens, echocardiography machine connections, wires and cables**: It may provoke accidents if attention is not paid (Image 3)
(E) **A protected IV access should be ensured**, and drugs/material required for resuscitation, as well as, emergency endotracheal intubation should be available.
(F) **Patients may suffer from iatrogenic arrhythmias**: due to the use of guidewires or the implantation of devices injuring the conduction system. Defibrillator paddles should be placed on the patient's chest and the defibrillator should be ready to be used.

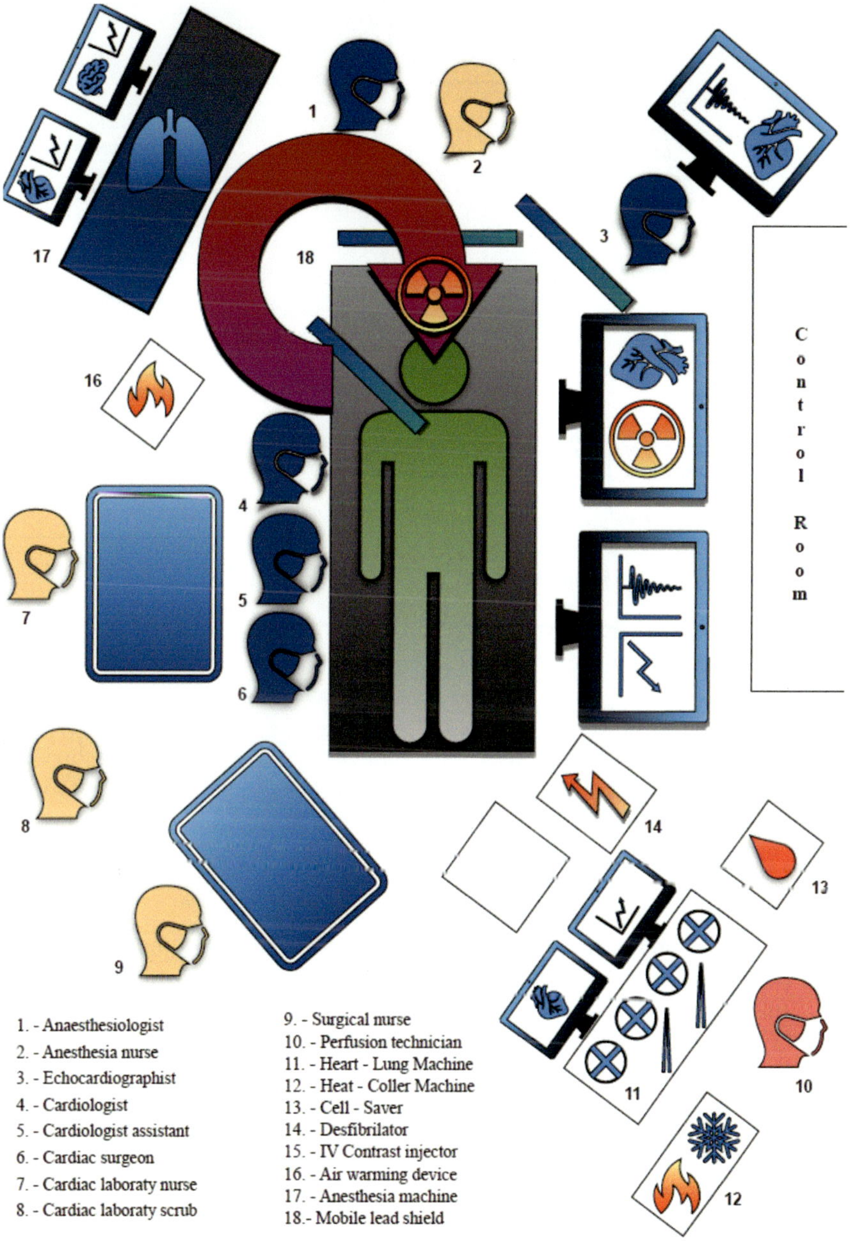

Fig. 3 HOR configuration

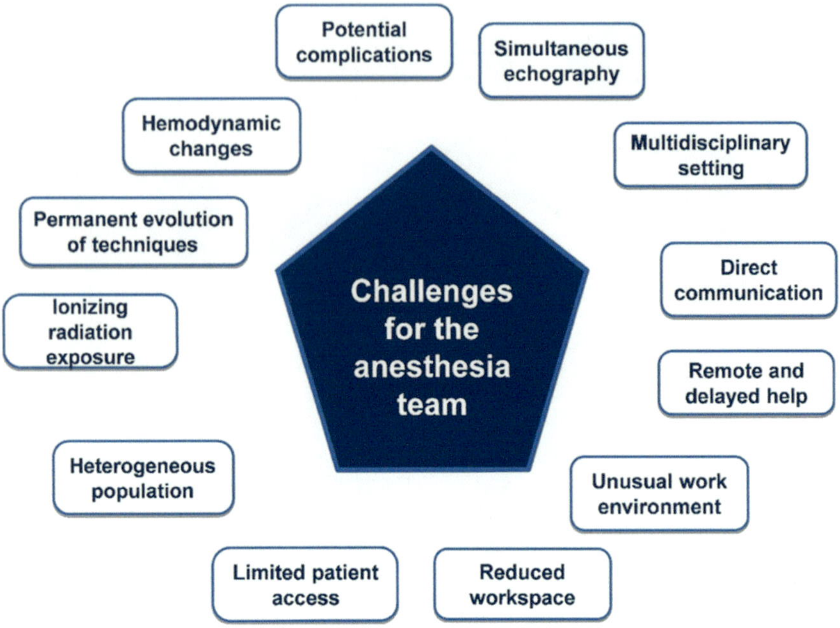

Fig. 4 Challenges for the anesthesia team HOR or CCL

(G) **Intra-arterial cannulation is indicated for**: patients undergoing high-risk procedures (on the heart left side procedures), patients with severe ventricular dysfunction, prolonged procedure or for blood gas control.
(H) **The use of local anesthetic (i.e. Lidocaine) by operators**: must always be taken into account to avoid exceeding the maximum dose recommended according to patient's weight.
(I) **Similar to the SOR**: the realization of the checklists recommended by the WHO, before start the procedure should be carried out to improve patient safety.
(J) **Crossmatch**: must be done before starting the procedure and blood products must be always available.
(K) **Anesthesiologists must be familiar with the difficult airway algorithm**: Respiratory depression is more frequent during sedation or anesthesia outside the OR.

Multidisciplinary Approach

If in the SOR the interlocution between operator and anesthesiologist is crucial, in the HOR this relationship must be even more intense, fluid and direct, the collaboration between all HT's members being essential to achieve good outcomes.

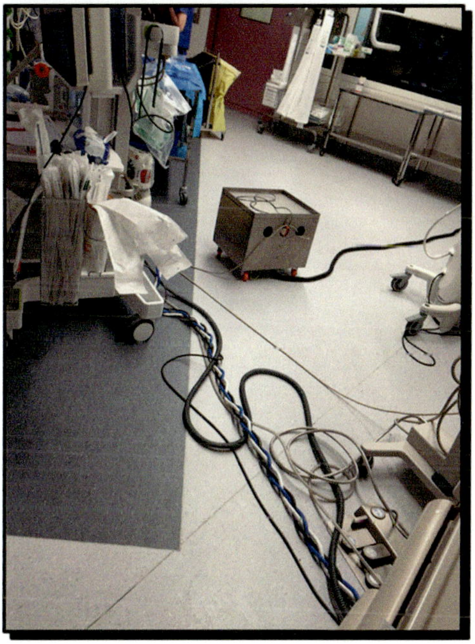

Image 3 Limited and dangerous free movement in Hybrid operating room

The selection of the anesthetic technique should be agreed among the operators, the patient and the anesthesiologist, although this will lastly be selected by the specialist.

Radiation protection

The work in the HOR or CCL implies the continuous exposure to the ionizing radiation which is used for the guidance of procedure. The anesthesiologist may be exposed even to greater radiation than the operators themselves if emergency intubation, during the administration of IV bolus or the verification of the neurological state of the patient.

To reduce the professional exposure to ionic radiation, the *ALARA principle* (*As Low As Reasonably Achievable*) should be follow. Table 1 shows the protective measures which should be implemented.

Table 1 ALARA principle (*As low as Reasonably Achievable*)

ALARA principle (As Low As Reasonably Achievable)	Prevention initiatives
Exposure time	• Reduce to the minimum • Restrictive access
Exposure distance	• It is recommended to keep a minimum distance of at least 90 cm • Doubling the source distance reduces exposure by 4 times
General measures (shielding)	• Lead aprons • Thyroid protection lead collar • Hats, gloves and lead glasses • Mobile lead acrylic screens to absorb ionic exposure by scattering
Continuous training	• Obligatory

Interventions

Transcatheter Aortic Valve Implantation (TAVI)

a. **Technical considerations**

Aortic stenosis is the most common valve heart disease requiring intervention and aortic valve replacement is the only effective therapy to reduce mortality. Since 2002, when the first TAVI was performed, this therapy has experienced a dramatic expansion, becoming one of the most frequent procedures performed in HORs and the first choice therapy for most patients with aortic stenosis.

In the last American and European Guidelines published in 2017, TAVI is recommended for patients who are at prohibitive risk or high surgical risk and is recognized as an alternative to surgery in patients considered at intermediate surgical risk. However, the recently published trials have proven the non-inferiority of TAVI in terms of mortality, stroke or rehospitalization at 1 year as compared to SAVR surgery in patients considered at low-surgical risk. Thus, TAVI will probably become the first choice therapy for aortic stenosis in a close future if the durability of transcatheter prostheses is proven to be not inferior to surgical bioprostheses.

TAVI consists of the insertion of a biological valve composed of a stent and pericardial leaflets using catheters on a beating heart. There are several types of bioprostheses;

1. Balloon-expandable valve prosthesis family (Image 4)
2. Self-expanding valves prosthesis family (Image 5)

Procedures are performed a retrograde access if the prosthesis is advanced towards the aortic ring from a peripheral arterial access, in the opposite direction to

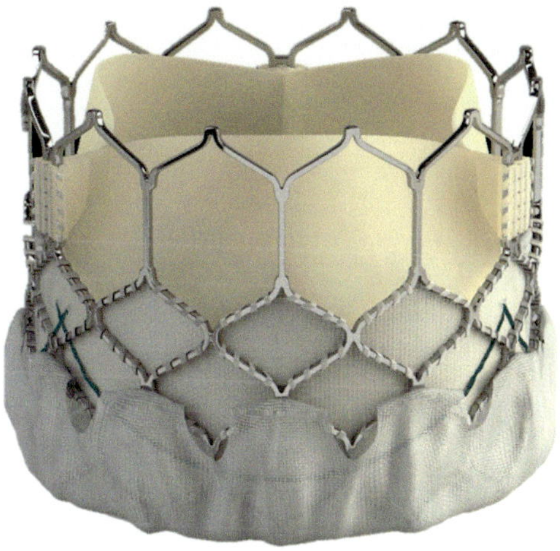

Image 4 Balloon-expandable valves family

the bloodstream, or anterograde access, in the direction of the bloodstream. In nowadays, the transfemoral access is the most frequently used (more than 90% of TAVI cases in Europe) due to its minimal invasiveness, the possibility to perform the procedure under local anesthesia/MAC and improved safety. Others retrograde accesses are the trans-subclavian, trans-carotid or trans-aortic, with greater invasiveness and therefore requires GA. The trans-apical access, which is performed using a left mini thoracotomy and puncture of the left ventricular (LV) apex, is only used in patients with no feasibility for others approaches, since it has been associated with increased mortality and morbidity.

Briefly, the steps of the procedure are as follows:

1. Obtaining the arterial access (femoral artery), which is used for pressure monitoring and IV injection of contrasts through a pigtail catheter.
2. Insertion of a temporary pacemaker through the femoral vein, positioned under fluoroscopic guide in the right ventricle (RV), which is used for the induction of pacing fast ventricular tachycardia (>160 beats/minute) during the procedure and to protect patients presenting conduction disturbances during the procedure.
3. Preparation of the primary access, which may be fully percutaneous or surgical approach.
4. Insertion of the arterial sheath, which dimensions are between 14 and 16 French
5. Crossing the aortic valve using a guidewire and a catheter and insertion of a stiff guidewire in the LV.
6. Aortic annulus dilation with balloon valvuloplasty to facilitate the insertion of the prosthesis, although this step is less frequently performed nowadays with most used prosthesis.

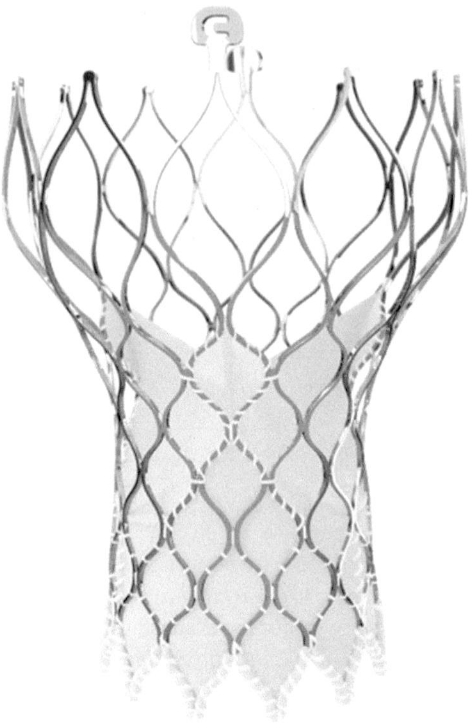

Image 5 Self-expanding prostheses family

7. Insertion of the transcatheter valve crimped on a catheter through the arterial sheath
8. Placement and deployment of the transcatheter heart valve at the level of the aortic annulus. Prosthesis are deployed:
   - With rapid and abrupt balloon swelling and rapid ventricular stimulation (more than 160 beats/minute), to decrease cardiac output and forward flow during valve deployment, in the case of balloon-self expandable prosthesis
   - Progressively in the case of the self-expanding variant; in general, without the need or minimum ventricular stimulation (less than 120 beats/minute)
9. Evaluation of results (gradients, leaks and prosthesis orientation) by echocardiography and angiography, identification of potential complications
10. Retrieval of material and closing of arterial accesses
11. Transfer to critical/intermediate care unit for monitoring for at least 24 hours

Even if TAVI has become a safe procedure, potential life-threatening complications may occur (Table 2), in this case, it's advisable to have always a cardiopulmonary bypass or an ECMO circuit prepared and available to use in the room. These complications should be anticipated and rapidly treated.

b. **Anesthetic considerations**

Different aspects are relevant for anesthesiologists involved in these procedures:

- These patients usually suffer from numerous concomitant diseases, which imply a high risk of complications.
- The age of patients undergoing TAVI is constantly increasing and it is no longer rare to face patients 85 years of age or older.
- Due to a minimalist approach to the TAVI procedure, the anesthetic management has also been progressively modified, going from a procedure that required a systematically GA towards a less invasive approach (without invasive monitoring, endotracheal intubation …) associated with moderate conscious sedation and subcutaneous infiltration of local anesthetics

The preferred anesthetic technique (Fig. 5) will depend on the patient's clinical status, access selected, expected complexity and duration of the procedure. In patients with no tolerance to supine decubitus position for a prolonged period (i.e.

Table 2 Perioperative complications of TAVI

Perioperative complications	Signs/symptoms	Image diagnosis
Severe aortic regurgitation	Low diastolic pressure	Echocardiography Fluoroscopy
Coronary occlusion	Thoracic pain, ventricular dysfunction	ECG Fluoroscopy
Stroke	Hemiplegia, aphasia, headache, vomiting and loss of consciousness	Positron emission tomography scan
Device embolization[a]	Hypotension	Echocardiography Fluoroscopy
Pericardial effusion/ Tamponade	Hypotension	Echocardiography
Rupture of the aortic annulus	Hypotension, Thoracic pain	Echocardiography Fluoroscopy
Atrioventricular conduction defects/ arrhythmias	High degree atrioventricular block, atrial fibrillation	ECG Fluoroscopy
Severe paravalvular leaks	Low diastolic pressure	Echocardiography Fluoroscopy
Vascular complications[b]	Hematoma, bleeding, abdominal pain, anemia,	Echocardiography Fluoroscopy

[a]Ventricular or Aortic ascending device embolization
[b]Aortic dissection, retroperitoneal bleeding or femoral arterial occlusion

decompensated heart failure or severe lung disease), non-collaborating patients or at high risk for periprocedural complications and pregnant women or patients with a programmed intervention through a surgical access, a GA with orotracheal intubation is indicated.

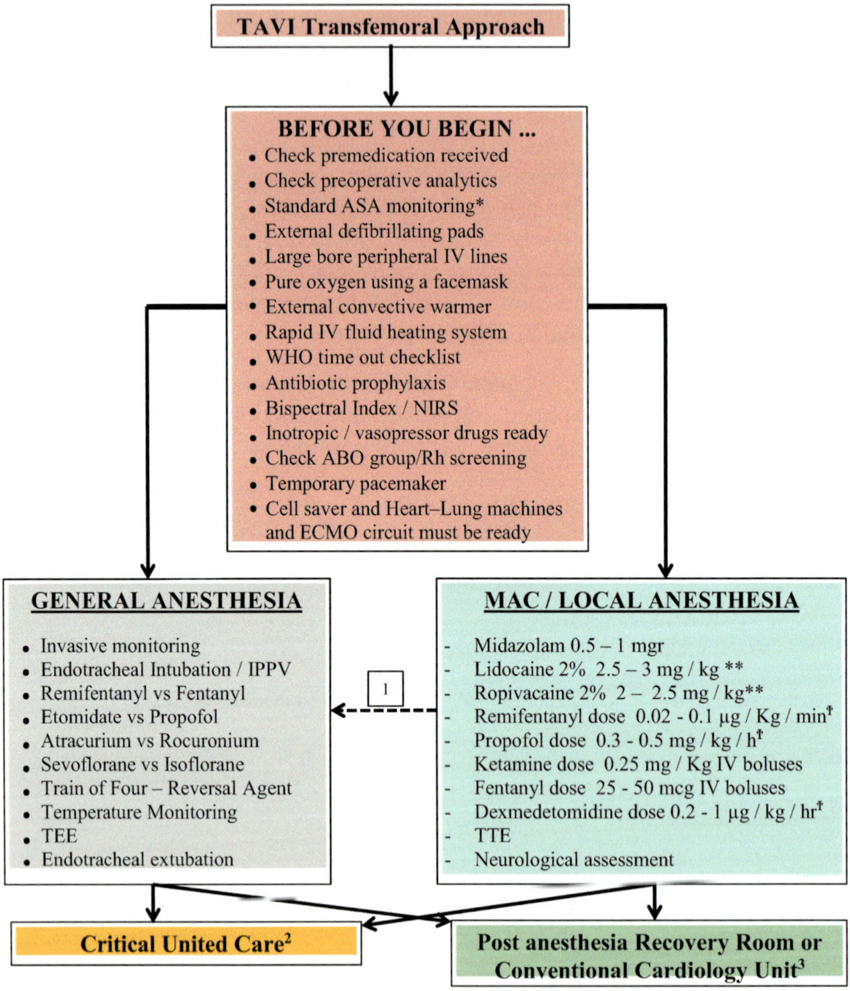

** Continuous peripheral pulse oximetry, heart rate, respiratory rate, exhaled CO_2 and noninvasive blood pressure every 3 – 5 minutes*

† Titrated to effect by TCI system

*** Ultrasound guided Ileo-inguinal and Ileo-hypogastric blocks and grow infiltration in the side arm of the femoral arterial sheath*

1 Emergency surgical conversion

2 In case of perioperative complications

3 Without perioperative complications

Fig. 5 Anesthetic's considerations for TAVI transfemoral approach

The usual anesthetic's drugs recommended are: Propofol or Etomidate as hypnotics, depending on the stability of the patient and ventricular function, Remifentanil as opioid and Atracurium or Rocuronium, for neuromuscular blockade at usual doses. Although the GA might have several advantages such as the protection of the airway, an increased comfort for the patient and the operator, facilitates the use of TEE and avoids potential movements of patients, MAC, conscious sedation and local or locoregional anesthesia are preferred for transfemoral approach in agreement with the current trend towards a minimalist approach of TAVI (Table 3). Ultrasound guided regional techniques, such as ileo-inguinal and ileo-hypogastric blocks with the use local anesthetic drugs, associated with infiltration subcutaneous in the puncture area of the catheters are frequently used.

Unlike GA, sedation allows for the immediate detection of acute neurological events, increases patient satisfaction, shortens the duration of the act and is less hypotensive requiring less frequently hemodynamic support with drugs. Indeed, in a recent study in the USA, sedation was associated with a shorter stay in the ICU, less inotropic requirements, lower 30-day mortality and lower risk of stroke compared to GA. However, the team should be ready to conversion to GA if necessary and this anesthetic technique does not allow for TEE for long time.

Regardless of the technique used, anesthetic management is similar to that of patients undergoing open-heart surgery. Briefly, the objectives are:

- To avoid prolonged tachycardia to allow an optimal coronary filling
- To ensure stable mean arterial pressure (>75 mmHg) with conserved peripheral resistance to favor coronary perfusion
- To ensure an accurate preload and ventricular contractility
- To keep sinus cardiac rhythm, reducing to minimum the duration of cardiac arrhythmias which may be poorly tolerated

Table 3 Minimalist approach of TAVI

Advantages	Disadvantages
– Use of MAC – Minimal conscious sedation – Verbal contact with the patient throughout the procedure – Transthoracic echocardiography – Minimal invasive devices[a] – Shorter length of procedure – Shorter length of hostipal stay – Same day ambulation – Lower cost – Increased patients satisfaction – Minimized use of inotropes	• Requires high HT's experience • Only in selected patients[b] • Favorable anatomic/technical aspects • No use of TEE • Worse evaluation of the degree of PVL[c] • Risk of oversedation/hypercarbia • Unprotected airway • Conversion to GA if complications • Patients with anticipated difficult airway • Patient discomfort/movement

[a]No Foley catheter, non-endotracheal intubation, no arterial or central line
[b]Contraindicated in extreme obesity, mental disorder, chronic backpain, inability to tolerate supine position, barriers to communication or pregnant patients
[c]PVL Paravalvular leak

- In our center, 70 IU/kg of unfractionated heparin is usually administered after the installation of the sheath; the patient is heparinized to obtain an ACT greater than 250 seconds. The anesthesiologist should regularly check that this value is maintained until prostheses implantation; after implantation of the prosthesis, the partial or complete reversion of heparin by protamine should be a decision agreed with the operator.

Finally, it is highly recommended to have a large-bore peripheral venous inserted, a rapid infusion heating system, several pacemakers devices, a cell-saver machine, air heating system and a defibrillator. NIRS might be useful if surgical access is performed, in particular, if trans-carotid approach is used.

Transcatheter Mitral Valve Implantation (TMVI)

Several studies have demonstrated the feasibility and safety of TMVI using transcatheter heart valves for aortic procedures in selected patients with failing previous bioprostheses (valve-in-valve) or rings (valve-in-ring) or mitral annulus calcification (valve-in-MAC).

This intervention may be performed using either the biatrial trans-septal approach, which is the prefered one, or through a trans-apical approach. GA with endotracheal intubation is necessary because this procedure is performed under 2D and 3D TEE guidance. Challenges of TMVI are the complexity of mitral anatomy, the close anatomical relationship with the LV outflow tract, valve positioning, valve sizing and the risk of valve thrombosis. Several potentially deadly complications may occur during these procedures. The risk of LV outflow tract obstruction and valve migration merit to be mentioned. Although this therapy is still at an early stage of development, this technology is expected to become a therapeutic alternative for the treatment of MR in the close future.

Percutaneous Mitral Valve Repair

The percutaneous edge-to-edge mitral valve repair with MitraClip® System (Abbott Laboratories, Menlo Park, California, USA) is commercialized in Europe since 2008 and in the USA since 2013 for the treatment of primary mitral regurgitation. Since 2019, it has also obtained the FDA approval for the treatment of secondary mitral regurgitation.

The MitraClip® system (Image 6) is a device for percutaneous edge-to-edge reconstruction of the mitral valve in patients with severe mitral regurgitation who are deemed at high risk for surgery. Usually, the procedure has low rates of periprocedural complications and generates a significant reduction in the degree of mitral regurgitation, as well as an improvement in the patient's functional capacity.

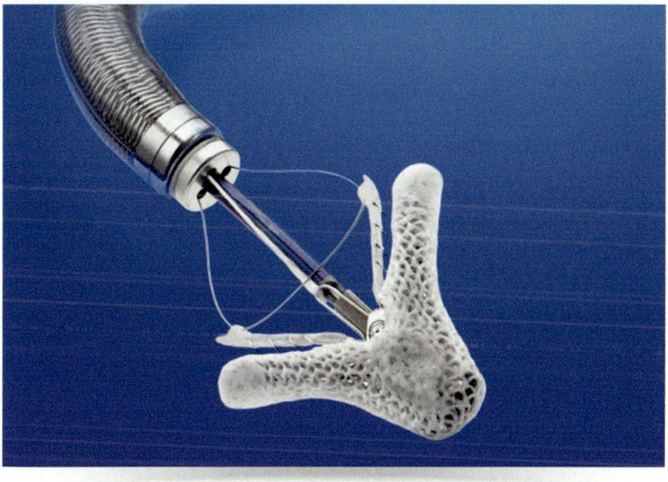

Image 6 MitraClip system

This device approximates the free edges of the median portions of anterior and posterior leaflets creating a double hole, likewise the Alfieri's surgical technique. A new device has been developed, although it has not yet been commercialized in most countries.

European Guidelines recommend percutaneous edge-to-edge mitral procedure to be considered in patients with symptomatic severe primary MR who meet the echocardiographic eligibility criteria and are judged inoperable or at high surgical risk by the HT. Although this therapy can improve symptoms and provide a reversal of LV remodeling, the rate of residual MR in the 5-years follow-up is higher in the percutaneous edge-to-edge repair group compared to the surgical repair group.

The procedure begins with the biatrial transeptal puncture, which is performed under TEE and fluoroscopic guidance. Once the access to the left atrium (LA) is ensured, the catheter on which the device is mounted is inserted and advanced through the inferior vena cava, the RA and the interatrial septum towards the LA. Then, the catheter is aligned with the mitral regurgitant jet and advanced through the mitral valve towards the LV, just below the edges of the leaflet intended to approach with the open arms oriented perpendicularly to the mitral leaflets coaptation plane. The system is progressively retrieved to the LA and free edges of the mitral leaflets, usually A_2 and P_2, are captured with grippers. When this is confirmed by 2D and 3D TEE, the clip is definitely closed. An extensive TEE evaluation is performed to confirm the reduction of mitral regurgitation, the absence of significant mitral gradient and the capture of both leaflets. If this is confirmed, the leaflet is released.

Usually, the anesthetic technique involves a GA with endotracheal intubation and controlled ventilation due to prolonged use of TEE, the poor clinical status of the candidates and the need for repeated and prolonged apneas, which may be required to favor the capture of the mitral leaflets. It is recommended low tidal volume ventilation, which is compensated with an increase of respiratory rate, to reduce lung movements and facilitate leaflets capture. An invasive arterial monitoring may be recommended.

The following technical points have to be kept in mind:

- MitraClip® system is performed by femoral venous access instead of arterial as TAVI, and, therefore, the risk of bleeding and hematoma at the puncture site is lower than TAVI.
- The biatrial transseptal puncture, despite it is performed under TEE guidance, may be complicated may be complicated with a cardiac tamponade.
- The procedure usually requires maximum muscle relaxation due to the prolonged use of TEE and to avoid any spontaneous movement during leaflets capture.
- Since a catheter is placed in the LA, it is required the administration of higher doses of unfractioned heparin than TAVI, to keep an ACT > 300 seconds.
- Sometimes, the operators may require a certain degree of bradycardia to more easily capture the mitral leaflets, which is achieved with the administration of adenosine that can generate extreme bradycardia or with Valsalva maneuvers; the anesthesiologist must ensure a preload, contractility and afterload preserved through the procedure.

Percutaneous Closure of Left Atrial Appendage

In patients with non-valvular atrial fibrillation, the left atrial appendage (LAA) is the most common source of thrombus formation, which may a which may cause a systemic embolism or a stroke. Chronic anticoagulation therapy is necessary to minimize the risk of neurologic ischemic events. However, in a significant proportion of patients, a prolonged anticoagulation may be contraindicated due to a high risk of bleeding, poor adherence to medical treatment or occurrence of neurological ischemic events despite an optimal level of anticoagulation. For these patients, the percutaneous exclusion of LAA may be recommended.

There are several types of LAA closure devices, most of them composed of nitinol. As for previous therapies, the closure device is folded into a catheter which is advanced endovascularly from the femoral vein towards the LA through the interatrial septum. Therefore, 2D and 3D TEE guidance is usually used for confirmation of the absence of thrombi in the LAA before procedures, determinate LAA size, guidance of the biatrial transseptal puncture, positioning of device, the evaluation of final result and the detection of peridevice leaks and complications. Potential complications are: cardiac tamponade, neurological events, transient myocardial ischemia due to gas embolism, transient arrhythmias and device embolization.

As previously describe, since TEE is used, GA is generally recommended, although in selected cases it can be performed with conscious sedation and non-invasive ventilation. Once the procedure is completed, most patients may be extubated on mobile table with no complications; the patients are transferred to the standard recovery room.

Percutaneous Closure of Patent Foramen Ovale and Atrial Septal Defects

Patent Foramen Ovale

The patent foramen ovale (PFO) is a residual opening of the secondary septum of the interatrial septum, which allows blood flow from the RA to the left side of the heart during fetal development. After birth, with the initiation of inspiration, the PFO is progressively closed, which is completed in the first year of life. However, in 25–30% of the population, the PFO can persist open. Although this mainly results in a left to right shunt, in conditions of increased pressure in the RA, a right to left shunt may occur which has been associated with cryptogenic stroke, arterial desaturation, and migraines.

TEE allows the diagnosis of PFOs employing the doppler-color mode through the defect in patients with larger PFOs or using agitated saline solution which is injected through a venous access with a simultaneous Valsalva maneuver. TEE is also used for procedural guidance, although the procedure may be guided by intracardiac echocardiography or by fluoroscopy. In our institution, we use TEE with a probe of small caliber which only allows for 2D images, with greater tolerance and comfort for patients (Image 7), using a using remifentanil by target controlled infusion (TCI) system at usual dose.

The PFO occluders are generally double disc self-expanding devices (Image 8). Catheters are advanced through a right femoral venous approach to the inferior vena cava until reaching the RA. After crossing the PFO, the preselected occluder device is implanted with the left disc in the left side of interatrial septum and the right disc in the right side. Once installed, the stability of the device is verified by slight traction of the device (Minnesota maneuver), and if it is confirmed the device is delivered. Then, a transthoracic echocardiography evaluation is performed to identify the presence of leaks or complications. The rate of perioperative complications is very low, with the most important ones: vascular complications, residual leaks, embolization of the device, arrhythmias, erosion or drilling of the interatrial septum and pericardial tamponade.

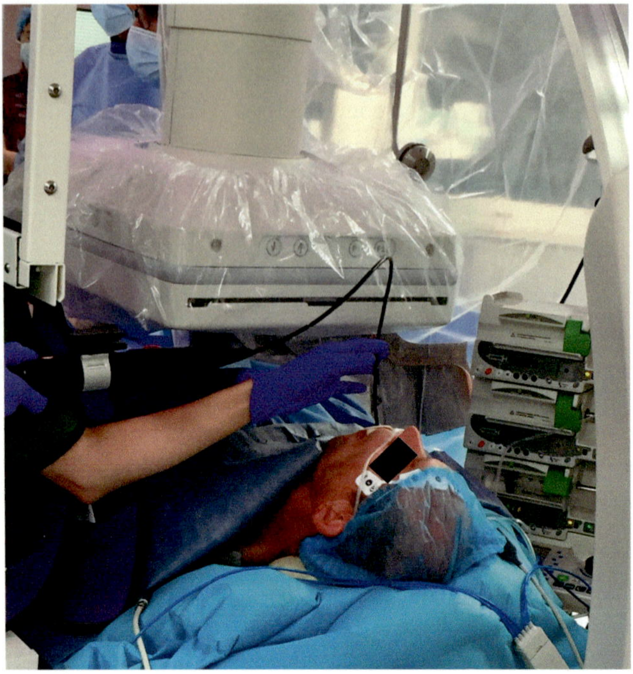

Image 7 TEE probe of small caliber

Percutaneous Closure of Atrial Septal Defects (ASD)

Indications for the ASD closure include an evidence of an overload of the RV volume with a pulmonary/systemic blood flow ratio >1.5 before the development of significant pulmonary hypertension, paradoxical embolism, orthodoxy, and platypnea.

Simple fluoroscopy, 2D and 3D TEE, or intracardiac echocardiography (ICE), all of them are used to guide the deployment of the ASD closure device and to confirm the results. Also, TEE allows determining the defect size inflating a very compliant balloon until complete flow occlusion, morphology, and localization of the defect. 3-D TEE may be more accurate for sizing the percutaneous closure device and reduce the risk of residual shunt after closure when compared with conventional 2-D TEE. Major complications, including arrhythmias and device embolism requiring surgical removal.

The technique of percutaneous closure of ASD is similar to that of PFO. Percutaneous PFO and ASD closures are usually performed under GA. Deep IV

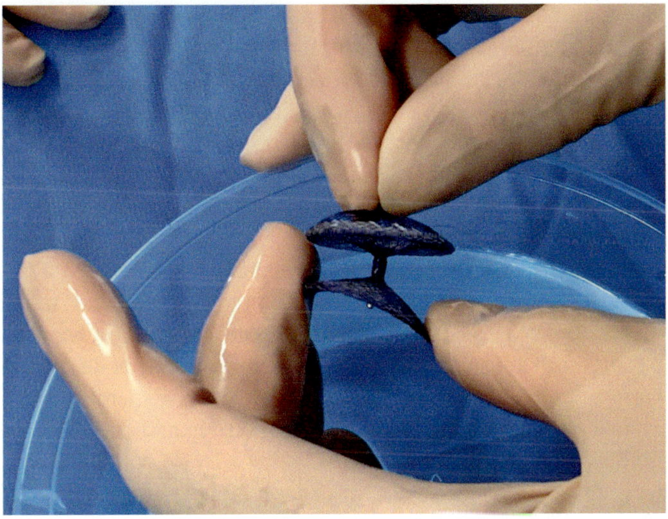

Image 8 Patent foramen ovale occluder

sedation by Propofol or Remifentanil by TCI system, with the adjuvant use of Midazolam may be used if ICE may be enough to guide the procedure.

When performing this procedure, the anesthesiologist should consider the following:

- Make a meticulous evaluation in the pre-anesthesia consultation with assessment of functional and clinical status and analysis of echocardiographic parameters including the size of the defect, the direction of blood through the shunt and its consequences: i.e. RV dilatation and dysfunction (left-to right shunt) or presence of arterial derangement and basal hypoxemia (right to left shunt)
- Ensure the absence of any air bubble in the IV lines due to the risk of systemic paradoxical embolisms. The use of filters in infusions is recommended, as well as the revision of the lines before induction.

The anesthetic management will depend on the shunt's directions:

- Right-to left shunts => it causes hypoxia. Circumstances increasing the pulmonary vascular resistances (i.e. acidosis, hypoxia, …) and reducing the systemic vascular resistances should be avoided since this would increase the degree of shunt
- Left-to right shunts => it causes RV overload. Circumstances increasing systemic vascular resistances (i.e. pain, awareness, arterial hypertension …) and reducing pulmonary vascular resistances should be avoided.
- Bidirectional shunt => right to left shunt should be minimized.

To reduce pulmonary vascular resistances, anesthesiologist should optimize perioperative ventilation, with hyperoxia and moderate hypocarbia as the objectives, since they are potent pulmonary vasodilators. Also, selective pulmonary vasodilators such as nitric oxide or prostaglandins may be administered.

In addition, a right to left shunt can be reduced by increasing the LA pressure with active support of systemic vascular resistances by using selective systemic vasoconstrictor drug assuming an adequate function of the mitral valve without increasing the pulmonary vascular resistances. It should be considered during anesthetic induction, maintenance and on awaking.

Both, systemic vascular resistances and pulmonary vascular resistances are extremely sensitive to the medications used, in particular, IV hypnotics and vasoconstrictors, to mechanical ventilation (pressure control mode generates more changes than volume control mode), and to the F_iO_2 (hyperoxia decreases pulmonary vascular resistances increasing right to left shunts) and the exhaled CO_2. The objective is to minimize changes in pulmonary vascular resistances while slightly increasing systemic vascular resistances. Therefore, drugs resulting in a prolonged increase in systemic vascular resistances should be avoided should be avoided, due the risk of increasing left to tight shunt. A certain degree of tachycardia is recommended to protect RV.

A judicious assessment of intravascular volume, the correct choice of anesthetics and avoiding hypoxia and hypercapnia, are some important management strategies in these patients.

Conclusion

The cardiac anesthetists are converting their habits to adapt to the increased demand generated by the development of the new percutaneous cardiac procedures. Despite the development of HOR has allowed that conditions are closer to SOR, the work in these rooms remain a continuous challenge due to the specific nature of the rooms, the interventions and patients treated.

To successfully work in these procedures, anesthesiologists must carefully plan his approach which must suit the needs of the patient and the operator, anticipate satisfactory solutions to complications, adapt to teamwork and follow each step of the procedure.

The knowledge and understanding of each step of these procedures and maintaining a fluid and direct communication with all HT's members are crucial to provide a high level of anesthetic care and maintain patient safety.

Different types of procedure may be performed and a wide variability of patients are treated. Thus, an initial anesthetic technique may vary from MAC, conscious sedation to GA, although the anesthesiologist must be always ready to convert to emergency GA at any time.

Recommended Readings

1. Braithwait S, et al. Anaesthesia in the cardiac catheterization laboratory. Curr Opin Anaesthesiol. 2010;23:507–12.
2. Apfelbaum JL, et al. Practice guidelines for management of the difficult airway: an updated report by the American Society of Anesthesiologists Task Force on Management of the Difficult Airway. Anesthesiology 2013;98:1269–77.
3. Hayman M, et al. Anesthesia for interventional cardiology. J Cardiothorac Vasc Anesth. 2012;26(1):134–47.
4. Hami H, et al. Anesthesia for cardiac catheterization procedures. Heart Lung Vessels. 2014;6 (4):225–31.
5. Iung B, et al. Recommendations on the management of the asymptomatic patient with valvular heart disease. Eur Heart J. 2002;23(16):1253–66.
6. Wolkmar F, et al. ESC/EACTS Guidelines for the management of valvular heart disease. Eur J Cardiothorac Surg. 2017;52(2017):616–64.
7. Mack MJ, et al. Transcatheter aortic-valve replacement with a balloon-expandable valve in low-risk patient. N Eng J Med. 2019;380:1695–705.
8. Popma JJ, et al. Transcatheter aortic-valve replacement with a self-expanding valve in low-risk patients. N Engl J Med. 2019;380:1706–15.
9. Tchetche D, et al. How to make the TAVI pathway more efficient. Interv Cardiol Rev. 2019;14(1):31–3.
10. Rajkumar DR, et al. In-hospital outcomes comparison of transfemoral vs transapical transcatheter aortic valve replacement in propensity-matched cohorts with severe aortic stenosis. Clin Cardiol. 2018;41:326–32.
11. Urena M, et al. Transseptal transcatheter mitral valve replacement using balloon-expandable transcatheter heart valves: a step-by-step approach. JACC Cardiovasc Interv. 2017;10 (19):1905–19.
12. Feldman T, et al. Randomized comparison of percutaneous repair and surgery for mitral regurgitation: 5-year results of EVEREST II. J Am Coll Cardiol. 2015;66:2844–54.

Postoperative Care

Basic Concepts of Critical Care Following Cardiac Surgery

Olga de la Varga Martínez, Mario Lorenzo-López, and Eduardo Tamayo Gómez

Introduction

Cardiac surgical critical care is emerging as an important sub-especiality in critical care medicine. The use of cardiopulmonary bypass (CBP) distinguishes cardiac surgery from other types of surgery, and it also introduces a unique set of potential postoperative complications. Some of them could be vasospasm, altered platelet-endothelial cell interactions, and a generalized inflammatory response.

As the population ages and care becomes more sophisticated, cardiac surgery is being performed on older, sicker and more complicated patients. At the same time, cardiac surgery has evolved introducing new techniques such as the mechanical circulatory support devices and the minimally invasive surgical techniques. Regardless of the procedure performed, successful outcomes depend also on optimal postoperative care in the ICU. Some of the avoidable deaths in cardiac surgery patients have been related to postoperative problems in the ICU. Currently, Fast-track protocols use short-acting anesthetics, judicious narcotics, and relative normothermia to facilitate rapid extubation and transfer out of the ICU in a relatively short time (24–48 h).

O. de la Varga Martínez (✉)
Department of Anesthesiology & Critical Care Medicine,, Infanta Leonor, Madrid, Spain

M. Lorenzo-López · E. Tamayo Gómez
Department of Anesthesiology & Critical Care Medicine, Clinico Valladolid, Valladolid, Spain
e-mail: eduardo.tamayo@uva.es

M. Vives and A. Hernandez (eds.), *Cardiac Anesthesia and Postoperative Care in the 21st Century*, https://doi.org/10.1007/978-3-030-79721-8_22

Monitoring and Initial Studies

The first critical phase of postoperative care stars during transfer from the operating room to the intensive care unit. During the transfer there are potential problems with airway and ventilation, sudden hypertension and hypotension, arrhythmias, bleeding, problems with the catheters and the drug infusion pumps. The patient must be monitored at all times, ventilation is provided by a manual resuscitator bag connected to a portable oxygen bank and cardiac medications should be available.

Upon arrival in the ICU, routine monitoring following cardiac surgery typically includes continuous ECG monitoring, pulse oximetry, invasive arterial blood pressure monitoring and temperature. A central venous catheter is necessary for administration of vasoactive medications and also allows measurement of central venous pressure (CVP). In the majority of patients, routine placement of a pulmonary artery catheter (PAC) is not required. PAC allows us to measure the pressures in the pulmonary artery, determine the filling of the left ventricle and the Cardiac Index (CI). Most PACs are removed within 12–24 h of surgery if significant vasopressor, vasodilator, or inotropic therapy is no longer required.

On arrival to the ICU, it is recommended to obtain a 12-lead ECG as it is more sensitive for the detection of ischemia. A chest radiograph is commonly obtained at ICU admission to exclude pneumothorax or hemothorax and to confirm endotracheal tube position, vascular catheter, and device placement such as intra-aortic balloon pump. The patient should be examined thoroughly (heart, lungs and peripheral perfusion) and the pacemaker should be checked.

Chest tubes are connected to a drainage system at -20 cm of H_2O. Active clearance of chest tube has been associated with reduced postoperative complications (including postoperative atrial fibrillation and pleural effusion) and costs after cardiac surgery in a prospective cohort study. Milking or stripping the tubes for preventing blood clotting is not recommended. Chest tubes can be removed when total drainage is less than 200 ml during the last 4 h. Urinary catheters are essential to monitor urine output (Table 1).

Initial laboratory studies should include arterial blood gas analysis, hemoglobin, platelet count, serum electrolytes, serum creatinine and coagulation parameters. The analysis of mixed venous saturation defines the balance between the supply of oxygen and its consumption, and together with lactic acid allows us to evaluate the adequateness of tissue perfusion. Immediate postoperative troponin levels are rarely informative, however, persistent troponin elevation 24 h postoperatively is associated with a higher cardiac mortality. Most experts maintain serum glucose between 140 and 180 mg/dL (7.8 and 10 mmol/L) during the period following cardiac surgery, since hyperglycemia is associated with worse outcomes in this population.

Table 1 Evaluation of the patient in the intensive care unit

1. Patient's data ______
2. Allergies ______
3. Surgical intervention ______
4. Monitoring: a. • Endotracheal tube connected to mechanical ventilation. b. • ECG, pulse oximetry, blood pressure, pulmonary artery pressure and cardiac output. Patient examination. c. • Raise the head of the bed 30°. d. • Intra-aortic Ballon pump. Check distal pulses. e. • Chest tubes placed to wall suction. Bleeding monitoring ______ f. • Urinary catheters. Output urine monitoring ______
5. Hemodynamic management: a. Vascular access ______ b. Intravenous fluid therapy ______ c. Inotrope and vasopressor support ______ d. Vasodilators infusions ______ e. Antiarrhythmics ______
6. Sedative infusions ______ 7. Analgesics ______
8. Anticoagulant therapy ______ 9. Antiplatelet therapy ______ 10. Thromboembolic prophylaxis ______
11. Gastrointestinal / Nutrition: a. Gastric protector ______ b. • Absolute diet c. • Oral tolerance d. • Nasogastric tube
12. Antibiotic prophylaxis ______
13. Pacemaker a. Mode: • Atrial • VVI • DDD • DVI b. Frequency ______ c. Sensitivity ______ d. • Off
14. • Chest radiograph
15. • Laboratory studies

Hemodinamic Management

The myocardial function after a period of cardioplegic arrest could be depressed temporarily due to ischemia and reperfusion injury, which may cause a reduction in the ejection fraction (EF) between 10 and 15%. The evaluation of the different pressures, cardiac index and systemic vascular resistance allows an appropriate

Table 2 Treatment of hemodynamic problems

Blood pressure	Pulmonary artery occlusion pressure	Cardiac index	Systemic vascular resistances	Treatment plan
↓	↓	↓	↓	Fluid
N	↑	N	↑	Venodilators/Diuretics
↓	↑	↓	↑	Inotropics
↑	↑	↓	↑	Vasodilators
↑↓	↑	↓	↑	Inotropic/Casodilators/ Intra-aortic balloon pump
↓	N	N ↑	↓	α-Adrenergic

selection of the fluids, inotropes and vasodilators, to optimize preload, afterload and contractility (Table 2).

Hemodynamic management of postoperative cardiac patients requires integration of hemodynamic, clinical, and laboratory data and interpretation of those data within the overall clinical context. Commonly targeted hemodynamic variables include blood pressure, indices of preload, and assessments of cardiac function and cardiac index. The overall goal for hemodynamic management is to maintain an adequate organ/tissue perfusion and oxygen delivery.

Blood Pressure

Blood pressure is a poor indicator of systemic perfusion and cannot be used as a hemodynamic goal in isolation. A mean arterial pressure (MAP) around 60–90 mmHg is a reasonable target. A lower MAP may be desirable in the face of poor ventricular function, mitral repair surgery, vulnerable aortic suture lines, or active bleeding. Postoperative hypertension is common and it may decrease stroke volume and increase myocardial oxygen demand. Hypertension may be caused by systemic vasoconstriction related to hypothermia induced during bypass.

Preload

Optimum cardiac function requires optimum cardiac preload. The best measure of left ventricular preload is the left ventricular end diastolic volume (LVEDV). It can be estimated by echocardiography or by pulmonary artery occlusion pressure. Left ventricular preload may be inadequate during the immediate postoperative period secondary to a loss of vasomotor tone, increased capillary permeability, intraoperative and postoperative blood loss, or high urine output due to hypothermia. For assessing fluid responsiveness, dynamic values of preload evaluation are most useful. These includes pulse pressure variation (PPV) on positive pressure ventilation and stroke volume variation (SVV), whose value above 11% is indicative of responsive to fluids. However, these techniques require controlled mechanical ventilation, normal right ventricle function, sinus rhythm, and they are inaccurate in patients with open chests.

Cardiac Output and Venous Oxygen Saturation

Thermodilution is the gold standard for cardiac output measurement along with the echocardiographic evaluation. The objective is to maintain a cardiac index more than 2.2 L/min/m^2 to ensure adequate tissue oxygenation, which can be assessed by mixed venous oxygen saturation (S_vO_2), based on the Fick principle. S_vO_2 greater than 65% is generally reassuring.

Laboratory Studies

Lactate is the best marker of impaired perfusion, levels above 2 mmol/L can identify patients with occult hypoperfusion, and its slow clearance is predictive of complications in the postoperative period.

Fluid Resuscitation

Fluid resuscitation is the first line treatment in hemodynamic instability. The need for volume replacement may be caused by blood loss, vascular permeability impairment secondary to ischemia–reperfusion injuries and increased vascular capacitance due to overheating. The fluids of choice for replacement are crystalloids, specially buffered balanced salt solutions such as Lactated Ringer's solution or Plasmalyte. Its administration must be done carefully, since in excess it can contribute to heart failure, pulmonary edema, hemodilution and increased requirements for transfusion, intestinal dysfunction and prolonged hospital stay. Hypotension refractory to fluid administration is a trigger for ruling out causes of low-cardiac output syndrome such as active bleeding, tension pneumothorax, cardiac tamponade or LV/RV systolic impairment.

Inotropes and Vasopressor Support

Many patients need inotropes or vasopressor support after separation of the CPB due to LV/RV systolic impairment and/or low systemic vascular resistance. Commonly used inotropic catecholamines include norepinephrine, dobutamine and epinephrine. Phosphodiesterase (PDEI) inhibitors, such as milrinone, amrinone, and enoximone, are another important type of inotropes, as well as the calcium sensitizer levosimendan, although current data do not yet support the beneficial effect on mortality. Levosimendan is not approved in the United States and there are cases associated with increased bleeding. Situations with excessive vasodilation or hypotension induced by inodilators, vasopressors may be useful. Inotropes may increase myocardial oxygen demand and they may be arrhythmogenic. High doses of vasopressors can cause ischemia in the peripheral and splanchnic areas.

Vasodilators

Vasodilators are useful for lowering blood pressure. Hypertension may increase cardiac afterload, enhance hemorrhage and threaten surgical anastomoses. They may also be used for cardiac preload (venodilators) or afterload (arterial vasodilators) reduction, for increasing stroke volume and for preventing coronary vasospasm. Given their short half-life, nitroglycerin and nitroprusside are first choice, although they may worsen hypoxemia by antagonizing hypoxemic pulmonary vasoconstriction. Nicardipine is an alternative, but it has a longer half-life, while clevidipine is a rapid-onset and ultra-short half-life calcium channel blocker that is rapidly hydrolyzed by plasma and tissue esterases.

Management and Prophylaxis of Arrhythmias

The trauma of cardiac surgery predisposes patients to atrial and ventricular arrhythmias, most commonly after valvular procedures. Atrial fibrillation can occur in 30–40% of patients, and may cause a 15–25% reduction in cardiac output due to atrioventricular asynchrony. Advanced age, sleep apnea, previous arrhythmias or congestive heart failure and long cardiopulmonary bypass (CPB) courses are risk factors for atrial arrhythmias. Hypothermia, electrolyte abnormalities, myocardial irritation, atrial distension and proarrhythmic drugs are also risk factors. Prophylaxis can decrease the prevalence of atrial fibrillation by almost 50%. In patients without the need for inotropic support, beta-blockers provide anti-ischemic and antiarrhythmic therapies. In patients with decreased cardiac function, agents with less negative inotropic effect, such as amiodarone, may be more adequate. Amiodarone is useful for pharmacological cardioversion, but hemodynamic instability requires immediate cardioversion. Ventricular arrhythmias are rare and may be caused by acute ischemia.

Bradycardia

Bradyarrhythmias are particularly common after valve surgery and are probably a consequence of direct surgical injury and local edema. If the bradycardia is symptomatic, temporary electrical pacing may be required. In some cases, permanent pacing may be necessary.

Sedation, Pain Control and Delirium

The adequate control of sedation and analgesia are fundamental elements in the postoperative care of cardiac surgery. The majority of patients arrive intubated in the ICU and usually remain anesthetized and under the influence of different drugs, such as neuromuscular blockers, with sedation remaining until the end or reversal of its effect. When early release of the respirator is anticipated, the use of short-acting sedatives such as propofol is indicated, which allows faster postoperative extubation than a combination of infusions of fentanyl and midazolam. Dexmedetomidine has both sedative and analgesic action, and also allows conscious sedation while the patient remains intubated, but should be used with caution because it can cause bradycardia and hypotension. Benzodiazepines should be avoided since they stimulate the appearance of delirium. Other causes of delirium include the use of fixations and invasive devices for a long time that impede the mobility of patients. Most deliriums are hypoactive and are often underdiagnosed. Early mobilization is one of the best prevention strategies along with conscious sedation with dexmedetomidine. Delirium may be treated with antipsychotic, but it should be used with caution due to its proarrhythmic effects. Since it is considered a preventable syndrome in 30% of cases, avoiding its appearance should be a priority. The use of prediction models such as DELIPRECAS for patients undergoing cardiac surgery makes it possible to detect preoperatively those with a higher risk of developing delirium and apply preventive measures to avoid its appearance.

The adequate control of pain allows to improve lung function, decrease delirium and reduce hospital stays. In the early postoperative phase, narcotics are the agents of choice, although intravenous paracetamol is an effective analgesic that may spare narcotics. Non-steroidal anti-inflammatory drugs should be used with caution due to adverse effects on renal and platelet function. The use of infusion pumps controlled by the patient is a method that achieves effective analgesia.

Hypothermia and Rewarming

Currently, cardiac surgery is aimed at maintaining normothermic CPB, which aims at temperatures above 34 °C. Cold pericardial irrigation, heat loss from open body cavities and the administration of cold fluids and blood products may cause hypothermia. Hypothermia favors the appearance of arrhythmias, causes vasoconstriction with greater resistance and decreases cardiac output, increases the peripheral O_2 consumption and the production of CO_2, prolongs the action of anesthetics with delayed extubation and increases the risk of wound infection. In the ICU, these situations should be avoided by rewarming the patients, with the air devices being the most effective, and taking special care with secondary vasodilation that may affect hemodynamics.

Ventilator Support and Respiratory Management

The majority of patients undergoing cardiac surgery arrive in the ICU intubated and mechanically ventilated. Almost all patients have restrictive physiology, pulmonary edema, decreased lung compliance and atelectasis, and some may have phrenic nerve lesions. Rapid extubation is associated with early discharge in the ICU and improved outcomes, although sedation and residual neuromuscular block may require controlled ventilation initially. As the patient warms up, the production of CO_2 increases and the lactate is emptied from the previously constricted vascular beds, which may cause a mixed metabolic and respiratory acidosis. This situation should be treated by increasing minute ventilation, preferably through increases in respiratory rate to maintain a low tidal volume to protect the lungs, since cardiac surgery constitutes a risk for acute respiratory distress syndrome (ARDS). The head of the bed should be raised to 45° to minimize the risk of aspiration and pneumonia associated with the ventilator.

Early-extubation is the best prevention for complications such as pneumonia associated with mechanical ventilation or prolonged dependence on the ventilator. Once the patient has reached a relative normothermia (35.5 °C), and hemodynamics allow it, the neuromuscular block is inverted and sedation is withdrawn. As the spontaneous respiration returns, the ventilator changes to a minimum pressure support (PS), being able to perform spontaneous breathing tests. CPB induces a systemic inflammatory response with increased capillary permeability and increased interstitial lung fluid, so fluid overload and blood transfusion should be minimized during resuscitation to avoid the onset of persistent respiratory failure. In these cases, the daily practices of spontaneous breathing, oral hygiene with chlorhexidine, raised head restraints, and daily sedation interruptions, are essential to minimize ventilation time mechanics and improve the results.

Management of Bleeding and Hematologic Dysfunction

Patients who undergo cardiac surgery have an increased risk of bleeding and thrombosis. The quantification of bleeding is performed by draining the chest tube, whose permeability should be confirmed periodically, although the definitions of excessive postoperative bleeding have varied substantially and there is no discrete value to identify clinically significant bleeding.

Extensive bleeding is usually due to one or more of the following factors: incomplete surgical hemostasis, residual heparin effect after cardiopulmonary bypass, clotting factor depletion, hypothermia, postoperative hypertension, hemodilution (dilutional thrombocytopenia and coagulopathy), or platelet abnormalities (platelet dysfunction and thrombocytopenia).

Postoperative bleeding frequently requires fresh frozen plasma and platelets to correct the coagulation abnormalities. Transfusion of packed red blood cells may also be necessary to replace blood loss and extensive bleeding can be mitigated by the administration of antifibrinolytic agent.

Transfusions are associated with an increased risk of mortality and adverse cardiac events, such as transfusion-related acute lung injury (TRALI), an increased risk of pneumonia, bacteremia and sternal wound infection, which is why we currently should perform restrictive transfusion strategies (transfusion trigger hemoglobin ≤ 7–8 mg/dL).

Recommended Readings

1. Frank E. Silvestry. Postoperative complications among patients undergoing cardiac surgery. June 2, 2017. http://www.uptodate.com. Accessed December 13, 2017.
2. Robert M. Bojar. Admission to the ICU and Monitoring Techniques. Manual of perioperative care in adult cardiac surgery. 5th ed. Wiley-Blackwell: 2011. p. 217–235.
3. R. Scott Stephens, Glenn J.R. Whitman. Postoperative critical care of the adult cardiac surgical patient, part I: routine postoperative care. Crit Care Med. 2015;43(7): 1477–97.
4. Robert M. Bojar. Early postoperative care. Manual of perioperative care in adult cardiac surgery. 5th ed. Wiley-Blackwell: 2011. p. 235–65.
5. O. de la Varga-Martínez, E. Gómez-Pesquera, M.F Muñoz-Moreno, et al. Development and validation of a delirium risk prediction preoperative model for cardiac surgery patients (DELIPRECAS): An observational multicentre study. J Clin Anesth. 2021;69:110158.

Issues in Cardiac Surgery

Alberto Hernandez and Mohamed R. El Tahan

Myocardial Revascularization

- Coronary artery bypass grafting (CABG) is the most common procedure in cardiac surgery. Minimally invasive coronary surgery and hybrid coronary revascularization have the potential for better short-term outcomes.
- The use of internal thoracic artery for CABG surgery has the best long-term patency of the graft. Harvesting the left internal thoracic artery is the graft of choice for the left anterior descending (LAD) coronary artery. Compared with the left internal thoracic artery, harvesting the right internal thoracic artery has slightly lower patency. The radial artery is left as the second choice for arterial conduit.
- The off-pump CABG "OPCABG", a surgical procedure performed without cardiopulmonary bypass (CPB), avoids of the systemic inflammatory insult associated with the use of CPB. The most important limitation of the OPCABG surgery is the longer time required for distal anastomoses which requires retraction and verticalization of heart to expose the target vessel adequately. It is crucial to maintain adequate preload to maintain stable hemodynamic parameters during this time.
- The minimally invasive direct coronary artery bypass grafting (MIDCAB) is performed through a mini-thoracotomy without using CPB. This procedure

A. Hernandez (✉)
Department of Anaesthesia and Intensive Care, Policlinica Ibiza Hospital, Ibiza, Spain
e-mail: albimar@yahoo.es

M. R. El Tahan
Cardiothoracic Anaesthesia, Anaesthesia, Surgical Intensive Care and Pain Medicine, College of Medicine, Mansoura University, Mansoura, Egypt

Imam Abdulrahman Bin Faisal University, Dammam, Saudi Arabia

M. Vives and A. Hernandez (eds.), *Cardiac Anesthesia and Postoperative Care in the 21st Century*, https://doi.org/10.1007/978-3-030-79721-8_23

requires placement of a double-lumen tube or a bronchial blocker for one lung ventilation to facilitate the surgical access. Anastomosis of a single internal mammary artery to the LAD is the commonly placed graft.

- The minimally invasive multivessel coronary surgery–coronary artery bypass grafting (MICS-CABG) through a small thoracotomy allows the surgeon to put several numbers of grafts. MICS-CABG may be performed with or without using CPB assistance.
- Hybrid coronary revascularization (HCR), an approach utilizing the best advances in both cardiology and cardiac surgery, allows successful revascularization through the least invasive approach ever. That is usually performed in a hybrid room as a one-stage technique including both surgical CABG and percutaneous coronary intervention (PCI) procedures, one immediately after another during the same session, or a two-stage procedure with either the CABG or PCI performed first, followed by the other intervention performed at another session few days or weeks later.

Concerns and Complications

- With harvesting the right internal thoracic artery, the flow may be inadequate if the right coronary artery is dominant and of good size.
- Retrograde administration of cardioplegia is a particular useful technique for adequate myocardial protection in case of placement of arterial conduits because cardioplegia cannot be delivered directly through the graft.
- During the OPCABG surgery, intravascular volume should be replenished to counteract the decreased venous return the heart was positioned for grafting of the circumflex coronary artery.
- There is a reported marked discrepancy from the left ventricle (LV) to the right ventricle (RV) impacting the ventricular function after CABG surgery. Several studies showed that the LV systolic function is well-maintained following CABG surgery especially in patients with reduced preoperative LV function. Contradictory, the LV diastolic function does not have similar changes. On the other hand, the RV systolic and diastolic functions are impaired during the early and mid-term postoperative follow up.
- Immediate postoperative impaired RV function is a well-known change after CABG surgery. The RV is highly dependent on the changes in intravascular volume. Hypovolemia as well as hypervolemia can compromise cardiac output and the perfusion of other organs.
- During circumflex coronary artery grafting, the heart is kept elevated retracted and the coronary sinus can be injured when coronary sinus pressure exceeds 50–60 mmHg.

Tips and Tricks in the Postoperative Care

- The use of transesophageal echocardiography (TEE) is usually required to rule out cardiac tamponade or acute myocardial ischemia in case of reported early-postoperative hypotension which is unresponsive to administering fluid challenges and increasing infusion rates of the vasopressor therapy.
- Immediate-postoperative myocardial ischemia after CABG surgery is a rare but troublesome finding that can be difficult to diagnose and to treat. Spasm of coronary artery or arterial conduit, mechanical issues such as kinking of a coronary artery graft, occlusion of the native coronary artery or coronary graft, or subendocardial ischemia are well-known causes for postoperative myocardial ischemia. An imbalance between myocardial supply/demand secondary to anaemia (haemoglobin concentration < 8.0 g/dl), hypotension, and tachycardia may predispose to myocardial ischemia. Coronary grafts related-issues with may require an urgent PCI or surgical exploration for reviewing of grafts.
- Although postoperative significant arrhythmia can occur, it is important to exclude poor RV function secondary to an occluded right coronary graft as a cause for persistent malignant ventricular arrhythmias.
- Massive haemothorax is a serious complication after CABG when the left internal mammary artery has been harvested.

Ascending Aortic and Aortic Root Surgery

- There are several challenges acknowledged during postoperative intensive care of patients undergoing aortic surgery particularly surgical repair of acute aortic dissection and aortic aneurysms.
- Aortic dissection occurs as blood flow is redirected from inside the true aortic lumen through an intimal tear into the false lumen in the aortic wall. This disruptive injury results in formation of an extending hematoma within the media towards the aortic root with distorting the aortic valve leaflets leading to aortic valve insufficiency, or narrowing of the ostia of the coronary arteries causing acute myocardial ischemia. In addition, acute aortic dissection can result in a rupture of the aorta into the pericardium and cause life-threatening cardiac tamponade.
- Aortic aneurysm, a localized enlargement and dilation of the aortic arterial wall, can affect any segment of the aorta but the ascending aorta is the most commonly affected segment. The aortic arch could be involved either as an isolated lesion or as an extension of the ascending aortic aneurysm. Progressive enlargement of the aneurysm is an indication for surgical resection of the

affected aortic segment and replacement with a synthetic tube graft can avoid inevitable rupture and death.

Concerns and Complications

- Neurological complications including ischaemic and haemorrhagic cerebral insults are the main concerns after surgery involving the aortic arch.
- Deep hypothermic circulatory arrest (DHCA) is the commonly used technique to provide cerebral protection during surgery on the ascending aorta and aortic arch. The majority of patients can tolerate up to a 30-min period of hypothermic circulatory arrest at 18 °C without significant neurological impairment., The incidence of transient neurologic insults rise to 60% with using DHCA for 60 min.
- Cerebral protection can be used using either selective antegrade or retrograde cerebral perfusion technique allowing using DHCA for a longer period of time than 30 minutes.
- Selective antegrade perfusion of the brain is accomplished through a cannula inserted into the innominate artery alone, the innominate and left common carotid arteries together, or the right axillary artery.
- Some surgeons prefer using retrograde cerebral perfusion through a cannula placed into the superior vena cava as a mean for cerebral protection, despite there is no conclusive data on the efficacy of this technique.
- The time needed for induction of hypothermia and rewarming for the DHCA can be the most critical stage of surgery. Cooling to 18°C usually takes about 20–30 min to be accomplished. However, rewarming must be done carefully and slowly to avoid overshooting normal body temperature.

Tips and Tricks in the Postoperative Care

- Hypothermia, hyperthermia, hypotension and hypoxaemia should be avoided during the first 6–8 postoperative hours to lessen the incidence of worsening of the neurological complications because of cerebral hypoperfusion or hypoxaemia.
- Bleeding is the commonest complication after aortic surgery using the DHCA. Massive postoperative bleeding can results in severe hypotension. Correcting coagulopathy, thrombocytopenia, and platelets dysfunction guided with thromboelastography (TEG) and rotational thromboelastometry (ROTEM) is essential after prolonged CPB and the use of DHCA. Surgical exploration

should be considered in case of significant postoperative bleeding despite of correction of medical cause.

- Caution should be exercised during waking-up and extubating the patients after surgery to avoid shooting up of the blood pressure and likely disruption of aortic anastomotic sutures.

Aortic Valve Surgery

There are some considerations regarding aortic valve surgery including;

Sutureless Aortic Valve Replacement (sAVR)

sAVR, a self-expanding bioprosthetic valve which does not require sutures during implantation, reduces the operative time, and the incidences of perioperative mortality and morbidity. sAVR surgery is followed with notable improved clinical conditions and decreased LV mass index at 1-year follow-up. A recent meta-analysis included 7 observational studies comprising 617 sAVR and 621 transcatheter aortic valve implantation patients demonstrates that the sAVR is associated with lower short-term mortality, less incidence of paravalvular leak and comparable rates of stroke and pacemaker implant.

Concerns and Complications

- Implantation of the sAVR in a patient with severely calcified aorta is challenging and could require considering DHCA without aortic cross-clamp.
- Early structural deterioration with failed sutureless valve function has been reported 4 years after surgery in a young patient with good functional conditions. Large longitudinal studies are needed to evaluate the long-term durability and hemodynamic performance of these valves particularly in a low-risk patient with excellent functional status.
- There other less frequent complications following sAVR including conduction abnormalities (e.g. new-onset left bundle branch block (38.1%), 3rd degree atrioventricular (AV) heart block (9.6%) requiring inserting permanent pacemaker, or right bundle branch block (2.5%)), intraoperative displacement, significant paravalvular leak, early or late postoperative endocarditis, thrombocytopenia, and delayed onset aorto-right ventricular fistula.

Conduction Abnormalities

In general, aortic valve replacement surgery has lower incidences of complete heart block and permanent pacemaker implantation than the transcatheter aortic valve replacement in patients with chronic heart failure.

sAVR is associated with higher risks of new onset AV conduction abnormalities (e.g. LBBB) and the need for permanent pacemaker than the conventional aortic valve replacement surgery. Prophylactic insertion of temporary pacing lead could be useful in these patients.

A recent meta-analysis including 13 studies with 40,447 patients who underwent aortic valve replacement with and without aortic annulus enlargement demonstrated similar overall unadjusted odds ratio for complete heart block and permanent pacemaker implantation.

Minimally invasive aortic valve surgery might be associated with risks for high-grade AV block but that does not require routine insertion of temporary epicardial leads in patients with normal rate and acceptable AV conduction.

Paroxysmal atrial fibrillation and other types of tachyarrhythmia are common in patients undergoing aortic valve replacement due to aortic stenosis.

Hypotension During and Following Aortic Valve Surgery

Hypotension following aortic valve surgery is multifactorial.

- First, vasoplegic syndrome, defined as mean arterial pressure < 50 mmHg or systolic blood pressure < 85 mmHg, low systemic vascular resistance (< 600–800 dyne s/cm^5, or systemic vascular resistances indices < 1800 dyne s/cm^5/m^2), cardiac index > 2.2 L/min/m^2, normal or reduced central filling pressures, and an increased need for vasopressors with normal intravascular volume, is a potentially life-threatening complication during the separation from cardiopulmonary bypass following aortic valve surgery. A combination of ascorbic acid (vitamin C), thiamine, and corticosteroids may mitigate vasoplegia via a number of mechanisms. Methylene blue with doses ranging from 0.5 to 2 mg/kg/h for 1- to 6-hour infusions or bolus doses of 2 to 3 mg/kg given preoperatively, intraoperatively, or postoperatively and hydroxocobalamin at doses of 5 g seems to improve the syndrome.
- Second, paravalvular leak (PVL), defined as a regurgitant jet originating between the outer margin of the prosthetic sewing ring and surrounding native tissues as diagnosed with echocardiography, is a possible complication after prosthetic valve implantation that might be associated with significant hypotension and hemodynamic perturbations. Sutureless aortic valve replacement surgery could be associated 4.2% overall rate of PVL. Percutaneous PVL closure has been introduced as an overall effective and safe procedure for postoperative correction of significant PVL.

- Third, there are other uncommon causes including immediate post bypass stuck valve, intracardiac thrombus formation, or Takotsubo cardiomyopathy.

Porcelain Aorta

Porcelain aorta has been used to address extensive circumferential or nearly circumferential calcification of the thoracic aorta such that precludes safe cross-clamping or entry to the ascending aorta. Aortic cross-clamping in patients with porcelain aorta who undergo open heart surgery is associated with high mortality and morbidity rates.

A useful four-types classification system for aortic arch calcification using non-contrast enhanced computed tomography to predict the possible solution for each patient has been described Table 1.

Possible Solutions for Operating on Porcelain Aorta

- Different techniques can be used for these high-risk patients including (1) a "no touch" technique that totally avoids manipulation of the ascending aorta with the use of off-pump technique, if applicable, (2) arterial cannulation into the axillary artery or the femoral artery or both for arterial return without clamping the aorta for heart valve surgery, (3) deep hypothermic circulatory arrest with antegrade cerebral perfusion for replacement of ascending aorta, (4) careful clamping the ascending aorta using a clamping forceps with a curved jaw to avoid injuring the calcified aortic wall, (5) bilateral axillary arterial perfusion with temporarily clamping of the left common carotid artery at the moment of aortic clamping to prevent debris flowing into the cerebral vessels or short-term moderate

Type	Incidence (%)	Description
Type 1	26	Single area of calcification at the origin of the brachiocephalic artery, left common carotid artery or left subclavian artery
Type 2	24	Calcification in at least two origins of the brachiocephalic artery, left common carotid artery
Type 3	11	Presence of non-annular, patchy clacifications in the ascending aorta in addition to calcifications at the origin of the brachiocephalic artery, left common carotid artery or left subclavian artery
Type 4	2	Extensive annular ascending aortic calcifications frequently accompanied by significant calcifications at other areas

Diken AI, et al Distribution of Thoracic Aortic Calcifications in Patients Undergoing Coronary Artery Bypass Grafting. Aorta (Stamford), 2017. 5(5): p. 132–138

hypothermic circulatory arrest to 30 °C, and (6) intraluminal balloon catheter occlusion as a substitute for external aortic clamping. However, the incidence of postoperative neurological complications is 12.5% with using most of these techniques.

- An alternative approach for those high-risk patients including initiation of total CPB through arterial cannulation of the distal aortic arch or femoral artery, longitudinal aortotomy, and slowly clamping of the aorta to remove the atherosclerotic material through the open incision has been described. However, postoperative stroke and transient ischemic attack have been reported in 7.1% of the studied patients precluding the wide acceptability of that technique.
- A novel clampless and sutureless hybrid technique for aortic arch debranching using prosthetic vascular grafts has been reported as an alternative solution for approaching a porcelain aorta and difficult anatomies.

Heart Valve Surgery with an Unclamped Aorta

Heart valve surgery without cross clamping aorta with beating heart or artificial evoked ventricular fibrillation under normothermic or hypothermic CPB has been described.
Minimally invasive aortic valve surgery with an unclamped aorta has been emerged as a feasible, effective, and safe alternative for the conventional redo surgery using cardioplegic arrest.
Simultaneous antegrade/retrograde warm blood perfusion with a beating heart with the aorta unclamped can be used for both aortic and mitral valve surgery.

Anticoagulation for Patients with Heparin Hypersensitivity

Hypersensitivity reactions after administration of unfractionated heparins or low-molecular-weight heparins are not uncommon. Four types of hypersensitivity are well known as shown in Table 2. The use of an alternative anticoagulant to heparin is required in patients with diagnosed heparin hypersensitivity during on-pump cardiac surgery.

Table 2 Types of heparin hypersensitivity reactions

Type	Characteristics
Type I "immediate-type" reactions (rare type)	A generalized urticaria, angioedema, bronchospasm, and severe anaphylaxis
Type II "classic" reaction	A severe adverse event of heparins is heparin-induced thrombocytopenia (HIT), induced by polyclonal antibodies, usually against the heparin–platelet factor 4 complex. Cutaneous manifestations of HIT type II include erythema and skin and mucosal necrosis
Type III "Arthus" reaction	It results from antigen–antibody complexes and is characterized by inflammation, erythematous induration, and edema at the injection site, which can result in subsequent hemorrhage and necrosis
Type IV allergic "delayed-type" reaction (commonest type)	It is characterized by itchy eczema and plaques at the injection sites

Table 3 Predictors of SAM

Measurement with TEE	Time of cardiac cycle	Echocardiographic view
Basal septal diameter > 1.5 cm	End diastole	ME LAX
C-sept distance < 2.5 cm	Onset of systole	ME LAX or ME 5 Chamber
PMVL length > 1.5 cm	Onset of systole	ME LAX or ME 5 Chamber
AMVL length > 2.0 cm	Onset of systole	ME LAX or ME 5 Chamber
AMVL:PMVL ratio < 1.3	Onset of systole	ME LAX or ME 5 Chamber
Mitral-aortic angle < 120°	Onset of systole	ME LAX or ME 5 Chamber

Possible Alternatives

- The published 2019 European Association for Cardio-Thoracic Surgery (ECTS)/European Association for Cardiothoracic Anaesthesiology (EACTA)/ European Board for Cardiovascular Perfusion guideline on CPB in adult cardiac surgery recommends using bivalirudin for anticoagulation in patients with contraindications to heparin usage during surgery requiring CPB. Pre-bypass administration of a loading dose of bivalirudin (1 mg/kg) followed with a continuous infusion of 2.5 mg/kg/h in conjunction with adding 50 mg to the prime solution has been shown to be a satisfactory alternative anticoagulant during CPB in patients with documented heparin hypersensitivity.
- Lepirudin, an anti-thrombotic recombinant DNA form of hirudin derived from yeast cells, provides effective anticoagulation but induces a higher postoperative blood loss than heparin, especially when effective coagulation test is unavailable. Lepirudin can be administered as a a loading dose of 0.5 mg/kg followed

with a maintenance infusion dose of 0.15 mg/kg/hour in addition to adding 25 mg (0.5 mg/kg) to the prime solution.

- A successful use of a challenge test can be a quick, safe and effective approach in patients with a history of hypersensitivity reactions to heparin with inconclusive diagnostic tests and/or whenever the use of alternative heparins is tricky.

Mitral Valve Repair Surgery

Systolic Anterior Motion of Mitral Leaflet (SAM)

Intraoperative use of TEE is very helpful in early diagnosis of SAM following (MV) surgery particularly following MV repair. SAM represents the dynamic anterior movement of the MV towards the interventricular septum during systole and results in hemodynamic perturbation secondary to LV outflow tract obstruction. SAM might be complicated with development of hemolytic anemia. MV repair can be complicated with development of junctional rhythm-induced SAM during the early postoperative period in the intensive care unit.

Predictors of SAM

Several preoperative predictors for development of SAM following MV repair have been identified including a low ratio of anterior to posterior leaflets heights, younger age, low end-systolic left ventricular volume, presence of bileaflet prolapse, and male sex (Table 3).

Management of SAM

Untreated SAM would negatively impact both short-term and long-term outcomes.

Medical therapy with aggressive volume-loading to keep an adequate preload, increasing afterload by using alfa agonists (e.g Phenylephrine), and reducing tachycardia using beta-adrenoceptor blockers are helpful in correcting mild to moderate degrees of SAM. Furthermore, avoid inotropic agents is mandatory.

Surgical revision with a second cross-clamping or a redo procedure are usually reserved for severe or persistent SAM.

Other Complications

MV repair surgery can be complicated with paravalvular leak, vascular injury, compartment syndrome in case of cannulation of femoral vessels for minimally invasive approach, hydropneumothorax and hydro-pneumopericardium, papillary muscles displacements after edge-to-edge repair, and chordal rupture.

A computational MV model to simulate functional mitral regurgitation by creating papillary muscle displacement has been developed. That model has the potentials to aid in the pre-procedural evaluation of possible complications such as chordal rupture and leaflet perforation following percutaneous edge-to-edge repair.

Unexpected Post-bypass Hypoxemia

Although the incidence of postoperative pulmonary complications is up to 10.9% of patients undergoing cardiac surgery, unexpected early hypoxemia after CPB is an uncommon finding.
TEE is required for surgical decision-making and to diagnose the likely underlying cause.

Causes for Unexpected Hypoxemia After CPB

- Severe pulmonary hypertension might be associated with signficant hypoxemia immediately after cardiac surgery.
- Pulmonary embolism, with an associated RV strain, is a common cause for unexpected hypoxemia in approximately 6% of patients undergoing cardiac surgery.
- Patent Foramen Ovale (PFO) is the most common cause of hypoxemia after CPB.

Right to left intracardiac shunt through a (PFO) has been acknowledged as a cause for unexpected postoperative hypoxemia.

The potential increase in right atrial pressure can lead to a right-to-left shunt through the PFO causing systemic hypoxia.

That could be induced with positive pressure ventilation, RV failure, pulmonary embolism with acute increase in the RV pressure, pericardial tamponade or effusion, localized pericardial hematoma with extrinsic compression of the RV, or myocardial infraction.

Diagnosis of the PFO

Diagnosis of the PFO can be challenging using color flow doppler study through the midesophageal four-chamber and bicaval views. Doppler and contrast echocardiography, with and without provocative maneuver might be needed to maximize the PFO detection rate.

To Close a PFO or Not?

A decision to close a PFO or not currently depends on the surgeons' personal preferences, the presence of hypoxemia and any anticipated deviation from the initial surgical plan.
Percutaneous closure of PFO provides an effective approach to the cases in which PFO is not closed during surgery with documented postoperative hypoxemia.

Redo Surgery

Redo cardiac surgery represents a clinical challenge due to a higher rate of perioperative morbidity and mortality.

Compared with the primary surgery, the redo CABG surgery is associated with higher in-hospital mortality, cardiac arrest, cardiogenic shock, and vascular and respiratory complications. The predictors of the higher mortality include history of heart failure and chronic kidney disease. Similar high mortality and complications rates are reported after reoperations on the proximal thoracic aorta.

In redo cases, adhesions may bring the ventricle close to the sternum. The sternal saw may cut through the RV or innominate vein resulting in massive hemorrhage.

In patients with a prior sternotomy and biventricular failure with a distended RV, the surgeon may expose the femoral artery and vein before opening the chest. If the RV is injured during sternal opening, expeditious femoral cannulation and CPB can be achieved.

In patients who have undergone previous CABG, it is important to identify the left internal thoracic artery and other conduits and to protect them during dissection of the heart. Any graft injury or manipulation leading to spasm or distal embolization of debris may result in hemodynamic instability.

Tips and Tricks

- Operating by an expert surgeon can potentially reduce chest tube drainage and needs for blood transfusions with improved patient outcomes.
- Meticulous surgical homeostasis should be considered.
- Aspirin should be discontinued at least 5 days before elective or urgent redo surgery.
- Prevention of fibrinolysis using tranexamic acid, aprotinin, or e-aminocaproic acid might be considered before the start of CPB.
- Routine use of cell salvage can avoid the need for perioperative transfusions however the re-transfusion of large volumes of cell salvaged blood (>1000 ml) may impair coagulation. Additionally, cell salvage is directly associated with higher infection rates. A meta-analysis including 15 studies demonstrates that the use of cell salvage during cardiac surgery does not have an impact on the rates of red blood cells, platelet and fresh frozen plasma transfusion; however, this should be interpreted in the light of the limitations of that study.
- The use of prothrombin complex concentrate might provide new merits for treating bleeding in patients undergo redo surgery.

Surgical Approaches:

- Avoidance of median sternotomy with the risk of right atrial and/or ventricular injury decreases the risk of bleeding. There is no consensus regarding the optimal surgical approach for patients requiring redo MV surgery either through right mini thoracotomy with or without peripheral cannulation or traditional re-sternotomy with central cannulation.
- A right mini thoracotomy approach is associated with reduced intensive care unit and overall hospital lengths of stay, less need for perioperative transfusion, and a trend towards faster postoperative extubation.
- Minimally invasive redo MV surgery using beating heart technique and peripheral cannulation through the right internal jugular vein, right femoral vein, and right femoral artery, under TEE guidances, has the potentials to reduce the operation time and CPB time, decreases the requirement for transfusion, shortens postoperative intensive care unit and hospital stays, and the time to extubation in the patients with giant LV.
- Minimally invasive MV surgery using either standard median sternotomy or mini thoracotomy has good mid-term results for re-repairing the degenerative MV disease.
- Minimally invasive aortic valve replacement surgery using percutaneous retrograde cardioplegia combined with antegrade cardioplegia and moderate hypothermia, without interruption of internal thoracic artery flow, is a safe and reliable technique in patients with previous patent internal thoracic artery grafts.
- Minimally invasive tricuspid valve repair can be useful in patients with previous MV replacement. Following induction of general anesthesia, the right femoral

artery and right internal jugular vein are cannulated percutaneously under combined ultrasound and TEE guidance. A limited right antero-lateral thoracotomy approach can be facilitated with deflating the right lung using a double lumen endobronchial tube or endobronchial blocker. Two saline-filled Fogarty catheters are inserted under echocardiography control to occlude the superior and inferior vena cavae before initiation of the CPB.

Persistent Left Superior Vena Cava

- Persistent left superior vena cava (PLSVC), the most common congenital malformation of thoracic venous return, can be find in 0.3 to 0.5% of the general population.
- The existence of PLSVC in addition to other congenital cardiac malformation increases the risk of perioperative mortality after cardiac surgery using CPB.
- Dilated coronary sinus is reported in 80% of patients presented with PLSVC and should be detected by TEE.
- In patients with the PLSVC, venous blood usually drains into: (1) the right atrium through a dilated coronary sinus (CS) (80–92% of patients), or (2) the left atrium, either directly or through an unroofed CS, causing right-to-left intracardiac shunt in approximately 10 to 20% of cases.
- Anomalous venous return secondary to the PLSVC may result in cardiac arrhythmias, palpitations, decreased exercise tolerance, progressive fatigue, chest discomfort, syncope or cyanosis.
- PLSVC is frequently diagnosed accidentally during invasive cardiac procedures like left-sided or right-heart catheterisation, cardiac surgical procedures, or cannulating the left internal jugular vein.
- Placement of a central venous catheter, or intracardiac leads for pacemaker or cardiac resynchronisation therapy implantation can result in incorrect positioning in the undiagnosed cases with PLSVC.
- Radiological detection of an anomalous route of a placed central venous catheter in the thorax raises the suspect of the presence of PLSCV.
- The presence of PLSVC is a relative contraindication to administering retrograde cardioplegia during cardiac surgery.
- Echocardiography can rule out the presence or absence of a left superior vena cava. Diagnosis by TEE is primarily based on detecting a dilated coronary sinus (greater than 1 cm)

- The volume of cardioplegia administered may be inadequate since it comes back through the PLSVC. Inadequate myocardial protection induced postcardiotomy cardiac dysfunction, cardiogenic shock, and arrythmias can be the consequences of unrecognized failed retrograde cardioplegia administration in patients with undiagnosed PLSVC. Therefore, the use of antegrade cardioplegia with infusing the cardioplegia solution directly into the coronary arteries ostia is preferrable in patients with the PLSCV.

Recommended Readings

1. Bilkhu R et al Sutureless aortic valve prostheses. Heart, 2019; 105 (Suppl 2): p. s1 s20.
2. Boultadakis V et al Sutureless aortic valve implantation in patient with porcelain aorta via unclamped aorta and deep hypothermic circulatory arrest. Ann Card Anaesth, 2017. 20(4): p. 447–449.
3. Mogilansky C et al New postoperative conduction abnormalities after the implantation of a rapid-deployment aortic valve prosthesis. Interact Cardiovasc Thorac Surg, 2019. 28(4): p. 581–586.
4. Falcetta G et al Intraoperative displacement of a Perceval sutureless prosthesis. Gen Thorac Cardiovasc Surg, 2019. 67(7): p. 633–636.
5. Mubashir T et al Transcatheter and Surgical Aortic Valve Replacement Outcomes for Patients with Chronic Heart Failure. J Cardiothorac Vasc Anesth, 2020.
6. Lam KY et al Conduction disorders and impact on survival after sutureless aortic valve replacement compared to conventional stented bioprostheses. Eur J Cardiothorac Surg, 2019. 55(6): p. 1168–1173.
7. Miyata K, Shigematsu S. Vasoplegic Syndrome after Aortic Valve Replacement. Masui, 2016. 65(1): p. 90–2.
8. Abramowitz Y et al Porcelain Aorta. Circulation, 2015. 131(9): p. 827–836.
9. Hartert M et al Cross-clamping a porcelain aorta: an alternative technique for high-risk patients. J Cardiovasc Surg (Torino), 2018. 59(5): p. 37 -745
10. Nishimori HM, Yamamoto K, Orihashi. Cerebral infarction occurs particularly in patients with porcelain aorta. J Thorac Cardiovasc Surg, 2015. 150(3): p. 744-5.
11. Diken AI, Yalçınkaya A, Özyalçın S. Distribution of Thoracic Aortic Calcifications in Patients Undergoing Coronary Artery Bypass Grafting. Aorta (Stamford), 2017. 5(5):132–138.
12. Okamura Y et al [Urgent coronary reoperation under the beating heart via the left thoracotomy]. Nihon Kyobu Geka Gakkai Zasshi, 1997. 45(6):p. 874–7.
13. Okamoto K, Fukui T. Bilateral axillary artery cannulation for severely calcified aorta and branches: a case report. J Cardiothorac Surg, 2016. 11(1): p. 98.
14. Cosgrove DM. Management of the calcified aorta: an alternative method of occlusion. Ann Thorac Surg, 1983. 36(6): p. 718–9.
15. Botta L et al The role of the minimally invasive beating heart technique in reoperative valve surgery. J Card Surg, 2012. 27(1): p. 24–8.
16. Pfőhler C et al Delayed-type heparin allergy: diagnostic procedures and treatment alternatives-a case series including 15 patients. World Allergy Organ J, 2008. 1(12): p. 194–9.
17. Kunst G et al 2019 EACTS/EACTA/EBCP guidelines on cardiopulmonary bypass in adult cardiac surgery. Br J Anaesth, 2019. 123(6): p. 713–757.

18. Gatt P et al Bivalirudin as an Alternative Anticoagulant for Cardiopulmonary Bypass During Adult Cardiac Surgery-A Change in Practice. The journal of extra-corporeal technology, 2017. 49(1): p. 49–53.
19. Parissis H Lepirudin as an alternative to "heparin allergy' during cardiopulmonary bypass. Journal of cardiothoracic surgery, 2011. 6: p. 44.
20. Pitsis A et al Mitral valve repair: moving towards a personalized ring. Journal of Cardiothoracic Surgery, 2019. 14(1): p. 108.
21. Nenna ANF, Spadaccio C et al Systolic Anterior Motion (SAM) Complicating Mitral Valve Repair: Current Concepts of Intraoperative and Postoperative Management. Surgical Technology International., 2020 Jun. 37.
22. Ashikhmina E et al Risk factors and progression of systolic anterior motion after mitral valve repair. J Thorac Cardiovasc Surg, 2020.
23. Toma M et al Effect of Edge-to-Edge Mitral Valve Repair on Chordal Strain: Fluid-Structure Interaction Simulations. Biology (Basel), 2020. 9(7).
24. Yeh YL et al Detection of right to left shunt by transesophageal echocardiography in a patient with postoperative hypoxemia. J Formos Med Assoc, 2006. 105(5): p. 418–21
25. Simon C et al Severe hypoxaemia after weaning from cardiopulmonary bypass: a case report. J Cardiovasc Med (Hagerstown), 2007. 8(11): p. 956–8.
26. Morales D, Williams E, John R. Is resternotomy in cardiac surgery still a problem? Interact Cardiovasc Thorac Surg, 2010. 11(3): p. 277–86.
27. Antoniou A et al Redo proximal thoracic aortic surgery: challenges and controversies. Gen Thorac Cardiovasc Surg, 2019. 67(1): p. 118–126.
28. Patel NC et al Reoperative mitral valve surgery via sternotomy or right thoracotomy: A propensity-matched analysis. Journal of Cardiac Surgery, 2019. 34(10): p. 976–982.
29. Aphram G et al Re-repair of the failed mitral valve: insights into aetiology and surgical management. Eur J Cardiothorac Surg, 2018. 54(4): p. 774–780.

Sedation, Pain Relief and Weaning from Ventilation

Anna Jarosz and Marcin Wasowicz

Introduction

Every patient undergoing cardiac surgical procedure is admitted to the intensive care unit (ICU) or post anesthesia recovery unit (PACU), which offer invasive monitoring and mechanical ventilation capabilities. Many cardiac surgical patients are temporarily in status of "controlled cardiogenic shock" caused by impact of surgical procedure, post-operative bleeding, vasoplegia, significant fluid shifts and/or systemic inflammatory response syndrome (SIRS). In order to facilitate smooth weaning from mechanical ventilation and transition from high dependency ward to surgical floor, ICU or PACU team must provide comprehensive care which includes pain and sedation management. Although the majority of patients can be weaned and extubated within the first 2–4 hours after operation (some on the operating table), adequate pain management needs to be continued for several days. Yet, 6–8% of cardiac surgical patients will require prolonged mechanical ventilation (>48 hours) and more complex treatment of pain, agitation and delirium (PAD).

A. Jarosz
Department of Anesthesia and Intensive Therapy, University Hospital Wroclaw, Wroclaw, Poland

M. Wasowicz (✉)
Department of Anesthesia and Pain Management, Toronto General Hospital/University Health Network, Toronto, Canada
e-mail: marcin.wasowicz@uhn.ca

Cardiovascular Intensive Care Unit, Toronto General Hospital/University Health Network, Toronto, Canada

Department of Anesthesia and Pain Medicine, Faculty of Medicine, University of Toronto, Toronto, Canada

M. Vives and A. Hernandez (eds.), *Cardiac Anesthesia and Postoperative Care in the 21st Century*, https://doi.org/10.1007/978-3-030-79721-8_24

Therefore, the main purpose of this chapter is to review current standards of pain and sedation management aiming at smooth weaning of mechanical ventilation of the cardiac surgical patient. Knowledge discussed is based on current guidelines and experience of both authors who had an opportunity to practice cardiac anesthesia and postoperative critical care on four different continents.

Pain Management

1. Introduction

Every cardiac surgical patient requires pain management. The intensity of pain post cardiac surgery depends on the location of the incision (s) (sternotomy vs. thoracotomy, vein harvesting, groin cannulation etc.). Most of the currently used pain medications have sedative properties, thus current guidelines on pain and sedation management put therapy of surgical pain in first place of their documents.

2. Pain assessment

Sternotomy and particularly thoracotomy are one of the most painful surgical interventions and commonly contribute to chronic pain syndromes, with an incidence of 7–66%, particularly after thoracotomy. Other causes of pain and discomfort in cardiac surgical population include chest tubes, indwelling catheters as well as all therapeutic and nursing procedures and even ambulation. Commonly, acute post-surgical pain is experienced in addition to preexisting chronic pain conditions. It is essential to monitor the severity of pain, its location and response to therapy. Use of Numeric Rating Scale (NRS), either verbal or visual provides the most reliable pain assessment for awake, cooperating patients. For patients with abnormal level of consciousness it is advocated to follow behavioral assessment tools. Purposely heart rate and systemic blood pressure are not part of the routine pain assessment, as these are very non-specific symptoms in cardiac population. Both Behavioral Pain Scale (BPS) and Critical Care Pain Observation Tool (CPOT) have been validated to assess pain in intensive care setting.

Critical Care Pain Observation Tool (CPOT)

Indicator	Description	Score
Facial expression	Relaxed, neutral	0
	Tense	1
	Grimacing	2
Body movements	Normal position, no movements	0
	Protection	1
	Restlessness	2
Compliance with ventilator (if intubated)	Tolerate ventilator	0
	Coughing but tolerating	1

(continued)

(continued)

Critical Care Pain Observation Tool (CPOT)		
Indicator	Description	Score
	Fighting ventilator	2
Vocalization (if extubated)	Talking	0
	Sigh, moan	1
	Crying out	2
Muscle tension	Relaxed	0
	Tense, rigid	1
	Very tense, rigid	2
CPOT ranges from 0 (no pain) to 8 (maximum pain), the goal is CPOT <2		

3. Multimodal analgesia

   A. Opioids

      Opioids should be given for pain greater than 4 in NRS and BPS scales and 2 in CPOT scale. Opioids are administered for surgical pain and additional doses could be prescribed as needed for procedural pain i.e. dressing changes or chest tubes removal. The choice of opioid is dependent on institutional protocols and practice, but routinely fentanyl, hydromorphone, morphine and oxycodone are used for their safe metabolism profiles and little impact on hemodynamics. Morphine may cause histamine release and its active metabolites may accumulate in renal impaired patients (very common comorbidity in cardiac surgical patients), but it is still widely used with no serious side effects. It is well described, that patient controlled analgesia (PCA) results in better pain control as well as overall less opioid consumption and less side effects, so should be considered in all patients capable of self-administering medications. Oral opioids are very effective in post-operative period and should be started as soon as patient can tolerate oral medications.

   B. Non-opioids

      Nonsteroidal anti-inflammatory drugs (NSAIDs) are analgesic, antipyretic and anti-inflammatory medications, adequate for mild-moderate pain or as adjuncts to opioids for moderate/severe pain. Their use in cardiac surgery patients is limited by their side effects, predominantly renal impairment, bleeding secondary to platelet dysfunction, prothrombotic properties in selective COX-2 inhibitors, gastro-intestinal bleeding and aspirin-sensitivity with bronchoconstriction. A lot of them are available in parenteral form.

      Acetaminophen has no known renal, cardiovascular and hematologic side effects. It is proven to be hepatotoxic in doses greater than 4g/24 hours, but with careful dosing it is a safe analgesic and antipyretic medication, routinely used in cardiac surgical patients, particularly in parenteral form, approved in many countries. This form of administration is a preferable one, as in critically ill patients the absorption (bioavailability) of rectal and oral doses may be variable.

Continuous ketamine infusion has shown to decrease the opioid requirement in general surgical patients, but its use and safety profile in cardiac surgical patients has not been validated.

Continuous lidocaine infusion is not recommended for post-operative pain management, as potential neuro and cardiac toxicity in critically ill patients outweighs its theoretical benefits. It should be mentioned that relatively new sedative, dexmedetomidine possesses strong opioid sparing capabilities.

C. Neuropathic pain adjuncts

Neuropathic pain medications (gabapentin, pregabalin, carbamazepine) are advocated for patients with known or likely neuropathic pain component. They are proven to reduce opioid consumption post cardiac surgery, although their use may be limited by possible sedative or cognitive effects in some patients. Some of them might have a role in ERAS protocols, which recently have been introduced to practice of cardiac anesthesia.

D. Regional anesthesia

Epidural analgesia reduces the incidence of pulmonary, cardiovascular and renal complications after cardiac surgery. Its well described complication—spinal cord injury from an epidural hematoma is estimated to occur in 1:1500–1:150000 cases, but is a deleterious condition, that precludes this technique from widespread use. Less invasive blocks—paravertebral and intercostal, with continuous local anesthetic infusion are more commonly used, particularly for thoracotomies and significantly decrease opioid consumption, being safe even in fully anticoagulated patients. Recently, newer blocks (Erector Spinal Plane block or Serratus Anterior Plane block) are gaining popularity since they are not contraindicated in patients receiving systemic heparinization and are characterized by high efficacy.

Sedation

1. Indication and principles

Routine sedation after elective cardiac surgical procedure is rarely required, majority of patients are adequately sedated as a result of proper pain management and residual effect of opioids used during surgery. Subpopulation of cardiac surgical patients who require routine use of sedatives are these who necessitate prolonged mechanical ventilation or who are experiencing post-operative delirium or agitation. In order to guide properly sedation requirements ICU staff must routinely monitor the depth of the sedation and occurrence of delirium.

2. Sedation scales

Use of sedation scales is mandatory as part of evidence-based critical care management. They are used to quantify the level of sedation and a degree of agitation. There are two well validated scales used in ICU setting, (Riker Agitation-Sedation Scale SAS, Richmond Agitation-Sedation Scale RASS). Regardless which scale is chosen, the most important is the continuous assessment of patient's sedation/agitation level, guiding the dose of sedatives being administered. This is important in context of fluctuating character of delirium, coordinating patient's activity and planning for nursing and therapeutic. Reporting of observed level of sedation, titrating sedatives and providing optimal comfort for critically ill patients always needs to consider these circumstances. Moreover, so far none of the neuromonitoring systems has proven to be superior than subjective scales in improving patient outcome and reducing consumption of health care resources. The most commonly scale used to monitor delirium is Confusion Assessment Method (CAM).

3. Medications

There are numerous randomized controlled trials (RCT) looking at the effectiveness of sedatives, including studies exclusively designed for cardiac surgical population. Cardiac patients are commonly electively admitted to intensive care department for early post-operative recovery, so their sedation requirement is different from general medical ICU population. There is evidence of shorter time to extubation with propofol over benzodiazepines infusions (−52 min to −1.4 hours), with no difference in adverse events. When looking into non-specific ICU population, this difference was even greater (−7.2 to −11.6 hours—comparable to one nursing shift), with 2.2 increase in risk in self-extubation in Propofol group, but without obvious harm in this course. The incidence of delirium seems to be similar. When dexmedetomidine was compared to benzodiazepines, there was even greater benefit for time to extubation (−1.9 days) and decrease in delirium incidence (RR 0.71) in the dexmedetomidine group, with more common, clinically insignificant bradycardia. Studies comparing propofol with dexmedetomidine showed no difference in time to extubation, favoring dexmedetomidine for less delirium incidence. Another alternative is to use volatile based sedation. This approach is allowing very precise control over the depth and length of sedation and has a minimal hemodynamic influence.

4. Fast-tracking

There is strong evidence that fast track early extubation post cardiac procedures (CABG or single valve) is safe and reduces the length of ICU stay. There are different models for post-operative early intensive care that show similar effectiveness. Successful fast tracking depends not only on post-operative management but also on low, but adequate opioid anesthesia and good surgical performance, particularly in terms of hemostasis and short CPB time. Overall, acceptable fast-track failure rate is described as 11% and identified risk factors of failure include: older age, poor left ventricular ejection fraction, extracardiac arteriopathy, preoperative intra-aortic balloon pump, raised serum creatinine, previous cardiac surgery, repeat cardiopulmonary bypass (CPB) during surgery and non-elective or complex surgery. Fast track approach (cardiac ERAS) is likely to be the future of modern, less invasive cardiac surgery.

Weaning from Ventilation

1. Introduction, weaning protocols

Successful weaning from mechanical ventilation is possible only when pain, agitation and delirium are all under control. Respiratory support should be adjusted along with sedation requirements and patient activity. Modern ventilation modes allow tailoring the level of support to individual patient's needs. Weaning is one of the most stressful and challenging moments in recovery of cardiac surgical patient, that can be associated with hemodynamic disturbances, that is why it should not be preceded by any aggressive weaning off inotropic support. It is known, that prolonged ventilation increases mortality and morbidity rate, including ventilator associated pneumonia and ventilator associated lung injury. On the other hand, failed extubation is also associated with increased mortality and length of hospital stay. Therefore, systematic approach to weaning is key to timely and safe extubation. Well validated models for prediction of prolonged mechanical ventilation after cardiac surgery were recently published, with history of previous cardiac surgery, lower left ventricular ejection fraction, shock, surgery involving repair of congenital heart disease and long cardiopulmonary bypass time being proven to be strong predictors.

2. Clinical criteria for weaning

There are no strict clinical criteria for successful weaning from mechanical ventilation. In case of cardiac surgical patient they usually include respiratory and circulatory component as well as the amount of chest tubes output. Early postoperative weaning meets different clinical criteria than long term ventilator weaning protocols. Regardless what weaning protocol is being followed, deterioration in any of the systems and organs impedes successful weaning.

3. Respiratory criteria for weaning

Spontaneous breathing trials (SBT) are intended to identify patients that are likely to have a successful extubation. These can be performed by providing a minimal ventilator settings support (PS 5–7 cmH_2O and PEEP =/<5 cmH_2O) to overcome the work of breathing, that is proven to be more beneficial in successful extubation than supplementing oxygen through an ETT with a T-piece. Long term ventilated patients should be subjected to special weaning protocols, where SBTs and sedation vacations are being introduced on a daily basis for longer, increasing periods of time, intervaled with resting from weaning with increased respiratory support.

Clinical and ventilatory predictors of successful weaning	
Neurological	Well controlled pain, agitation and delirium
	Alert, awake and able to follow commands, some protocols indicate GSC >10 (>8) (early post op extubation criteria)
	Stable neurologic deficit (patients with chronic brain/nerve injury of whatever origin)
Cardiovascular	No or minimal cardiovascular support (most protocols mention a maximal dose of dopamine 5 mcg/kg/min)
	Patients post even elective cardiac procedures may require higher inotropic/ vasopressor support but still be good candidates for ventilator weaning as long as they are hemodynamically stable and the requirement for cardiovascular support is stable or decreasing
Respiratory	Adequate cough and gag reflex present
	Improvement of condition that lead to respiratory failure
Other Bleeding? Fluid balance	Temperature <38.5 °C
	Metabolic and electrolyte stability
Ventilatory	RSBI (rapid shallow breathing index—spontaneous frequency of breathing/ tidal volume (L)) f/Vt <105
	PaO_2/FiO_2 >200
	FiO_2 <0.5
	PEEP <5 cmH_2O
	f <35 breaths/min
	SpO2 >92%

4. Failure to wean

Failure to wean is defined as the failure to pass a spontaneous-breathing trial or the need for reintubation within 48 hours following extubation. The incidence of extubation failure is 4–13% and reintubation is associated with a 7–11 fold increase in hospital mortality. Positive SBT over 30–120 min does not guarantee successful extubation. Risk factors of early extubation failure post cardiac surgery include old age, severe preoperative comorbidities, need for preoperative intra-aortic balloon pump, multiple transfusions (>10 units) usually leading to fluid overload, surgery of thoracic aorta and prolonged CPB. Depending on a reason for failed weaning a few approaches can be advocated. Non-invasive ventilation is likely to be useful for patients with COPD and other chronic respiratory disorders, particularly in patients with exacerbation. Systemic steroids are indicated only in patients with known laryngeal oedema, however there is no benefit in using prophylactic steroids in general population. Finally tracheostomy can be considered in patients with prolonged (>7–14 days) ventilation, or earlier, if the patient's condition makes timely weaning unlikely (for example massive stroke or neurological injury). It is also indicated in patients, who do not require mechanical ventilation, but who are unable to maintain or protect their airway. The main advantage of tracheostomy is better patient's comfort and autonomy. As mentioned before, worsening of cardiac function should always be ruled out first as a possible cause of failure in weaning.

Summary

Every patient who is undergoing cardiac surgical procedure requires intensive care management during early postoperative recovery phase (6–10 hours). Majority of patients can be extubated within first postoperative hours, therefore they need only comprehensive pain management facilitating smooth weaning of mechanical ventilation. Approximately 6–8% of cardiac patients require prolonged mechanical ventilation (>48 hours), therefore they need more complex management of pain, agitation and delirium and long-term plan of discontinuation of mechanical ventilation. Presented review briefly discussed aforementioned topics.

Recommended Readings

1. Sharma V, et al. A derived and validated score to predict prolonged mechanical ventilation in patients undergoing cardiac surgery. J Thorac Cardiovasc Surg. 2017;153(1):108–15. https://doi.org/10.1016/j.jtcvs.2016.08.020. Epub 2016 Aug 29.
2. Devlin JW, et al. Clinical practice guidelines for the prevention and management of pain, agitation/sedation, delirium, immobility and sleep disruption in adult patients in the ICU. Crit Care Med. 2018;46(9):e825–73. https://doi.org/10.1097/CCM.0000000000003299.
3. Bainbridge D, et al. Current evidence on fast track cardiac recovery management. Eur Heart J Suppl. 2017;19(suppl A):A3–7. https://doi.org/10.1093/eurheartj/suw053.
4. Teboul JL. Weaning-induced cardiac dysfunction: where are we today? Intensive Care Med. 2014;40(8):1069–79. https://doi.org/10.1007/s00134-014-3334-4. Epub 2014 May 27.
5. Jerath A, et al. Volatile-based short-term sedation in cardiac surgical patients: a prospective randomized controlled trial. Perioperative Anesthesia Clinical Trials Group. Crit Care Med. 2015;43(5):1062–9.
6. Wasowicz M, Jerath A. Expanding the use of volatile anesthetic agents beyond the operating room. Can J Anesth. 2014;61(10):905–8. https://doi.org/10.1007/s12630-014-0211-0.
7. Subira C, et al. Effects of pressure support vs. t-piece ventilations strategies during spontaneous breathing trials on successful extubation among patients receiving mechanical ventilation. A randomized clinical trial. JAMA 2019;321:2175–82.

Haemodynamic Complications

Marc Giménez-Milà, Purificación Matute, and Marc Vives

Introduction

Cardiothoracic intensive care is becoming more obviously a sub-speciality of Intensive Care Medicine, relying on a good understanding of surgical procedure and skills to diagnose and treat eventual complications. Complications that affect cardiovascular system are the most frequent complications after cardiac surgery.

Typically, patients undergoing heart surgery may present themselves with ischaemic heart disease, hypertension, valve disease and atrial fibrillation. Also, the type of surgical procedure and anaesthetic approach can be related with appearance of complications such as Atrial fibrillation in patients undergoing mitral valve surgery, complete heart block in valve replacements, vasoplegic status after Infective endocarditis surgery, risk of major bleeding after complex aortic procedures, pneumothoraces after central line insertion and Fluid overload or hypovolemia depending on intraoperative fluid administration.

Depending on the severity, they may prompt to invasive monitoring such as pulmonary artery catheters, echocardiography, computed tomography pulmonary angiogram (CTPA) scan and coronary angiography. They will provide diagnostic information that can orientate us towards the best treatment restoring the adequate oxygen delivery to organs.

Although academic classification is seldom made, most of the times they are presented together. Following, the most frequent haemodynamic complications are presented in three big families: systemic hypertension, hypotension and rhythm disturbances.

M. Giménez-Milà (✉) · P. Matute
Department of Anaesthesia and Critical Care, Hospital Clínic de Barcelona, University of Barcelona, Barcelona, Spain

M. Vives
Department of Anesthesiology and Critical Care, Hospital Universitari de Girona Dr J Trueta. University of Girona, Girona, Spain

M. Vives and A. Hernandez (eds.), *Cardiac Anesthesia and Postoperative Care in the 21st Century*, https://doi.org/10.1007/978-3-030-79721-8_25

Hypertension

Systemic arterial hypertension is defined by systolic blood pressure >130 mm Hg or diastolic blood pressure > 80 mm Hg and is one of the main determinants of cardiac afterload.

It increases cardiac workload and metabolic consumption, posing the myocardium at risk of ischaemia. Risk of postoperative surgical bleeding is increased likewise the risk of haemorrhagic cerebrovascular accidents, being a relevant entity during the postoperative period.

Causes of systemic hypertension are overdosage of inotropic or vasopressor drugs, poor pain control, delirium, hypothermia, essential hypertension and secondary hypertension (Table 1). Treatment may include analgesic drugs, antipsychotic agents, cessation of vasopressors or antihypertensives agents.

Commonest used agents are nitrovasodilators, which produce mainly venodilation via NO formation. Examples of this family are Glyceril trinitrate (GTN), sodium nitroprussiate and nitric oxide. They all produce tolerance and prolonged administration of sodium nitroprussiate has been linked to cyanide poisoning. Other drug families are: beta-blockers, Angiotensin converting enzyme inhibitors (ACEi), angiotensin II receptor blockers (ARBs), alpha-blockers, Calcium channel blockers, Prostaglandin analogues and diuretics (Table 2). They have different mechanism of action and exhibit different side effects that will affect on the decision of which agent should we start with. As a general rule, drugs with short life time that are administered via intravenous infusions are preferred.

Hypotension

Low blood pressure is the manifestation of different clinical syndromes. Of note, not all hypotension is accompanied by low cardiac output, but truly enough, all hypotension should trigger further investigation. The key point is to understand whether this hypotension is accompanied by low cardiac output and therefore hypoperfusion to vital organs. Physical examination, measurement of urinary

Table 1 Common causes of secondary hypertension

Cause	Clinical presentation
Renal artery stenosis	Worsening renal function after ACEi and ARBs
Coartation of Aorta	Differential blood pressure >20 between arm and leg
Phaeocromocytoma	Sweat, palpitations, headache
Cushing syndrome	Obesity, haemorrhagic dyastasis
Thyrotoxicosis	Tremor, heat intolerance
Hyperaldosteronism	Hypopotasemia

Table 2 Commonest anti-hypertensives

Group	Agents	Relevant features
Nitrovasodilators	GTN, NO, Nitroprussiate	Venodilator, produces tachyphylaxis Nitroprussiate induces coronary and cerebral steal phenomenon
Beta-blockers	Labetalol, Esmolol	Decreases Oxygen consumption. Produces bradycardia and bronchospasm
ACE inhibitors, ARBs	Ramipril, Enalapril, Losartan	Careful administration in renal dysfunction
Calcium channel blockers	Amlodipine	Periheral oedema, liver dysfunction
Alpha-blockers	Doxazosine	Orthostatic hypotension
Others	Hydralazine, Magnesium	Safe for pregnant patients
Diuretics	Furosemide, thiazides	Produces ototoxicity, electrolites disturbances
Prostanglandin analogue	Prostacyclin	iv and nebulised. Improves RV performance
Inodilators	Enoximone, Milrinone	Decreases pulmonary vascular resistance and systemic vascular resistance

output, plasmatic lactate, intracavitary pressures (CVP and PAOP) and systemic and pulmonary vascular resistances (SVR and PVR) could all help us clarifying the situation. Moreover, either transthoracic or transoesophageal echocardiography will provide information about preload status, contractility, valve function and signs of vasoplegia.

(A) Hypovolemia

Hypovolemia is the commonest cause of hypotension seen in ICU in patients after cardiac surgery. Preoperative fasting and depletive treatment with diuretics altogether with long lasting operations with limited administration of intravenous fluids promote that many patients will require administration of crystalloids upon admission in ICU. Inadvertent surgical bleeding or iatrogenic Aortic dissection needs a quick diagnosis with immediate correction of associated possible coagulopathy with transfussion of blood and products. Surgical advice should be considered to assess need of re-sternotomy for surgical revision.

Trends on intracavitary pressures may indicate lack of correction if intravascular volume. Moreover, the following echocardiographic features are indicators of hypovolemia: kissing papillary muscles, small end-diastolic diameter (EDD) of LV, collapse and diameter of IVC during inspiration in spontaneously breathing patients.

(B) Vasoplegia

Prevalence is 5–25% with no risk factors and 30–50% with risk factors. Inflammatory response after cardiopulmonary by-pass (CPB), in some patients, implies a drop in SVR. Vasoplegic syndrome is characterised by moderate to profound hypotension (mean BP < 50 mmHg), normal or elevated Cardiac Index (CI > 2.4 L min^{-1} m^2), reduced systemic vascular resistance (less than 800 dynes cm^{-5}) and marked attenuated response to vasoconstrictors. Patients with a preoperative infection like infective endocarditis or prolonged runs of CPB induce a higher cytokine release that can lead to loss of the vascular tone. Other known risk factors are the use of preoperative iv heparin (lowers ionised calcium), LVEF < 35%, diabetes mellitus and preoperative inflammatory state. Diagnosis consists on the use of pulmonary artery catheter and calculation of SVR. Echocardiography will give us indirect signs such as hyperdynamic LV and a small End systolic LV but with a normal EDD. Treatment include administration of vasopressors such as Noradrenaline and Vasopressin. Suprarenal insufficiency should be suspected in refractory vasoplegia, and if clinical setting compatible hydrocortisone may be helpful (Table 3). Metilene blue has been described in cases of refractory vasoplegic syndrome after CPB.

Differential diagnosis should be made with sepsis through a thorough physical examination, review of laboratory results such as white blood cells formula, C-reactive protein (CRP) and Pro-calcitonin. If clinical suspicion is maintained further examinations like image studies (CT scan, Chest X- Ray) may be prompt while microbiological cultures are obtained, broad-spectrum antibiotics started and judicious intravenous fluid resuscitation commenced (3). Bowel ischaemia due to athero-embolic events is a possible complication after major cardiovascular procedures. It can also induce a sepsis-like haemodynamic profile with persistently increased serum lactate. CT-abdomen or Angiography will reveal the occlusion point and an emergent laparotomy may be the treatment in selected patients after consultation with general surgery team.

(C) Low Cardiac output

Low Cardiac output due to LV dysfunction or RV failure is a well-defined cause of hypotension. RV is extremely sensitive to increases in afterload leading to RV distension, decreasing output and compromising performance of LV. Pulmonary hypertension needs careful attention and treatment to preserve systolic function of RV. Phosfodiesterase inhibitors (milrinone, enoximone), NO and Prostaciclin decrease PVR reducing RV afterload.

Decreased contractility can be due to reperfusion injury after surgical revascularisation, myocardial ischaemia due to coronary vasospasm or thrombosis or due to inadequate cardioprotection intraoperatively. In valvular surgery a significant paravalvular leak or prosthetic valve malpositions can all lead to valve regurgitation or stenosis and heart failure. Also an undiagnosed ventricular septal defect (seen in complex cases of Aortic valve replacement) can lead to intra-cardiac left to right shunting. Systolic Anterior Motion (SAM) is an entity that needs attention specially

Table 3 Treatment of vasoplegic shock

Agents	Comments
Noradrenaline	–1st line therapy –Dose: 0.03–1.5 mcg/kg/min –At high dose may cause tachyarrhythmias and adverse cardiac events –Intracelular acidosis or ATP deplection causes inhibition of voltage gated calcium channels—no vasoconstriction –The need for high-dose catecholamines should prompt the clinician to consider adding, a non-catecholaminergic agent
Vasopressin/ Terlipressin	–2nd line therapy –Dose terlipressin: 0.5–1.5 mcg/kg/h. Vasopressin: 0.01–0.06 IU/min –V1/V2 ratio: 1 for vasopressin. V1/V2 ratio 2.2 for terlipressin (higher vascular selectivity) –Recommended if refractory vasoplejic shock with noradrenaline > 0.5 mcg/kg/min –PVR and RV afterload is not increased –Afferent renal artery is not affected –Data suggest may be associated with better renal outcomes and less atrial fibrillation
Epinephrine	–Dose: 0.01–0.3 mg/kg/min continuous infusion –Recommended if mixed shock (ventricular disfunction associated) with CI < 2.2 L min^{-1} m^2 –May induce glycolysis and pyruvate generation, which result in lactic acidosis, via β2-adrenergic receptor
Metilene blue	–It directly competes with NO for activation of guanylyl cyclase, the enzyme responsible for synthesizing cGMP from guanosine triphosphate (GTP) and it inhibits inducible NO synthase, potentially reducing the upswing in NO concentration –Dose: Continuos infusion 1–1.5 mg/kg over 1–2 h –Contraindicated if moderate to severe pulmonary hypertension and mixed shock with a Cardiac Index < 2.2 L min^{-1} m^2 –PVR and RV afterload is increased –May cause RV failure if baseline severe PHT –May precipitate serotonergic syndrome, hemolytic anemia (especially in patients with G6PD deficiency) and interferes with pulse oximetry
Hydrocortisone	–Dose: 50 mg/6 h –Recommended if refractory vasoplejic shock with noradrenaline >0.5 mcg/kg/min –May hasten reversal of post-CPB shock, as they do in sepsis, but fail to reduce mortality rates –None of the studies performed focused explicitly on postoperative vasoplegic shock
Vitamin C (ascorbic acid)	–Has known anti-inflammatory effects and may improve autoregulation of microcirculatory blood flow –Dose: 6 gr per day
Vitamin B12 (hydroxocobolamin)	–Mechanism: ability to bind the vasodilatory compound hydrogen sulfide

(continued)

Table 3 (continued)

Agents	Comments
	–Dose: 5 mg over 15 min –Only described in case reports
Angiotensin II	–Endogenous hormone that makes up a component of the renin–angiotensin–aldosterone axis and is a direct, potent vasoconstrictor –Dose: Continuous infusion starting at 20 ng/kg/min –Limited data

after mitral repair and in very hypertrophic LV submitted to Aortic valve replacement. Echocardiography will show regional wall motion abnormalities, prosthetic abnormalities and evidence of SAM. Treatment varies depending on aethiology and may be inotropic drug administration, re-sternotomy for surgical revision and percutaneous coronary intervention in cases of coronary thrombosis. Catecholamines (Dobutamine, Dopamine, Adrenaline) are the commonest inotropic drugs acting through AMPc path differing to Levosimendan that increases sensibility of Troponin to Calcium.

Medical treatment of SAM include optimisation of preload, betablocker for heart rate control and discontinuation of inotropes while promoting a relative high afterload. Intra-aortic balloon pump and mechanical circulatory support (ECMO and ventricular assist devices) are therapeutic option for advanced reversible cardiogenic shock, indications and contraindications are beyond the scope of this chapter being discussed previously in chapter "Anaesthesia for Heart Transplantation".

(D) Obstructive

Pericardial tamponade, tension pneumothorax and acute pulmonary embolus are possible complications after cardiac surgery. They share physiopathologic mechanisms with resistance to blood through heart with compression of cavities and impaired chamber filling due to occupation of pericardial space, mediastinum shift due to pneumothorax or obstruction of flow through pulmonary vessels. High suspicion is key for diagnosis in all.

Pericardial tamponade is presented with evidence of organ dysfunction (oliguria, metabolic acidosis, hyperlactacidaemia, hypotension) with elevated CVP and tachycardia (Table 4). If not diagnosed timely it can lead to cardiac arrest. Echocardiography is key showing collapse of right sided chambers (RV in end diastole and RA in early systole). Fluid resuscitation is mandatory until drainage of collection is performed either surgically or percutaneously.

Tension pneumothorax can occur in patients with end-staged COPD which are under mechanical ventilation or patients after central access insertion (jugular or subclavian vein). Unexplained hypotension in a patient with unilateral absence of ventilatory sounds may raise all alarms. Although Chest X-ray may provide confirmation, if suspicion index is high insertion of chest drain should not be delayed due to high risk of further deterioration if left untreated.

Table 4 Features of pericardial tamponade

Clinical features	Tachycardia, hypotension, high CVP > 13 and signs of organ hypoperfusion Pulsus paradoxus, loss of "*y*" in CVP trace
ECG	Low voltage, electric alternant pattern
Chest X-ray	Enlarged cardiac silhouette
Echocardiography	Diastolic collapse of RV, IVC dilation > 21 mm with a collapse < 50% in inspiration
Doppler	Mitral flow (Max E wave–Min E wave/mean E wave) decreased > 25% and Tricuspid flow increased > 40% during inspiration (spontaneous breathing). Inverse with mechanical ventilation

Table 5 Features of acute pulmonary embolism

Clinical features	–Tachycardia, hypotension and high CVP and hypoxemia, usually associated with a peripheral vein thrombosis
Chest X-ray	–Normal lung
Lung and vascular US	–Normal lung (sliding present, A lines, no B lines, no consolidation) associated with a lack of collapse of common femoral vein or deep femoral vein or popliteal vein in the fossa
Echocardiography	–Dilated RV (basal diameter > 35 mm or RV to LV end-diastolic area ratio >1) –Flattened IV septum –60/60 sign: Acceleration time < 60 ms of RVOT flow and PASP < 60 mmHg –TAPSE < 16 cm –TAPSE/PASP ratio < 0,4 (high risk patients) –TDIs' < 9.5 cm/s. Thrombus in right heart cavities may be observed

Acute pulmonary embolus is an infrequent situation after heart surgery with CPB. Haemodynamic and/or unexplained respiratory compromise are typical presentations (Table 5). CTPA scans will show thrombotic material in pulmonary vessels but if the patient is unstable bedside echocardiography may be an alternative diagnostic option. Dilation of both RA and RV with a paradoxical septum motion, evidence of thrombus in IVC, RA, RV or Pulmonary artery can be seen, which they may push clinician towards thrombolytic therapy.

Rhythm Disturbances

Loss of sinus rhythm can precipitate a clinical deterioration with a decreased cardiac output in patients with compromised diastolic function (i.e. concentric LV hypertrophy due to severe Aortic stenosis). Supraventricular tachycardias are the commonest rhythm disturbances with Atrial fibrillation (AF) and atrial flutter at the top. > 65 years old Hypertension, valve surgery, previous history of AF, COPD and inotropic drug administration are known to be risk factors for presenting with AF and is associated with heart failure, stroke and death.

Aims for treatment include control of Heart rate, maintenance of sinus rhythm and prevention of thrombotic events. Discontinuation of inotropic drugs, normalisation of electrolytes and consideration of undiagnosed infection source are measures to be considered in first place. Administration of sulphate of Magnesium is a possible intervention for both treatment and prophylaxis with limited evidence and controversial studies.

Amiodarone, Class III antiarrythmic, is used for both rate control and pharmacological cardioversion. Other options for heart rate control include short acting betablockers like esmolol and nondihyhydropyridine Calcium blocker like Diltiazem. Digoxin is a valid options for patients with normal kidney function bearing in mind the narrow therapeutic index with risk of cardiotoxicity.

Institution of anticoagulation needs to be balanced against the risk of surgical bleeding specially while chest drains are not removed. CHADS-VASc is a stablished risk score that helps on decision of anticoagulation.

Electrical cardioversion is reserved to patients haemodynamically unstable. Ideally, in patients with AF >48 hours that have not reached anticoagulation levels, thrombus should be ruled out with TOE prior cardioversion.

Certain patients undergoing valve replacement and septal myectomy are at risk of complete heart block due to reversible or irreversible damage of conduction system. Heart block will improve within days is the vast majority but in some a permanent pacemaker will have to be inserted before removal of transient epicardial pacing wires.

Recommended Readings

1. Whelton PK, et al. High blood pressure clinical practice guideline, hypertension; 2017, p. 22.
2. Mehaffey JH, Johnston LE, Hawkins RB, et al. Methylene blue for vasoplegic syndrome after cardiac operation: early administration improves survival. Ann Thorac Surg. 2017;104(1):36–41.
3. Maack C, Eschenhagen T, Hamdani N, et al. Treatments targeting inotropy. Eur Heart J. 2018. https://doi.org/10.1093/eurheartj/ehy60.
4. Jedwab RM, Hutchinson AM, Redley B. Magnesium sulphate replacement therapy in cardiac surgery patients: a systematic review. Aust Crit Care. 2019;32(5):421–33.

Cardiac Surgery-Associated Acute Kidney Injury

Marc Vives

Defining Cardiac Surgery-Associated

Acute Kidney Injury

See Tables 1 and 2.

Renal Protective Strategies

Preoperative Strategies

Delaying elective surgery for renal function optimization in patients with reversible AKI, by avoiding nephrotoxics (such as non-steroidal anti-inflammatory agents, aminoglycoside antibiotics, radiocontrast agents, ACE inhibitors and ARBs), optimizing cardiac output and intravascular volume depletion for congestive heart failure treatment, should be considered.

Current data show that preoperative aspirin therapy may be associated with a significant decrease in the risk for 30-day mortality and postoperative renal failure. Subgroup of patients with eGFR <60 ml/min may have further benefit from using preoperative aspirin.

However, due to the increase risk of bleeding, aspirin should be stopped 3–5 days before non-CABG surgery. Still controversial, whether to stop aspirin, as well, in CABG surgeries with no symptoms of unstable angina or main stem disease.

Recent trials show no benefit from starting statins preoperatively.

However, continuation of statins until the day of surgery should be considered.

M. Vives (✉)
Department of Anesthesiology and Critical Care, Hospital Universitari de Girona Doctor Josep Trueta, Avinguda de França, S/N, 17007 Girona, France

M. Vives and A. Hernandez (eds.), *Cardiac Anesthesia and Postoperative Care in the 21st Century*, https://doi.org/10.1007/978-3-030-79721-8_26

Table 1 KDIGO Acute kidney injury definition

AKI is defined as one of the following:
• An increase in serum creatinine by > = 0.3 mg/dL (26.5umol/l) within 48 h
• An increase in serum creatinine to > = 1.5 times from baseline within the previous 7 days
• Urine volume < = 0.5 ml/kg/h for 6 h

Table 2 KDIGO staging of Acute Kidney Injury

Stage	Serum creatinine	Urine output
I	1.5–1.9 times baseline or > 0.3 mg/dL (26.5umol/l) increase	< 0.5 ml/kg/h for 6-12 h
II	2–2.9 times baseline	< 0.5 ml/kg/h for > 12 h
III	3 times baseline or > 4 mg/dL (353.6 umol/l) increase or initiation of RRT or in patients < 18 years a decrease in eGFR < 35 ml/min/1.73m^2	< 0.3 ml/kg/h for > 24 h or Anuria > 12 h

It is reasonable to use preoperative erythropoietin (EPO) plus iron (especially if ferritin is <100 mg/L), given several days before surgery, in patients with preoperative anemia (hb < 12.5), candidates for operation who refuse transfusion (eg, Jehovah's Witness) and in patients who are at high risk for postoperative anemia. However, chronic use of EPO is associated with thrombotic cardiovascular events in renal failure patients suggesting caution for this therapy in individuals at risk for such events (eg, coronary revascularization patients with unstable symptoms).

Intraoperative Management Strategies

There is evidence to suggest that low preoperative and intraoperative haemoglobin levels are associated independently with CSA-AKI, but unfortunately, there is also evidence to suggest that intraoperative transfusion is independently associated with CSA-AKI.

2017 EACTS/EACTA Guidelines on patient blood management for adult cardiac surgery recommends that one transfuse PRBCs on the basis of the clinical condition of the patient rather than on a fixed haemoglobin threshold with a class I and level B. It is also stated that a haematocrit of 21–24% may be considered during CPB when an adequate DO_2 (>273 ml O_2/min/m2) level is maintained.

Transfusion to keep the Hb > 7 g/dL during CPB, on patients at risk for end-organ ischemia/injury, may be considered (IIb).

TRICS-III trial showed no difference in primary outcome (a composite outcome of death from any cause, myocardial infarction, stroke, or new-onset renal failure with dialysis) comparing hemoglobin 7.5 versus 9.5 g/dL as a trigger for transfusion of RBC intraoperatively and postoperatively in the ICU.

Hyperglucemia (>180 mg/dL) should be avoided during the perioperative period, with caution to avoid also hypoglucemia.

The initiation of a program on blood management decreases the rate of RBC, platelets and FFP transfusion, as well as the rate of AKI (34% relative risk reduction; p 0.039) and the associated healthcare cost. This program consists of transfusion TEG-guided, preoperative anemia optimization, restrictive threshold for intraoperative transfusion, retrograde autologous priming, reduced volume of the bypass circuit and increase use of cell saver and tranexamic acid.

Based on current data, use of mini-CBP and zero-balanced ultrafiltration during CPB, especially for patients with eGFR < 60, may be also considered.

A goal-directed perfusion initiative aiming for DO_2 > 300 ml with MAP > 70 mmHg during CPB plus zero-balanced ultrafiltration, was associated with a significant reduction of AKI at 72 h (23.9% vs. 9.1%). Hence, based on current data, MAP > 70 mmHg and DO_2 > 300 ml O_2/min/m during CPB should be considered.

Surgical Strategies

The CORONARY trial suggests that OPCABG was associated with no significant differences in RRT requirement [hazard ratio (HR), 1.04 (0.61–1.76), P = 0.59]. However, a definition for initiation of RRT was lacking. Hence, patients with the same clinical situation might have been managed differently. Furthermore, OPCABG was associated with a significant decrease in mild AKI, defined by RIFLE-risk [HR, 0.87 (0.76–0.98), P = 0.02] or AKIN stage 1 [HR, 0.87 (0.80–0.96), P = 0.01]. The CORONARY trial at 1 year and 5-years follow-up showed no difference in RRT requirements. However, mild AKI was not analysed.

Pharmacological Renal Protection

A large recent multicenter RCT, the Myriad trial, on 5,400 patients showed no decrease risk of AKI associated with the use of volatile.

Hence, based on current data, the use of volatile anesthetics are not associated with a decrease risk of AKI.

The Renal RIP trial showed a significant reduction on the incidence of major adverse kidney events (death, RRT and persistent renal dysfunction) at 90 days

(14.2% vs. 25%, p = 0.034), associated with the use of rIPC in high risk patients with Cleveland Score >= 6. Moreover, AKI patients in rIPC group recover faster. They observed that the effect of rIPC is attenuated by propofol. Hence, based on current data, use of remote Ischemic pre-conditioning in high risk patients with Cleveland Score ≥ 6, without using propofol, may be considered.

The LICRA trial on 1,136 patients showed no differences in AKI -KDIGO II and III- at 5 days, comparing 0.9% Saline with buffered salt solution. However, in our opinion, given the existing data showing increase risk of AKI with 0.9% saline in ICU patients, balanced crystalloid solutions should be used, unless hyponatremia is present.

It has been suggested that the use of prophylactic fenoldopam, a selective dopamine receptor-1 agonist, during cardiac surgery, might have a renoprotective effect. Unfortunately, a definitive recent multicenter RCT on 667 patients was stopped for futility in the interim analysis.

Natriuretic peptide may induce natriuresis and vasodilatation by opposing the RAAS and vasopressin system. Several multicenter trials and meta-analyses show benefit by decreasing RRT and AKI. Data from 7 systematic reviews showed a significant decrease of RRT rate associated with atrial NP (NNT = 22) and cerebral NP (NNT = 11), with no effect on mortality. Hence, based on current data, use of natriuretic peptide, especially in high risk patients, may be considered.

It has been suggested that the use of sodium bicarbonate might be renoprotective. A higher tubular pH could be protective by inhibiting the hydroxyl radical generation and lipid peroxidation. A multicentre RCT on 427 patients in 2013 was negative. More recently, a meta-analysis of 3 RCT, on 877 patients, observed a benefit in a sub-group analysis on patients undergoing CABG (adjusted OR for RRT 0.38 (0.25–0.58) and OR for AKIN grade 3 0.45 (0.43–0.48). However, imbalances in prognostically important characteristics were observed. Henced, based on present data, prophylactic use of bicarbonate should not be considered.

Levosimendan has predominant renal afferent vasodilatation, rather than efferent. It has been suggested that its use might be renoprotective. A metanalysis on 1,345 patients from 13 RCT, which 87.5% have LVEF < 40%, showed a reduction of AKI rate (OR 0.51, 95% CI 0.34–0.76) and AKI requiring RRT (OR 0.43, 95% CI 0.25–0.76), associated with the use of levosimendan. A recent metanalysis on 2,243 patients from 14 RCT, which included 2 recent large RCT, showed that levosimendan was associated with a significant reduction in 30-day mortality (RR = 0.71, 95% CI = 0.53–0.95; P = 0.023). Subgroup analysis showed that this benefit was confined to the moderate and low ejection fraction studies (RR = 0.44, 95% CI = 0.27–0.70; P < 0.001), whereas no benefit was observed in the preserved ejection fraction studies (RR = 1.06, 95% CI = 0.72–1.56; P = 0.78). Levosimendan also reduced the risk of renal replacement therapy (RR = 0.66, 95% CI = 0.47–0.92; P = 0.015) and low cardiac output (RR = 0.40, 95% CI = 0.22–0.73; P = 0.003). Based on current data, levosimendan still may have a role if use preoperatively, especially for patients with LVEF < 30% and mainly CABG patients.

Dexmedetomidine, is a highly selective alfa-2 agonist with short half-life. Ratio Alfa-2 to alfa-1 1,600:1. Inhibits renin release and attenuates sympathetic activity and vasoconstriction. It causes sympathetic stabilization, anti-inflammatory effect and Ischemic/Reperfusion injury attenuation. Data from a RCT on 200 patients, showed a significant AKI reduction rate (14% vs. 33%) associated with dexmedetomidine compared to placebo. A retrospective single-center on 1,133 patients, using propensity score matching and logistic regression, observed an association between dexmedetomidine and a decrease in AKI rate (26.1% vs. 33.75%; adjusted OR 0.7; 95% CI 0.54–0.91, $p = 0.008$).

Vasopressin binds to AVPR1a to promote vasoconstriction through several pathways, including modulation of adenosine triphosphate–sensitive K + channel function and nitric oxide production and enhancement of the vascular response to catecholamines. Since vasopressin acts on renal efferent arterioles, as opposed to Noradrenaline which acts mainly on the renal afferent arteriole, might have nephroprotective effects. A single double-blind RCT on 330 patients on vasoplejic shock after cardiac surgery, showed a lower composite primary end-point (30-day mortality or stroke, AKI, Mech Vent > 48 h, reoperation), with the use of vasopressin —2% versus 49%, $p = 0.0014$- compared to norepinephrine. Use of vasopressin was also associated with less AKI (10.3% vs. 35.8%, adjusted OR 0.26, 95% CI 0.15–0.46, $p < 0.0001$), less AF with vasopressin (63.8% vs. 82.1%; $P = 0.0004$), no difference in digital or mesenteric ischemia and myocardial infarction. Hence, based on current data, use of vasopressin to protect the kidney in patients with vasoplejic syndrome after cardiac surgery, should be considered.

A recent RCT, on 96 patients, showed that nitric oxide administration (40-ppm during the entire cardiopulmonary bypass period) to patients at moderate risk of renal complications (Cleveland Score, median 3.8 vs. 3.7) undergoing elective cardiac surgery with CPB was associated with decrease in acute kidney injury incidence (20.8% vs. 41.6%; RR 0.5 (95% CI 0.26–0.95; $p = 0.023$) and a higher urine output during cardiopulmonary bypass: 2.6 [2.1;5.08] versus 1.7 [0.80;2.50] mL/kg/h; $p = 0.0002$. Urinary neutrophil gelatinase-associated lipocalin levels 4 h after surgery were significantly lower in NO- treatment group: 1.12 [0.75;5.8] versus 4.62 [2.02;34.55] ng/mL; $p = 0.005$. Significant increase in the urine output during CPB and the decreases in CK and CK-MB in NO-treatment group during postoperative period may suggest an improvement of splanchnic and tissue perfusion potentially preventing DAMPs production.

Cardiopulmonary bypass is associated with changes in intrarenal hemodynamics with local nitric oxide (NO) deficit and vasoconstriction possibly due to local oxygen delivery impairment and renal medullary hypoxia eventually resulting in ischemia–reperfusion injury. Administration of CPB may result in hemolysis and generation of free hemoglobin, which scavenges endotheliocyte-produced NO so a decrease in NO bioavailability causes microcirculatory disorders. Nitric oxide is essentially involved in the nephroprotective mechanisms in animal models of ischemic-reperfusion injury. Nitric oxide is considered a pluripotent molecule and a key mediator of the protective effects in renal ischemia–reperfusion preconditioning. Decrease in NO bioavailability leads to persistent multifocal vasoconstriction potentially triggering vasoactive nephropathy and ischemic injury. Nitric oxide homeostasis and aberrant NO interactions with platelets and coagulation factors significantly contribute to thromboses and abnormal microcirculation including those in renal glomerulus.

Therefore, based on current data, use of intraoperative NO in moderate-high risk patients for developing AKI should be considered.

Therefore, based on current data, the most promising drugs are the following: Natriuretic peptide, Dexmedetomidine, Vasopressin and nitric oxide.

Postoperative Strategies

Data from a RCT on 276 high risk patients showed that KDIGO bundle decrease AKI rate after cardiac surgery. AKI defined by KDIGO 1 or worse at 72 h postoperatively (71% vs. 55%, OR 0.48; 95% CI 0.29–0.79). KDIGO bundle consist of avoiding ACEi/ARB first 48 h postoperatively, avoiding hyperglycemia first 72 h postoperatively, using alternatives to radiocontrast agents and lastly optimizing hemodynamics (goal of Cardiac Index > 3L/min/m2) guided by PiCCO first 48 h (consequently, more dobutamine and similar amount of fluid was used, compared to standard of care).

The early use of RRT after cardiac surgery has been suggested to be associated with improved in-hospital survival in patients with CSA-AKI. Data from a meta-analysis on 847 patients, including 2 RCT and 9 observational cohorts, showed a decrease of 28-days mortality associated with use of early RRT after cardiac surgery (OR 0.29, 95% CI 0.16–0.52, $p < 0.0001$).

A recent well-designed single center RCT on 231 patients (50% of them were post cardiac surgery patients), showed that early use of RRT (within 8 h of diagnosis of KDIGO stage 2) was associated with a decrease in 90-day mortality (39.3% vs. 54.7%), a decrease in RRT duration, mechanical ventilation time and length of hospital stay and increase rate of renal recovery by day 90 (53.6% vs. 38.7%), compared to late use of RRT after cardiac surgery (within 12 h of KDIGO stage 3).

Therefore, based on current data, use of early RRT should be considered.

KDIGO guidelines suggest the use of Continous Renal Repalcement therapy (CRRT) in unstable patients (grade 2B). However, Extended Daily Dialysis (EDD) may also be suitable for treatment in this setting. EDD provides hemodynamic tolerability and is significantly cheaper. No difference in renal function, mortality, renal recovery and hospital stay has been shown. Hemodynamic measurements, including HR, SBP and DBP were comparable. A summary of current Renal protection strategies in cardiac surgery may be found in Table 3.

Table 3 Renal protection strategies in cardiac surgery

Preoperative	Intraoperative	Postoperative
Aspirin	Avoid RBC unless Hb < 7 gr/dL	Keep Hb > 7.5gr/dL
Continue statins	Avoid hemodilution and keep Hb > 7gr/dL	Avoid ACEi/ARB 48 h
Anaemia optimization	Off-pump CABG	Early RRT
Avoid volume deplection	DO_2 > 300 ml/min/ with MAP > 70 mmHg during CPB	Avoid Glycemia > 180 and large glucose variability
Avoid nephrotoxics	Vasopressin/Terlipressin	Avoid nephrotoxics
Iron if Hb < 12.5 and ferritin < 100 mg/L	Avoid Glycemia > 180 and large glucose variability	To optimize CO individually by thermodilution first 2 days
Exogenous albumin if level < 4gr/dL in OPCABG	PBM (TEG, cell saver and tranexamic acid)	Dexmedetomidine
	rIPC in Clev Score > 6 with no propofol	
	Levosimendan for CABG if LVEF < 40%	
	Zero-balanced UF duringCPB for patients with eGFR < 60	
	Use of Nitric Oxide in moderate-high risk patients for CSAKI	

Early Detection of Acute Kidney Injury

The Role of Biomarkers

The use of serum and urinary biomarkers is an additional and promising new approach for the early diagnosis of CSA-AKI. However, the use of biomarkers remains more cumbersome than other diagnostic approaches and is not widely available. The serum creatinine level is traditionally used as a biomarker for renal impairment, but its usefulness can be affected not only by physiological processing (for example, urinary clearance of creatinine, or muscle mass) but also by drugs that block the tubular secretion of creatinine and by some underlying medical conditions, such as diabetes and liver disease.

Given the limitations of serum creatinine as a biomarker, there has been increasing interest in the last decade in the identification of new serum and urinary biomarkers for the early diagnosis and prognostication of AKI following cardiac surgery. New biomarkers could aid early diagnosis of AKI, even in the absence of concurrent renal dysfunction. In response to ischaemic or nephrotoxic injury, tubular cell proteins are released into the urine. Thus, measurement of urinary biomarkers may be more specific and more sensitive than the measurement of serum biomarkers for the detection of AKI.

Novel biomarkers seem to improve risk stratification of CSA-AKI. However, the superiority of one biomarker over another, and the superiority of biomarkers over clinical models, are uncertain. At this stage, the use of biomarkers should not replace thorough clinical assessment of patients with AKI. Finally, the cost-effectiveness of using novel AKI biomarkers in clinical practice remains unclear.

Conclusion

AKI after cardiac surgery is a major perioperative complication that is associated with significant morbidity, mortality and associated costs. Preventive strategies are limited and the evidence for most interventional therapies is as yet not substantive. As our understanding of the pathogenesis of AKI after cardiac surgery grows, we will be able to direct preventive and therapeutic strategies better.

Current approaches include deferring elective surgery until there is adequate recovery following pre-existing renal injury, careful preoperative risk stratification of patients and consideration of less invasive procedures in those at greatest risk. Intraoperatively, the aim should be 'haemodynamic optimization' with goal-directed therapy that includes volume enhancement and judicious use of blood transfusion and inotropic support. We should attempt to avoid renal injury associated with prolonged aortic cross-clamping, prolonged CPB, intravascular haemolysis or contrast dye exposure. The most promising prospects for pharmacological renal protection appear to lie with atrial natriuretic peptide, vasopressin, dexmedetomidine and nitric oxide but much more data are needed. Finally, early treatment by RRT of patients early diagnosed by panels of biomarkers may improve outcomes.

Conflict of Interest None declared.

Recommended Readings

1. Vives M, Hernández A, Parramon F, et al. Acute kidney injury after cardiac surgery: prevalence, impact and management challenges. Int J Nephrol Renovasc Dis. 2019;12:153–66. https://doi.org/10.2147/IJNRD.S167477.
2. Lei C, Berra L, Rezoagli E, et al. Nitric oxide decreases acute kidney injury and stage 3 chronic kidney disease after cardiac surgery. Am J Respir Crit Care Med. 2018;198(10):1279–87. https://doi.org/10.1164/rccm.201710-2150OC.

3. Meersch M, Schmidt C, Hoffmeier A, et al. Prevention of cardiac surgery-associated AKI by implementing the KDIGO guidelines in high-risk patients identified by biomarkers: the PrevAKI randomized controlled trial. Intensive Care Med. 2017;43(11):1551–61. https://doi.org/10.1007/s00134-016-4670-3.
4. Bollinger D, et al. Avoiding acute kidney injury after cardiac surgery: simple and easy? J Cardiothorac Vasc Anaesth. 2018;32:223–4. https://doi.org/10.1053/j.jvca.2017.09.045.

Neurocognitive Dysfunction and Delirium

Lucillia Bezu and Bernard Cholley

Abbreviations

AF	Atrial fibrillation
CABG	Coronary artery bypass grafting
DSM	Diagnostic and Statistical Manual of Mental Disorders
EUROSCORE	European System for Cardiac Operative Risk Evaluation
NIRS	Near-infrared spectroscopy
PCI	Percutaneous coronary intervention
POAF	Postoperative atrial fibrillation
POCD	Postoperative cognitive decline
STS	Society of Thoracic Surgeons
TAVR	Transcatheter aortic valve replacement
TTE	Transthoracic echocardiography

L. Bezu (✉) · B. Cholley
Assistance Publique-Hôpitaux de Paris, Hôpitaux Universitaires Paris Ouest, Hôpital européen Georges Pompidou, service d'anesthésie 20 rue Leblanc, 75015 Paris, France
e-mail: lucillia.bezu@aphp.fr

L. Bezu · B. Cholley
Université Paris Descartes, Sorbonne Paris Cité, France

L. Bezu
Equipe 11 labellisée Ligue contre le Cancer, Centre de Recherche des Cordeliers, INSERM U 1138, Paris, France

L. Bezu
Service d'Anesthésie-Réanimation, Hôpital Européen Georges Pompidou, AP-HP 20 rue Leblanc, 75015 Paris, France

B. Cholley
UMR S1140, INSERM, Paris, France

M. Vives and A. Hernandez (eds.), *Cardiac Anesthesia and Postoperative Care in the 21st Century*, https://doi.org/10.1007/978-3-030-79721-8_27

Introduction

Postoperative neurological complications such as ischemic strokes, cognitive decline, seizure and delirium are a major cause of morbidity and mortality after cardiovascular surgery. Strokes occurring within a month after cardiac surgery increase the mortality rate to 20%. The incidence of perioperative neurological injuries is estimated between 6 and 28%. This incidence is certainly underestimated as evidenced by modern neuroimaging technique such as MRI, which allows to diagnose brain ischemia in asymptomatic patients. The use of minimally invasive surgical procedures like percutaneous coronary artery interventions or off-pump coronary artery bypass grafting has not decreased the incidence of neurological injuries. Patient-related risk factors and comorbidities seem to be more impacting and have to be taken into account by surgeons and cardiologists to choose the type of procedure and apply perioperative preventive care whenever possible. It is clear that the number of cardiac surgical procedures may increase in the future with population ageing. Evaluating the preoperative risk of neurological injuries, recognizing as well as managing these complications is a mandatory requirement for clinicians working in the cardiovascular theater.

In this chapter, we will review the different types of neurological complications occurring after cardiac surgery and their risk factors. We will also discuss perioperative anesthetic management and postoperative treatment strategies to decrease the risk of incidence and to optimize the recovery of patients with brain disorders after cardiac surgery.

Types of Postoperative Neurological Complications

Type I: Ischemic Stroke

Type I complications are well-recognized after cardiovascular surgery and represent the most lethal problems with a mortality of up to 21%. Stroke events represent the first cause of disability and the second cause of death after cardiac surgery. They complicate 1–7.4% of all procedures with cardiopulmonary bypass and up to 9.7% of multi-valve surgeries (Table 1).

Table 1 Perioperative stroke incidence according to cardiac surgery

Cardiac surgery	Stroke incidence (%)
CABG	3.8
Beating heart CABG	1.9
Combined CABG and valve surgery	7.4
Aortic valve surgery	4.8
Mitral valve surgery	8.8
Double or triple valve surgery	9.7

CABG, coronary artery bypass grafting

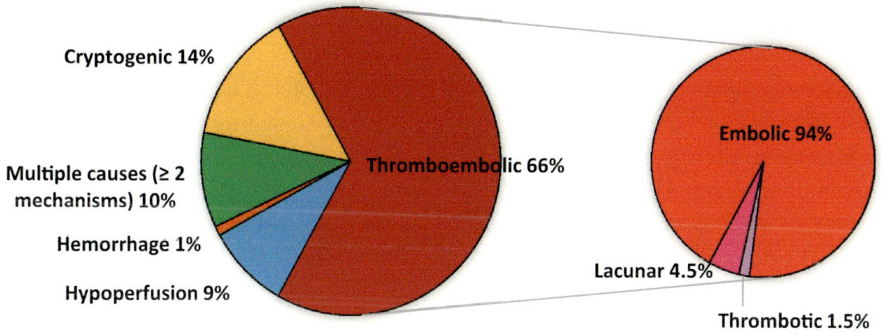

Fig. 1 Stroke etiology

Most often, these focal lesions are due to thromboembolic events occurring during the procedure (40%) after the direct manipulation of the heart and the aorta, or after material projection by the extracorporeal pump. Intraoperative strokes are usually diagnosed at the time of extubation or at day 1, but 58% of ischemic strokes occur later ($\geq$ day 2) and are linked to post-operative atrial fibrillation.

Emboli can be solid, composed of cell fragments, lipid particles and debris from atheromatous plaques, and more rarely gaseous, especially after open heart surgery, when air bubbles can remain trapped within the left heart chambers. Cerebral hypoperfusion, facilitated by hypotension or anemia, is a common aggravating factor. Intracerebral hemorrhage is uncommon (Fig. 1).

Type II: Cognitive Disorders and Encephalopathy

Type II complications encompass all cognitive declines without focal sign defined for instance by language, memory, attention disturbance or psychomotor retardation. Cognitive disorders are more linked to old age and preexisting vascular disease than intraoperative events or technique. Indeed, type II disorders incidence is the same with or without cardiopulmonary bypass. The incidence of cognitive disorders is greater than that of ischemic stroke (28–60%) and these complications are most often reversible. However, a controversial syndrome of postoperative cognitive decline (POCD) associated with a deleterious impact on quality of life and increased 1-year mortality has been described in the literature. Definition and diagnosis of this syndrome are tricky. First of all, this syndrome is not included in the DSM-V (Diagnostic and Statistical Manual of Mental Disorders-V) classification. Very often, the studies have used different tests to describe POCD. Preoperative cognitive evaluation of patients is rarely performed, and quantifying the extent of cognitive decline after surgery represents a difficult challenge.

Seizure

Incidence of seizures after cardiac surgery is close to 0.4%. The causes are multiple: focal lesion, air embolism, toxic encephalopathy resulting from medications administered during the surgery (i.e.: tranexamic acid, beta-lactamines…), or metabolic disorders (hypoxemia, hypoglycemia, hypocalcemia…). Seizures appear in various ways: generalized tonic-clonic seizures, focal seizures, or behavior arrest. In the presence of postoperative seizures, it is important not to miss possible gaseous emboli, since hyperbaric oxygen therapy may represent an effective curative treatment if performed early.

Delirium

Delirium consists of fluctuation in mental status with confusion, attention disorder, memory and psychomotor decline, as well as circadian disruption. It concerns 20–30% of patients after cardiac surgery. Postoperative delirium may be associated with type II complications and agitation is also common. Delirium is correlated with poor outcomes: higher mortality, cognitive disorders and decreased quality of life. Delirium is more frequent after 60 years of age. Perioperative stress, drugs (benzodiazepines), alcohol withdrawal and hypoxia-anemia are the main precipitating factors. Major clinical trials are conducted to try to identify sedation strategies that reduce the incidence of postoperative delirium. To date, no specific treatment has demonstrated a clear ability to reduce this complication.

Risk Factors

Procedures

Coronary Artery Bypass Graft Surgery

Strokes occur at a frequency ranging between 0.8 and 5.2% after CABG surgery. Even in asymptomatic patients, MRI performed in the postoperative period detects strokes in 18 to 26% of the low-risk patients and in more than half of the high-risk patients. Recent data suggest that the type of revascularization procedure does not significantly impact on stroke incidence. Off-pump CABG was initially developed to decrease the rate of cerebral injuries due to pump-related embolic events. However, no significant difference in terms of stroke rate, long-term cognitive dysfunction, and 30-day mortality was found in patients who benefited from off-pump compared to on-pump CABG. Similarly, percutaneous coronary interventions (PCI) are increasingly performed instead of on-pump CABG. Three trials

(SYNTAX, FREEDOM and ASCERT) comparing CABG and PCI observed more strokes in the CABG group but a lower mortality rate. Finally, the choice of revascularization procedure is determined mainly by local expertise, since stroke risk is not clearly affected by the technique itself. It has been demonstrated that the use of epiaortic ultrasound examination in patients undergoing CABG is superior to manual palpation and TTE to detect aortic atherosclerosis, modify the surgical plan and reduce the risk of stroke. This is probably one of the areas where changes in the current practices of many centers could have a significant impact in the reduction of "preventable" strokes.

Aortic Surgery

The rate of stroke after aortic surgery ranks between 5% and 10%. This type of surgery is often performed under hypothermic circulatory arrest. During this procedure, cerebral flow may be maintained with the use of retrograde or antegrade cerebral perfusion. Retrograde cerebral perfusion (via the superior vena cava) has not demonstrated a reduction in postoperative neurological complications. Antegrade perfusion (after cannulation of the left carotid artery and clamping of the left subclavian artery) is commonly used but requires a patent Willis circle to provide a homogeneous brain perfusion. Otherwise, a bilateral antegrade perfusion with cannulation of both primitive carotids can be performed. Currently, there is no evidence supporting one technique for cerebral protection over another. In addition, severity of aortic atherosclerosis is directly correlated with stroke.

Valve Surgery

Minimally invasive transcatheter aortic valve replacement (TAVR) was initially indicated for high risk and fragile patients. Recent studies are suggesting noninferiority or even better results from TAVR over surgical replacement even in low-risk patients with respect to incidence of death and stroke. Multivalvular replacement risk is significantly higher than isolated valve implantation and surgical treatment is exclusively recommended for symptomatic patients unless there is myocardial or pulmonary arterial repercussion.

Atrial Fibrillation

Preexisting atrial fibrillation is also a potential source of emboli and a major risk factor of stroke. Moreover, 30–50% of patients present post-operative atrial fibrillation (POAF) after CABG procedure and this incidence is even higher after valvular surgery. Some authors even reported 100% of POAF after surgical aortic valvular replacement when an implantable loop recorder was used for detection of arrythmia. Prevention of POAF is therefore of paramount importance to try to reduce the incidence of postoperative stroke. Nowadays, the guidelines recommend the use of beta-blockers as a first-line treatment. Perioperative withdrawal of these agents has been recognized as a major risk factor for POAF. Some surgeons advise to perform posterior pericardiotomy during the procedure to reduce POAF. Ligation of the left atrial appendage may be proposed for patients with permanent atrial fibrillation to reduce the risk of thrombus formation. Surgical treatment of atrial fibrillation (Maze procedure, cryoablation, radiofrequency) is sometimes associated in the hope of restoring sinus rhythm in patients with permanent or persistent atrial fibrillation.

Occlusive Cerebrovascular Disease

Patients with carotid stenosis of 50 to 99% present a 7.4% perioperative risk of stroke. It is recommended to screen patients before cardiac surgery using echo and Doppler duplex examination to detect significant carotid stenosis (Class I, Level C). Combined carotid and coronary surgery may be considered in the case of symptomatic carotid disease (Class IIa, Level C).

Patient-Related Factors

Type I complications are mainly due to cerebral macro-embolism promoted by direct manipulation of atherosclerotic plaques during the procedure (surgical palpation, or cannula jet against atheromatic wall of the ascending aorta). Atherosclerosis of the ascending aorta, ischemic stroke history, internal carotid stenosis, diabetes, hypertension, dyslipidemia, female gender and age are also major risk factors for Type I complications.

Age, hypertension, arrhythmia, anemia, drug and alcohol dependence are the common risk factors linked to type II complications and POCD (Tables 2 and 3).

Genetic Factors and Biomarkers

Genetic and proteomic approaches tend to explain cognitive disorders occurring after cardiac surgery. Recent data suggest that some single nucleotide polymorphisms of C-reactive protein may be associated with a decrease in cognitive troubles. Contradictory results imply that "apolipoprotein E-e4", a molecule associated with Alzheimer's disease could be a potential screening factor. Cerebrospinal fluid biomarkers such as S100β, tau and β-amyloid are well-correlated with cognitive

Table 2 Risk factors of stroke after cardiac surgery

Patients factors	Procedure factors
Age>70 years Female sex Hypertension Left cardiac insufficiency (Ejection fraction< 40%) Diabetes Dyslipidemia Chronic renal insufficiency History of stroke or transient ischemic attack Valvulopathy Atherosclerosis in ascending aorta Atrial fibrillation Carotid stenosis	Emergency surgery Type of surgical procedure Duration of cardiopulmonary bypass Aortic cross-clamp time Manipulation of proximal aortic with atherosclerosic lesions Arrhythmia

Table 3 Risk factors of delirium after cardiac surgery

Patient factors	Procedure factors
Age > 60–70 years Gender male History of cerebrovascular disease Delirium in history Comorbidities Atrial fibrillation Withdrawal (alcohol, opioids…) Metabolic disorders (hypoxia-anemia…) EUROSCORE (> 5)	Blood transfusion in the first 48 h Procedure type (excepted isolated CABG) Longer aortic clamping time (> 120 min) Mechanical ventilation (> 24 h) Drugs (anesthetic agents: fentanyl, benzodiazepine) Postoperative atrial fibrillation Length of stay in the ICU > 24 h

disorders. Neuron-specific enolase and glial fibrillary acidic protein showed interesting results as eventual diagnostic and prognostic factors for postoperative delirium.

Perioperative Management

Cerebral Monitoring

Intraoperative cerebral monitoring provides anesthesiologists with insights on brain perfusion (Doppler velocities of middle cerebral arteries), brain tissue oxygenation (NIRS), and even function (electroencephalography, BIS®, or Sedline®). It is undoubtedly very relevant to have regional indicators of the adequacy of perfusion, or to be able to detect the occurrence of asymmetry in the electrical cortical pattern in situation where the brain is exposed to the risk of stroke. However, data showing that interventions targeting the various parameters of cerebral monitoring in order to reduce the incidence of complications are lacking. Continuous electroencephalographic monitoring can detect ischemia and seizure but is seldom available during cardiac surgery. Cerebral oximetry monitoring using near-infrared spectroscopy (NIRS) can detect cerebral oxygen desaturation events, which are directly correlated with cognitive disorders severity, but only if they occur in the very limited volume of brain tissue monitored by the device. Finally, transcranial Doppler can detect the microemboli signals in the middle cerebral arteries. Twenty percent of cardiac surgical patients have a loss of cerebral autoregulation, which is associated with increased stroke rate.

Hypothermia

Hypothermia decreases cerebral metabolism and inflammatory response, which allows to perform procedures under circulatory arrest without major neurological side effects. However there is no evidence that hypothermia prevents cognitive function decline after cardiac surgery. Moreover, hypothermia prolongs the duration of procedures and cardiopulmonary bypass, which in turn increases the risk of postoperative neurological disorders of all types. Finally, the rewarming period exposes the brain to additional damage if performed too quickly. Neurological consequences are directly proportional to the decrease of jugular vein saturation during the rewarming. Hypothermia does not yield additional reduction in postoperative neurological complications but remains a very useful strategy to perform procedures under circulatory arrest.

Secondary Cerebral Stress of Systemic Origin

As for brain trauma, secondary cerebral stress of systemic origin (hypotension, hypertension, hypoxemia, hypercapnia, hypocapnia, anemia, hyperthermia, hypothermia and hyperglycemia) has to be controlled. Indeed, cerebral autoregulation is particularly disturbed in case of severe hypothermia (<25 °C), pH-stat management of PCO_2 during bypass (leading to respiratory acidosis and increased cerebral blood flow), or diabetes. During cardiopulmonary bypass, cerebral autoregulation is best preserved as long as mean arterial pressure $\geq$40 mmHg, temperature $\geq$28 °C, and when normocapnia is maintained.

An association was found between intraoperative hypotension and postoperative neurologic complications in particular for patients with severe aortic atherosclerosis. A systolic blood pressure of less than 50 mmHg for at least 10 minutes increases the incidence of neurologic complications. It is recommended to target a mean arterial pressure greater than 80 mmHg.

Severe hemodilution with a hematocrit lower than 18% increases stroke rate especially in elderly patients after coronary bypass. Hemoglobin has to be maintained at least above 7 g/dl (Class IIa, Level C). Antifibrinolytic therapy used during cardiac surgery decreases blood loss, but aprotinin was associated with a higher rate of stroke and encephalopathy. This drug was subsequently withdrawn from the market, but its reintroduction is currently evaluated with regards to a potential positive benefit/risk balance. Tranexamic acid induces seizures but has been less studied than aprotinin.

Perioperative hyperglycemia increases neurocognitive disorders especially in non-diabetic patients. Current STS guidelines recommend maintaining glycemia lower than 180 mg/dl in the perioperative period (Class I, Level B).

Epiaortic Ultrasound

As mentioned in paragraph 2.1.1, epiaortic ultrasound examination prior to aortic cannulation, may help to detect atheromatous plaques more effectively and safely than by using TTE or manual palpation of the aorta. By locating the plaques at risk of producing emboli, it has been suggested that as much as one third of postoperative strokes could be avoided. Whenever plaques are detected, the surgeon can modify his cannulation plan in order to choose a safer approach (using femoral or subclavian artery) and reduce cerebral embolization (Class IIa, Level B).

Cardiopulmonary Bypass Management

Cardiopulmonary bypass management (pH-stat versus alpha-stat) has a moderate impact on neurologic outcome. During pH-stat acid-base management, the perfusionist aims at achieving a PCO_2 of 40 mmHg and a pH of 7.40 at the patient's actual temperature. On the other hand, when using alpha-stat, pH is not temperature-corrected. Thus, pH-stat management leads to higher PCO_2 values, respiratory acidosis, and increased cerebral blood flow as a consequence of cerebral vasodilation. In a prospective study involving 52 patients randomized to alpha-stat versus pH-stat management, the authors showed that pH-stat management led to increased jugular venous oxygen saturation, suggesting increased cerebral blood flow. A study by Murkin et al. comparing pH-stat to alpha-stat suggested that alpha-stat management was associated with a decreased incidence of cognitive dysfunction in patients undergoing prolonged cardiopulmonary bypass. The authors concluded that pH-stat management might increase cerebral blood flow, but also the embolic load to the brain. Type II complications are also less frequently observed under alpha-stat management.

Postoperative Treatment

If a patient presents with postoperative neurological disorders, it is mandatory to eliminate metabolic or pharmacologic etiologies and to rule out confounding factors. Some neurological complications require emergency management whereas others just need monitoring and prevention of aggravating circumstances. Neurological symptoms deserve neuroimaging (brain MRI or CT-scan) to confirm the underlying diagnosis and guide treatment. Modern neuroimaging technologies such as MRI with diffusion-weighted imaging or functional imaging serve as supplement to identify micro-embolism, acute cerebral events, asymptomatic ischemic attack, and to target patients at risk from neurocognitive decline after cardiac surgery. When an acute ischemic stroke is suspected, the patient has to undergo computerized tomography or magnetic resonance angiography in emergency to localize the intra-arterial occlusion. Thrombo-aspiration (thrombectomy) or catheter disruption techniques are the only therapeutic maneuvers available in the immediate postoperative period and can be performed at specialized centers. Intravenous thrombolysis cannot be performed within 14 days following major surgery. The delay to perform thrombectomy after a perioperative strokes should be less than 3 to 8 hours, according the vessel involved. Ischemia may be associated with cerebral edema and secondary brain hemorrhage. The control of secondary cerebral stress of systemic origin is absolutely mandatory.

Treatment of seizure is based on benzodiazepine administration combined with exclusion of precipitating factors.

Some data suggested that new neuroleptics such as olanzapine, risperidone, or dexmedetomidine, an alpha-2-agonist could be of interest. Dexmedetomidine has been widely investigated and initially raised hopes that it would help reduce postoperative delirium. However, the alleged benefits in terms of cognitive function, delirium, days off ventilator, and ICU length of stay have not been confirmed by recent large-scale studies. The proportion of patients developing hypotension, bradycardia, and even asystole is far greater with dexmedetomidine than with usual sedation.

Prevention

Pharmacologic Therapies

Aspirin is commonly administered in the perioperative period for patients undergoing cardiac surgery. Aspirin decreases stroke incidence by 50% if initiated within 48 hours after CABG. The use of aspirin before surgery does not reduce the incidence of cerebrovascular events.

Inhibitors of 3-hydroxy-3-methylglutaryl coenzyme A reductase (statins) are also routinely administered in the perioperative period of CABG surgery. These agents significantly reduce atrial fibrillation occurrence, hospital duration, stroke incidence and mortality, probably through their anti-inflammatory and neuroprotective effects that are part of their pleiotropic properties. Therefore, maintenance of their administration perioperatively is recommended (Class 1, Level A Recommendation).

A meta-analysis including 58 studies showed that amiodarone or betablockers given 5 days before surgery decrease the incidence of POAF. However, no guidelines recommend the systematic preventive use of these agents 5 days before surgery yet. Beta blockers should be administrated 24 hours before CABG to reduce POAF incidence.

a. **Preoperative carotid disease treatment**

According to the American College of Cardiology/American Heart Association guidelines, it is recommended to perform carotid screening in patients over 65 years, smokers, with left coronary stenosis, with peripheral vascular disease, with transient ischemic attack or stroke history or with carotid bruit on examination (Level C). Carotid endarterectomy "before CABG or concomitant to CABG" is thus advocated in case of high-risk asymptomatic disease (80% stenosis) or with symptomatic stenosis (Level C).

b. **Preoperative risk predictors**

In 2003, Charlesworth et al. proposed a predictive model for perioperative strokes after CABG integrating the different patient- and procedure-related risk factors.

Some online calculators such as EUROSCORE II (EUROpean System for Cardiac Operative Risk Evaluation) or STS Adult Cardiac Surgery Risk Calculator or the NSQIP surgical risk calculator based on demographic variables, comorbidity, cardiac data and procedure type may help the physicians to calculate mortality risk after cardiac surgery. However none of these models estimates the risk of neurologic complications specifically.

http://www.euroscore.org/calc.html
http://riskcalc.sts.org/STSWebRiskCalc273/.
https://riskcalculator.facs.org/RiskCalculator/

Concluding Remarks

Neurocognitive dysfunction and delirium still represent very frequent complications after cardiac surgery with significant impact on mortality, despite the technical improvement in surgical procedures. Patient risk factors, especially cardiovascular and atherosclerosis diseases, represent the main potential etiologies for these complications and have to be recognized before the procedure. Aspirin and statin introduced in preoperative proved to be a good option to decrease neurologic complications occurrence. Epiaortic ultrasound is a simple, noninvasive procedure that may potentially modify the surgical plan and reduce the risk of aortic arch embolism when atheroma is detected prior to aortic cannulation. During the perioperative period, anesthesiologists must pay attention to any information on neurological symptoms and should focus on evicting factors such as atrial fibrillation, hypotension, anemia or psychoactive medications. In case of neurological injury, early diagnosis with appropriate modern neuroimaging and early thromboaspiration associated with rehabilitation represent the best strategy to optimize recovery.

Recommended Readings

1. Popma JJ, et al. Transcatheter aortic-valve replacement with a self-expanding valve in low-risk patients. N Engl J Med. 2019;380(18):1706–15.
2. Mack MJ, et al. Transcatheter aortic-valve replacement with a balloon-expandable valve in low-risk patients. N Engl J Med. 2019;380(18):1695–705.
3. Jorgensen TH, et al. Temporal changes of new-onset atrial fibrillation in patients randomized to surgical or transcatheter aortic valve replacement. Int J Cardiol. 2017;1(234):16–21.
4. Couffignal CAJ, Ait-Hamou N, Cholley B, Fellahi JL, Duval X, et al. Timing of b-blocker reintroduction and the occurrence of postoperative atrial fibrillation after cardiac surgery. Anesthesiology. 2020;132(2):1–13.
5. Mufti HN, Hirsch GM. Perioperative prediction of agitated (hyperactive) delirium after cardiac surgery in adults—the development of a practical scorecard. J Crit Care. 2017;42:192–9.
6. Gailiusas M, et al. Association between serum biomarkers and postoperative delirium after cardiac surgery. Acta Med Litu. 2019;26(1):8–10.
7. Wu M, et al. Perioperative dexmedetomidine reduces delirium after cardiac surgery: a meta-analysis of randomized controlled trials. J Clin Anesth. 2018;50:33–42.
8. Shehabi Y, et al. Early sedation with dexmedetomidine in critically Ill patients. N Engl J Med. 2019;380(26):2506–17.

Resuscitation in the Cardiac Intensive Care Setting

Tim Strang, Syed Faisal Hashmi, Joel Dunning, and Adrian Levine

Introduction

The Cardiac Surgery Advanced Life Support (CALS) course was developed in response to recognized differences required for management of arrested patients post sternotomy as an addendum to standard ERC ALS guidelines. CALS form the European ACTS and US STS guidelines [1]. This methodology has now been taught in interactive simulation courses worldwide with e learning and formal certification—www.csu-als.org These modifications to standard ALS have now been incorporated by the ERC and incorporated into the 'Special Situations—post cardiac surgery' section, which applies only to patients up to 10 days post sternotomy, who arrest on a cardiac intensive care unit. The "10 day rule" has been adopted due to a number of reasons.

Firstly, the disease processes that cause cardiac arrest after day 10 are unlikely to be those for which emergency re-sternotomy will be beneficial. Secondly, that by this time intra-pericardial adhesions are forming which makes emergency re-sternotomy and internal cardiac massage extremely difficult for all but the most experienced cardiac surgeons.

T. Strang (✉)
Anaesthetist, Manchester Foundation Trust, Wythenshawe Hospital, Wythenshawe, England
e-mail: timstrang@doctors.org.uk

S. F. Hashmi
Cardiothoracic Surgeon, Manchester Foundation Trust, Wythenshawe Hospital, Wythenshawe, England

J. Dunning
Cardiothoracic Surgeon, James Cook Hospital, Middlesborough, England

A. Levine
Cardiothoracic Surgeon, Royal Stoke University Hospital, Stoke-on-Trent, England

M. Vives and A. Hernandez (eds.), *Cardiac Anesthesia and Postoperative Care in the 21st Century*, https://doi.org/10.1007/978-3-030-79721-8_28

How It is Different from Standard Ward Arrest I.E ALS Protocol

In the intensive care setting many more skilled member of staff are available and the patient is often highly monitored and intubated. In case of a cardiac arrest, the unresponsive patient or abnormal rhythm is recognised immediately and CPR commenced. There are a much wider range of possible therapies then available for the resuscitation team. Chest re-opening is a standard part of resuscitation—indeed when considering the 4 h's and 4 t's in the post sternotomy setting all these pathologies are resolved by chest opening. This is because the cause of arrest on the cardiac ICU is often mechanical eg tamponade, blown graft, loss of pacing, unrecognised tension pneumothorax.

What Are the Key Components of Arrest Management

Early identification of patient pre-arrest.

Key specific roles for team members on arrival at scene (Fig. 1).

Adoption of modified protocol regarding defibrillation /drugs see Fig. 2.

Use of simplified chest opening kit (Fig. 3).

Use of 'all in one' sterile drape (with a central adhesive window)—no prep to wound.

Successful outcome in 48% if chest opened rapidly [2].

Key Specific Roles and Modifications from 'Standard' ALS

1. Identification of Arrest—do not be sidetracked by monitor traces!
Defibrillate or pace before massage if equipment present at bedside.
Efficacy of massage can be judged from A line trace.
Switch IABP to pressure mode.

2. Airway role: confirmation of ET tube position, exclude or treat tension pneumothorax (may be difficult in a noisy ICU environment) Please note how the 'traditional' protocol has been modernised in the light of the CV 19 pandemic. Accent has been placed on the wearing of full PPE, avoiding aerosol generation particularly from inadvertently disconnected airway equipment. SAFE DOFFING OF PPE IN AN AREA SO AS NOT TO FURTHER SPREAD VIRUS IS MANDATORY. This is easily forgotten after the drama of an emergency.

3. Defibrillation –in VF 3 shocks if required are administered before chest opening, anticipate the need for internal paddles to be attached and used with defibrillator.

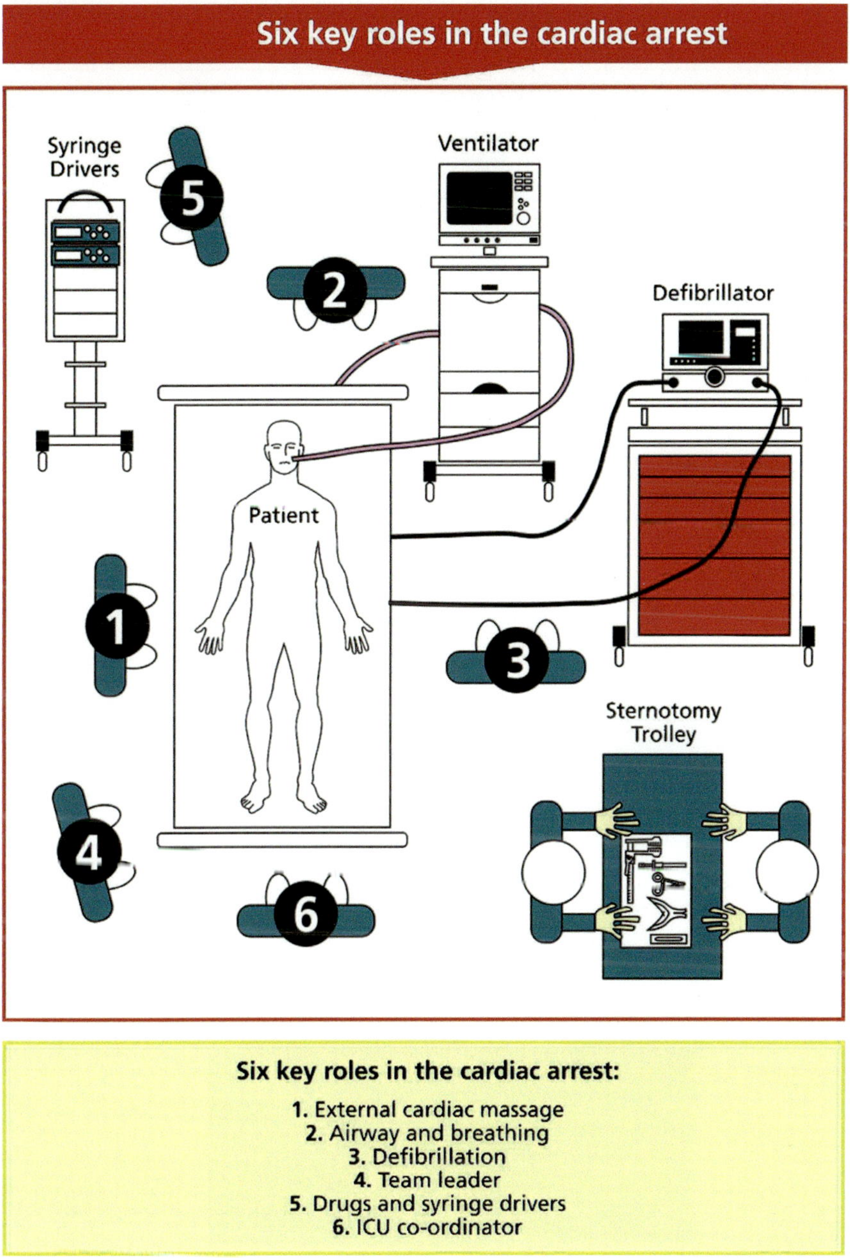

Fig. 1 The chest opening team

CARDIAC ARREST IN POST -OP CARDIAC SURGICAL PATIENT WITH RECENT STERNOTOMY

POTENTIAL OR CONFIRMED COVID 19 POSITIVE FULL LEVEL 3 PPE BEFORE APPROACHING PATIENT

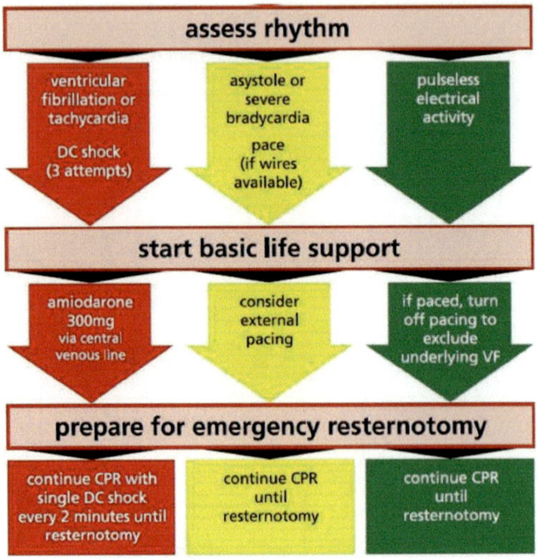

AIRWAY AND VENTILATION

IF INTUBATED / VENTILATED

100% O_2 AND GIVE MUSCLE RELAXANT

SUCTION ETT WITH **CLOSED SUCTION** IF CONNECTED; **DO NOT DISCONNECT FROM VENTILATOR UNLESS HIGH VENTILATOR PRESSURE / ETT PROBLEM SUSPECTED**

CLAMP ETT; PLUS PUT VENTILATOR ON 'STAND BY' IF DISCONNECTING VENTILATION CIRCUIT AT ANY TIME

LISTEN FOR BREATH SOUNDS BILATERALLY TO EXCLUDE PNEUMOTHORAX OR HAEMOTHORAX

IF TENSION PNEUMOTHORAX SUSPECTED , IMMEDIATELY PLACE LARGE BORE CANNULA IN THE 2ND RIB SPACE ANTERIOR MID-CLAVICULAR LINE

IF NON-INTUBATED

BAG / MASK VENTILATION WITH 2 PERSONS / 2 HANDS + AIRWAY ADJUNCTS + HME ATTACHED, TO iGel / LMA , LEADING TO RE-INTUBATION BY **MOST SENIOR ANESTHETIST / INTENSIVIST PRESENT**

DO NOT GIVE ADRENALINE / EPINEPHRINE UNLESS A SENIOR DOCTOR ADVISES IT

IF AN IABP IS IN PLACE CHANGE TO PRESSURE TRIGGER

DO NOT DELAY BASIC LIFE SUPPORT FOR DEFIBRILLATION OR PACING FOR MORE THAN **ONE MINUTE IF ALL IN ATTENDANCE WEARING LEVEL 3 PPE**

AFTER ARREST REMOVE PPE AS APPROPRIATE AND REMOVE / THROW AWAY ALL EQUIPMENT AS LOCAL COVID POLICY

Fig. 2 Arrest protocol

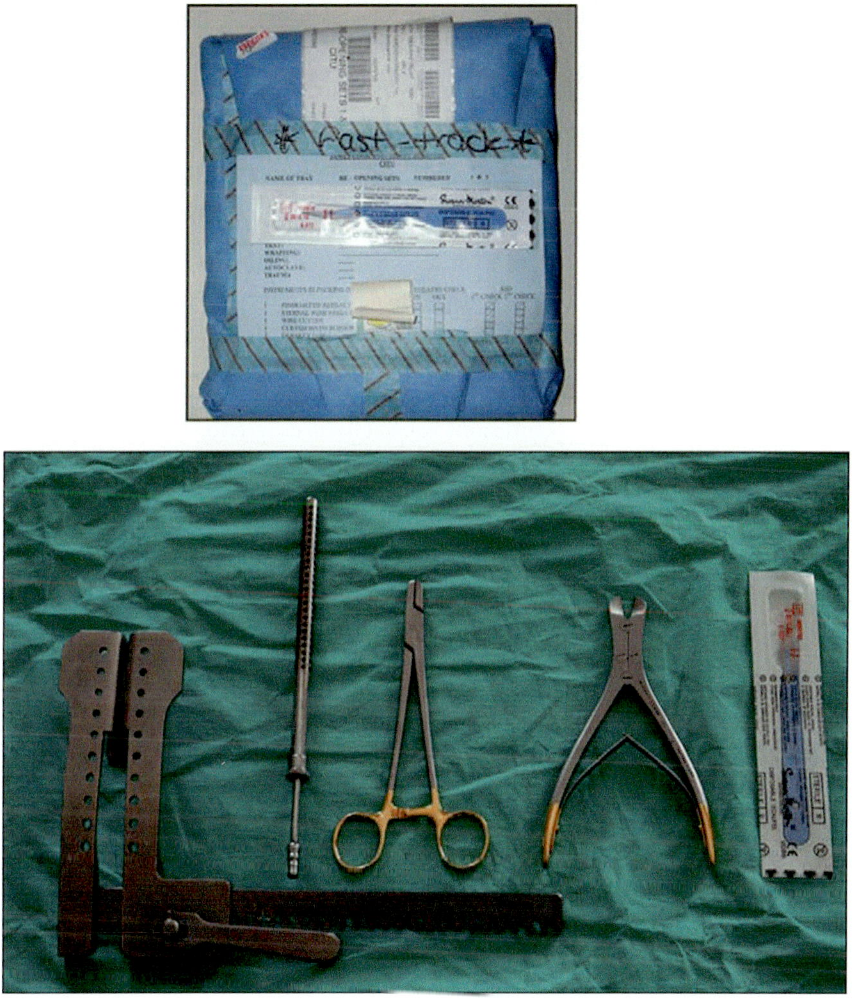

Fig. 3 Simplified chest opening kit

Asystole—attach pacer (then another if required)—DDD, rate 90, maximum output, check connections anticipate the need for internal wires.

PEA—turn off pacer to unmask covert VF.

4. Team Leader—Make Early Decision to Open Chest. (Do not Delay by Phone Calls to Senior)

Gown and glove rapidly minimal (if any) hand wash.

Do not apply cleaning agents to wound—these work by drying and delay opening.

Apply 'all in one drape' to patient after massager has removed wound dressing.

Massage over sterile dressing until chest opening kit delivered.

Open chest (another sterile assistant can help), deliver internal massage/shocks, identify cause of arrest.

Communication can be challenging particularly if CV 19 respirator PPE masks are worn –practise using 'silent cockpit ' drills and local visual aide memoirs can be useful.

5. Drugs—do NOT give epinephrine (will cause catastrophic hypertension once tamponade relieved). Stop all infusions especially if drug error a possibility.

6. Coordinator sends for additional help. Assist others to rapidly gown and deliver opening kit.

What are Pitfalls of Chest Opening

Note scalpel cannot be packaged in a hospital assembled sterile kit—use a disposable scalpel or preferably the complete disposable CALS opening kits (available www.csu-als.com).

Chest opening itself is harmless—even without sternal retraction tamponade may be resolved.

Internal massage can carry hazards—avoid dislodging LIMA, grafts and pacing wires.

Only use 2 handed technique—one placed gently posterior to LV.

Single handed technique may result in thumb through RV or annular disruption!

Is the Protocol Intended to Credential Nurses to Open the Chest Independently?

The protocol is intended to teach all members of the team the indications for opening the chest, how to open the chest safely and efficiently as a team. Even though it is unlikely CALS accredited nurses will open the chest independently without a surgical provider present. More often they may play a role in assisting the providers who are doing so. Having a good understanding of the process and the equipment makes the overall procedure more efficient and more likely to be successful.

What do we do in Patients that have not had a Sternotomy but have had Cardiac Surgery via Another Approach (Mini-Thoracotomy)?

The protocol is designed for patients who have had a sternotomy only BUT the ethos of the training teaches the need to prepare for every eventuality which can occur post-operatively with such patients. Simply put the operating surgeon must ensure that the staff members are fully aware of how an emergency reopening should be performed should cardiac arrest occur in these patients. Further guidance on how emergency access to such patients hearts and the performance of internal cardiac massage can be found on the document CALS AND MINIMAL ACCESS CARDIAC SURGERY.

Further information to help with regular training

www.csu-als.org

Full EACTS guidelines http://webapp.doctors.org.uk/Redirect/dx.doi.org/10.1016/j.ejcts.2009.01.033

CALS manual

http://webapp.doctors.org.uk/Redirect/www.lulu.com/content/442826

Demonstration of chest opening

https://www.youtube.com/watch?v=PHgYZDgQJgc.

References

1. Dunning J, et al. Guideline for resuscitation in cardiac arrest after cardiac surgery. Eur J Cardio-thoracic Surg. 2009;36:3–28.
2. Mackay JH, Powell SJ, Osgathorp J, Rozario CJ. Six-year prospective audit of chest reopening after cardiac arrest. Eur J Cardio-thoracic Surg. 2002;22:421–5.

Management of Mechanical Circulatory Support on the Intensive Care Unit

M. Charlesworth and R. Templeton

Acute Heart Failure on the Critical Care Unit

Acute heart failure is a state of 'cardiogenic shock', where the performance of either the right, left or both ventricles leads to inadequate end-organ perfusion and eventually, multi-organ failure syndrome. It should not be confused with chronic heart failure and its exacerbations, but is heterogenous in its presentation and with variable precipitants and severity. Early diagnosis and recognition are key to optimise delivery of oxygen to tissues and avoid the spiral towards refractory cardiogenic shock. This includes persistent systemic hypotension and signs of impaired end-organ perfusion, but definitions in the literature vary and clinical history taking together with examination are arguably of the most utility. It can be classified according to echocardiographic and clinical features (Box 1).

Box 1: Classification of cardiogenic shock by ejection fraction.

- Heart failure with reduced ejection fraction (< 40%)
- Heart failure with mid-range ejection fraction (40–49%). Must also have elevated brain natriuretic peptide and at least one of: structural heart disease, such as left ventricular hypertrophy or left atrial enlargement; or diastolic enlargement.
- Heart failure with preserved ejection fraction (> 50%). Must also have elevated brain natriuretic peptide and at least one of: structural heart disease, such as left ventricular hypertrophy or left atrial enlargement; or diastolic enlargement.

M. Charlesworth (✉) · R. Templeton
Consultants in Cardiothoracic Anaesthesia, Critical Care and ECMO, Wythenshawe Hospital, Manchester University NHS Foundation Trust, Manchester, UK
e-mail: michael.charlesworth@mft.nhs.uk

R. Templeton
e-mail: rtempleton7@doctors.org.uk

M. Vives and A. Hernandez (eds.), *Cardiac Anesthesia and Postoperative Care in the 21st Century*, https://doi.org/10.1007/978-3-030-79721-8_29

Causes include, but are not limited to: acute coronary syndrome and its complications; myocarditis; arrhythmogenic right ventricular cardiomyopathy; and other cardiomyopathies. The selection of patients for mechanical circulatory support is complex, and depends on: baseline patient demographics; aetiology of cardiogenic shock and its severity; technical limitations; resources and training; and in some cases, whether the patient would be a candidate for heart transplantation following recovery from any associated multi-organ failure. This is further complicated by the range of available devices and their management on the critical care unit (Fig. 1).

After cardiogenic shock has been recognised and before the need for referral to a specialist heart team, there are several management strategies that must be considered. First, invasive arterial blood pressure monitoring must be available, as must central venous access (and ideally access for renal replacement therapy, if needed). Although echocardiography allows the performance of the heart to be evaluated more generally, it may also reveal: inflammation; pericardial disease; structural/valvular heart disease; pulmonary artery pressures; and shunting. It allows for dynamic measurements to be taken to assess the response to certain interventions, such as a fluid bolus, vasopressors or inotropes. Vasopressors might be used for systemic hypotension, with noradrenaline the first line agent followed by vasopressin and then other agents for refractory vasoplegia, such as methylene blue or high dose hydroxocobalamin. Next, in a patient with cardiogenic shock and systemic hypotension, escalating vasopressor requirements are seldom enough alone to restore end-organ perfusion, and inotropes should be considered. These may help to improve stroke volume, and the choice of which drug to use (dobutamine, milrinone, dopamine, adrenaline, levosimendan etc.) is usually dependent on the treating centre, with no ideal inotrope suitable for all cases. Fluids might then be used to treat hypovolemia, but fluid balance must be carefully monitored and renal replacement therapy initiated early in the overloaded or acidotic patient. In subacute cases, significant fluid overload is commonly seen, which can result in venous congestion and exacerbate poor organ perfusion.

Haemodynamic monitoring might be achieved with a pulmonary artery catheter, and although these have fallen out of favour in some centres, they might still have a role when titrating therapy for the patient with cardiogenic shock. They enable the measurement of pulmonary artery pressures, right atrial and ventricular pressure, pulmonary artery wedge pressure, mixed venous oxygen saturations, oxygen delivery, oxygen consumption and oxygen extraction. Such values will be of interest to the heart team, should the patient be referred for mechanical circulatory support. Transpulmonary thermodilution might also allow for variables to be determined, such as: cardiac output; pulse pressure variation; stroke volume variation; global end-diastolic volume; pulmonary vascular permeability index; and extravascular lung water.

Ultimately, the patient should be discussed early with the local heart team, more so if the patient is young and a possible candidate for heart transplantation in the long term. The heart team might then takeover care of the patient and consider the

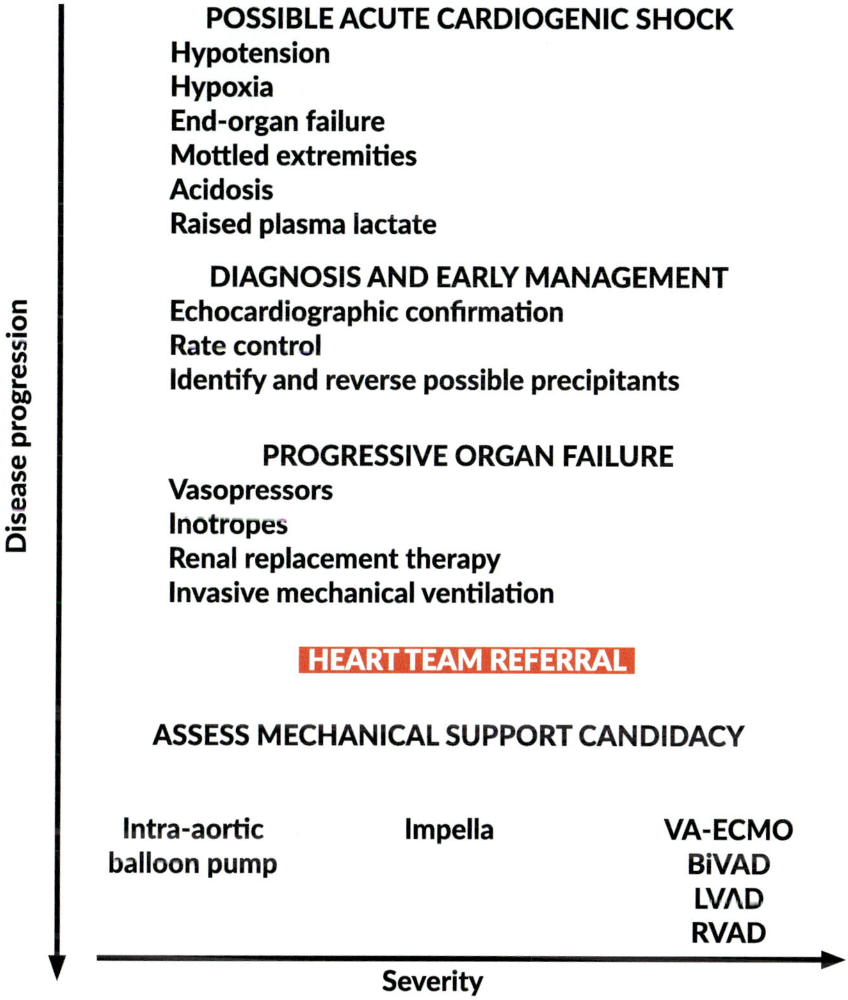

Fig. 1 The management of cardiogenic shock in the UK. Patients with cardiogenic shock might present or be cared for at a hospital without access to a heart team, in which case these patients should be discussed with the nearest heart team hospital. There is no agreed consensus on which to select patients for mechanical support or on which device should be used, and each case is assessed on a case-by-case basis

use of mechanical circulatory support, which can take various forms. Mechanical circulatory support can be as: a bridge to decision; a bridge to candidacy; a bridge to transplantation; a bridge to recovery; or destination therapy.

Venovenous Extracorporeal Membrane Oxygenation

Venovenous extracorporeal membrane oxygenation (VV-ECMO) is indicated for certain patients with severe respiratory failure and is centrally commissioned in England, with five centres providing the service. Patients with acute heart failure have variable clinical presentations, but acute hypoxia is usually a feature. It is common for patients with acute heart failure to be referred for VV-ECMO early in their management, and if the aetiology is thought to be cardiogenic shock, they should instead be discussed with the heart team for assessment of mechanical circulatory support candidacy.

Intra-Aortic Balloon Pump Counterpulsation

Intra-aortic balloon pumps (IABP) consist of a balloon filled with helium (in case of balloon rupture, helium is absorbed fully into the blood without a risk of gas emboli) which inflates in time with the cardiac cycle. Once the aortic valve closes, the balloon inflates, displacing blood within the aorta. The displaced blood is directed preferentially into the coronary arteries, thereby improving myocardial oxygen delivery. Secondly, when the balloon deflates, a negative pressure is created in the aorta, which reduces afterload and causes a suction event into the left ventricle, again reducing left ventricular workload and helping prevent left ventricular wall distension. The IABP-SHOCK II randomised controlled trial included 600 patients with cardiogenic shock after acute myocardial infarction with early revascularisation, and found no difference between IABP and control groups. Although the IABP was downgraded by several institutions for cardiogenic shock thereafter, and with no evidence for benefit reported in a recent meta-analysis, it still arguably has an important role to play as an initial device for heart failure at our centre. It augments cardiac output by ~ 0.5 l min^{-1}, decreases afterload, increases mean arterial pressure, decreases LVEDP, decreases pulmonary artery wedge pressure, has no effect on preload and increases coronary perfusion.

Impella 2.5, CP and 5.0

Impella (Ambiomed, USA) is a device inserted percutaneously into the femoral artery, with the catheter threaded up into the left ventricle through the aortic valve. A rotatory impeller at the end of the catheter suctions blood from the left ventricle, which is ejected back into the ascending aorta, reducing left ventricular end diastolic pressure and thereby wall tension as well as augmenting forward blood flow. Impella 2.5 and CP can achieve a flow of 1.0–2.5 l min^{-1} and 3.7–4.0 l min^{-1}, respectively, and can be used for 7–10 days. Impella 5.0 (which requires a surgical cut down for insertion) achieves a maximum flow of 5.0 l min^{-1} and can be used for 2–3 weeks. They decrease afterload, LVEDP and preload. They increase mean arterial pressure and coronary perfusion pressure. The cost of a single-use Impella 2.5 is £15,000, and the reusable control unit is also £15,000. The cost of an IABP is £600. They are seldom used at our institution. There has not yet been conclusive evidence to show they are associated with a survival benefit versus other management strategies.

Tandem Heart

Tandem Heart (Cardiac Assist, UAS) is sometimes known as a peripheral ventricular assist device. A catheter is placed in the femoral vein and threaded up into the right atria. The interatrial septum is punctured and the tip of the catheter sits in the left atria. Blood is suctioned from the left atria and reperfused back into the femoral artery via the second catheter. This can allow for almost total augmentation of the left side of the heart and again can reduce left ventricular end diastolic pressure and thereby wall tension and myocardial oxygen demand. They can achieve a flow of 2.5–5.0 l min^{-1}, can be used for 2–3 weeks, and increase mean arterial pressure and afterload. They decrease preload and have no effect on coronary perfusion. Again, the evidence is uncertain as compared with other therapies, and they are seldom used at our institution.

Venoarterial Extracorporeal Membrane Oxygenation

Venoarterial extracorporeal membrane oxygenation (VA-ECMO) is a form of extracorporeal circuit which can be initiated either via a central (e.g. post-cardiotomy) or peripheral (e.g. used during or peri-cardiac arrest) configuration. A large bore vein is cannulated and an arterial return cannula is inserted into a central artery. The right atrium and the ascending aorta are commonly used for a central configuration, and the femoral vessels are typically used for a peripheral configuration. That said, it is possible to mix the two and/or other vessels, such as the subclavian artery. Blood is extracted from the venous system, oxygenated and pumped back into the arterial system. An oxygenator is required within the circuit to prevent massive systemic hypoxia resulting from total shunt.

Quick to initiate, patients can be placed on peripheral VA-ECMO in less than 10 min from a decision to cannulate. This allows for so called ECMO-CPR or ECPR situations where VA-ECMO is used in cardiac arrests, as an alternative to traditional CPR and a bridge to further therapy, such as primary percutaneous coronary intervention. VA-ECMO is best utilised for short-term support over a few days, as blood flow to the pulmonary system is reduced drastically by the VA-ECMO circuit, and significant systemic anticoagulation is required to prevent clot formation in the pulmonary vasculature. If long-term mechanical circulatory support is needed, conversion to a more medium-term ventricular assist device configuration, such as a biventricular assist device, is undertaken.

Due to the configuration of peripheral VA-ECMO, Harlequin syndrome can develop. This is characterised by a return of myocardial function but with poor pulmonary function. In these cases, as the heart starts to eject, deoxygenated blood is diverted preferentially to the upper limbs and head. An increase in minute ventilation (or FiO_2), or reconfiguration to VV-, VV-A- or V-AV-ECMO may be required to prevent this issue. In recovering hearts on VA-ECMO, left ventricular dilation can become problematic. This occurs due to the retrograde supply of blood into the aorta by the ECMO circuit; this configuration requires the damaged heart to eject any blood reaching the left ventricle against the afterload pressure generated by the pump. In a recovering heart, this can cause severe left ventricular dilation and further damage to the myocardium. Devices such as an IABP or Impella can be used with VA-ECMO to offload the left ventricle and prevent distention.

A further issue with peripheral VA-ECMO is the possibility of ischemia to the leg in which cannulas are placed. A large bore arterial cannula may completely obstruct and prevent flow distally, resulting in limb ischemia. This can be overcome with the use of a reperfusion cannula; a smaller cannula placed distally to the large bore ECMO arterial line facing towards the foot. Oxygenated blood is infused into this cannula from the ECMO circuit to reperfuse the leg.

Postcardiotomy cardiogenic shock describes the syndrome of refractory cardiac performance following cardiac surgery. The use of VA-ECMO for the management of postcardiotomy cardiogenic shock is controversial, and there are at least three scenarios where it may be necessary. First, pre-emptive postoperative VA-ECMO, where the decision for postoperative mechanical support is made prior to surgery, for example in the context of poor pre-operative cardiac function. Second, early yet unplanned post-cardiopulmonary bypass VA-ECMO following a long duration of cardiopulmonary bypass due to, for example, unexpected surgical complications. Third, late rescue VA-ECMO following several attempts at weaning, either immediately following cardiopulmonary bypass or following transfer to the intensive care unit. The use of mechanical circulatory support for postcardiotomy cardiogenic shock is further complicated by the wide range of available devices, the availability of VA-ECMO in different centres, variations in experience and expertise as a function of local VA-ECMO workload, and regional variations in the diagnosis and management of postcardiotomy cardiogenic shock. Furthermore, survival appears to be low for such patients and it is not yet possible to predict who will survive. Many questions remain, however, such as those in relation to practices around patient selection, how best to study long-term outcomes, the ethics and efficacy of ECMO in such patients, and on all aspects of clinical decision-making. Results from our centre are reasonable (Table 1), yet there remain many questions about the management of acute heart failure following cardiac surgery that require addressing (Fig. 2).

Table 1 Several key studies reporting outcomes for patients treated with VA-ECMO for PCCS. Our own results from Manchester are highlighted at the bottom of the table

	Number of patients; n	30-day survival; %	Hospital discharge survival; %	1-year survival; %	2-year survival; %	Comment
Distelmaier et al. [13]	385	–	56%	40%	–	Included transplant and ECPR patients
Fux et al. [14]	105	–	44%	–	–	The most comprehensive analysis in the literature
Liden et al. [15]	33	–	45%	36%	–	Included heart transplant patients
Loforte et al. [16]	155	–	46%	–	–	High rate of peripheral VA ECMO (52.5%)
Luo et al. [17]	36	–	42%	–	–	Low mean age (49 years)
Mikus et al. [18]	14	–	43%	35%	–	Only 14 patients
Wang et al. [19]	62	–	55%	52%	–	Included heart transplant patients
Yang et al. [20]	12	–	67%	–	–	Only 12 patients
Charlesworth et al. [12]	39	51.3%	41%	37.5%	38.5%	No cannula- or ECMO-related complications

VA-ECMO can achieve flows of 3.0–7.0 l min^{-1}, can be used for 3–4 weeks, increases afterload and mean arterial pressure, and reduces preload. It has no effect on coronary perfusion.

Temporary Ventricular Assist Devices

Patients are eligible for a ventricular assist device if they have more than one of the following: ejection fraction <25%; more than two heart failure hospitalisations in the previous 12 months without an obvious cause; dependence on inotropic therapy; progressive end-organ dysfunction; and deteriorating right ventricular function. Acute right ventricular failure can be a challenging diagnosis to make, but

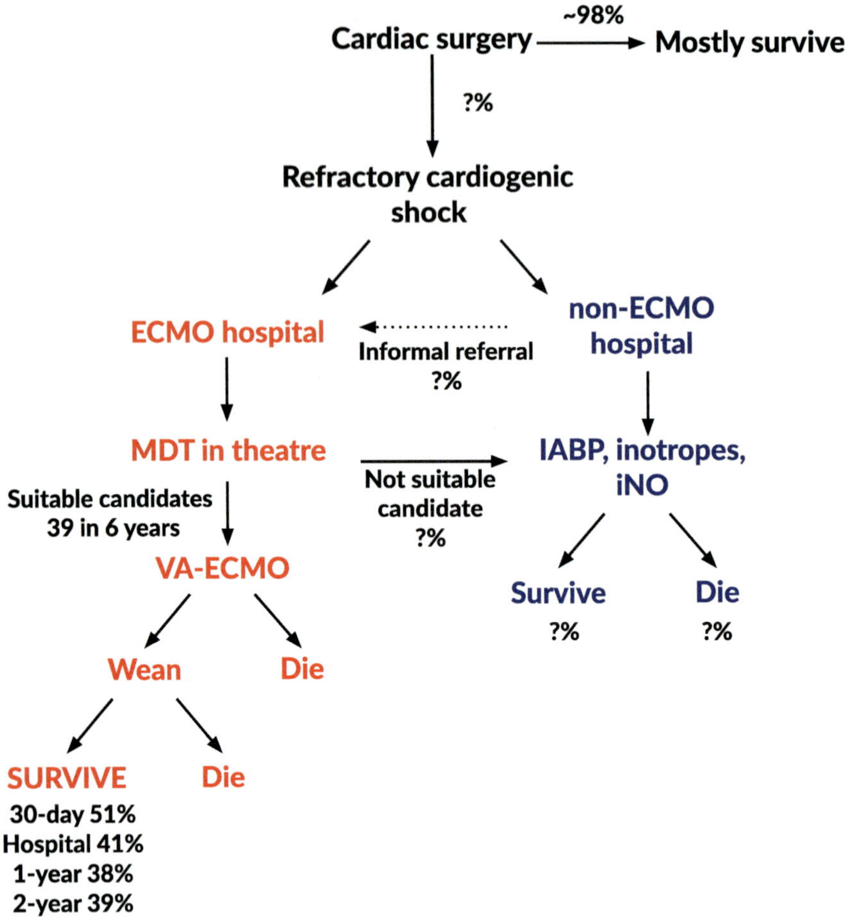

Fig. 2 A flow diagram of the referral pathway for VA-ECMO for PCCS at our centre. One of the key aims for the future is to determine the missing data marked by a '?' MDT, multidisciplinary team; IABP, intra-aortic balloon pump; iNO, inhaled nitric oxide

should be considered in all patients with clinical features of cardiogenic shock and/or respiratory failure. It may be associated with: acute coronary syndromes; myocarditis; pulmonary embolism; acute respiratory failure; postcardiotomy; post-transplantation; and following left ventricular device implantation. Medical management begins with addressing reversible causes, but later involves: optimisation of right ventricular preload; reducing right ventricular afterload; and inotropic therapy with either a phosphodiesterase inhibitor or a β1-agonist.

Mechanical circulatory support options for isolated right ventricular failure include: Impella RP; tandem RVAD; Protek Duo; or indirect right ventricular bypass with VA-ECMO. The Protek Duo (Cardiac Assist Inc., Pittsburgh, PA) is a dual lumen cannula with inflow from the superior vena cava and right atrium, and the outflow lumen delivering blood into the main pulmonary artery. The cannula is attached externally to an extracorporeal circuit with a centrifugal pump that may incorporate an oxygenator. This differs from VV-ECMO, as the right heart function is assisted. In our institution, we also use a Centrimag (Levitronix LLC, Waltham, MA, USA) device for short- or medium-term support, with surgically placed cannulae. Cannulae are inserted through a midline sternotomy, though they can be tunnelled to allow for chest closure, or inserted percutaneously. It allows for bridging to heart transplantation, a long-term mechanical support option or recovery. It can also be used after cardiac surgery as a bridge to recovery [21]. Likewise, a Centrimag left ventricular device can be used for short term support or bridging to longer term support, transplant or recovery.

A biventricular assist device utilises two extracorporeal circuits, two Centrimag pumps and with the option of adding in an oxygenator, although this may not be necessary if pulmonary function is preserved. Such devices can be used for longer-term mechanical circulatory support and patients can be fully awake, which enables neurological assessment and optimisation prior to transplantation or recovery. They must, however, be cared for in a critical care environment as the risk of sequalae from all type of mechanical support complications remains, such as bleeding, stroke, thrombosis and multi-organ failure syndrome. That said, a BiVAD is recommended in certain patients with acute heart failure despite optimal pharmacological and device management and who are otherwise suitable for heart transplantation, to improve symptoms and reduce the risk of hospitalisation, and to reduce the risk of premature death while awaiting transplantation.

Implantable Left Ventricular Assist Device

Implantable left ventricular assist devices (LVADs) are an increasingly common therapy for advanced heart failure (NYHA IIIb/IV) despite optimal medical management. They allow for long-term support of a failing heart whilst maintaining patient autonomy, independence and quality of life by allowing patients to leave hospital and resume normal day-to-day activities.

Implantable LVADs are small devices which are grafted directly to the left ventricle and ascending aorta. Devices have been through multiple generations and evolved significantly, initially mimicking normal, pulsatile blood flow, but near-continuous flow is now almost universal. The most common LVAD implanted in the UK today is the Heartmate III (Thoratec, USA), a centrifugal pump with magnetic levitation of the impeller. Although many other VADs have been manufactured, the only other device in common circulation within the UK is the HVAD (Heartware, USA), a centrifugal pump with hydrodynamic bearings.

Implantable LVADs work in a similar fashion to Centrimag VADs; they are placed at the apex of the heart with an inflow cannula facing towards the mitral valve, and a core of cardiac muscle is removed to allow room for the inflow cannula. Modern devices sit at the apex itself, with an outflow return cannula traversing across the heart ending in the aorta. Bloods is suctioned from the left ventricular apex and pumped towards the aorta, thereby augmenting cardiac output and offloading the left ventricle. Flows can reach 8 L per minute and it can, therefore, fully support the systemic circulation.

One of the main differences between implantable and Centrimag VADs is the power supply and control console. Once implanted, a long-term LVAD has a drive line tunnelled under the skin and exits the patient via the abdominal wall. This line allows an external console to be attached (Fig. 3), either as a box at the bedside, or smaller device which can be carried by the patient on a belt or in a backpack. Along with the external console are two batteries, these allow for the device to be powered whilst the patient is away from an external power source. The main long-term complications of implantable LVADs are bleeding and infection. Gastrointestinal or neurological bleeding are most common, as long-term Warfarin therapy is required to prevent pump thrombosis. Antibiotic prophylaxis is initiated oftenly for drive line infections. Many of these patients present for elective non-cardiac surgery, which should ideally be undertaken at VAD centres, but with all having an appreciation of the issues involved [22].

Anticoagulation

Although decisions on anticoagulation are determined by the underlying pathophysiology, patient factors, and the device used, they are usually on a case-by-case basis. For anticoagulation on the critical care unit, heparin is the drug of choice, and is monitored using APTT ratios or anti Factor Xa levels. In such patients, the possibility of heparin induced thrombocytopenia must be considered and investigated if clinically likely, as it is likely to result in paradoxical thrombotic events. For patients who have undergone cardiac surgery, the threshold for anticoagulation is high. For those undergoing ECPR, a bolus (usually around 5000 units) is given on cannulation, and an infusion of heparin started thereafter. Stable patients on a BiVAD are commonly prescribed a heparin infusion, whereas those with an IABP might not always require it. Patients with an implantable LVAD are usually prescribed warfarin long-term.

Weaning

The role of echocardiography for weaning is key, and decisions are usually made on a case-by-case basis. Some patients will require escalating (e.g. adding an oxygenator or temporary RVAD) and some patients will be successfully weaned to recovery. Patients without multi-organ failure syndrome might be transplanted.

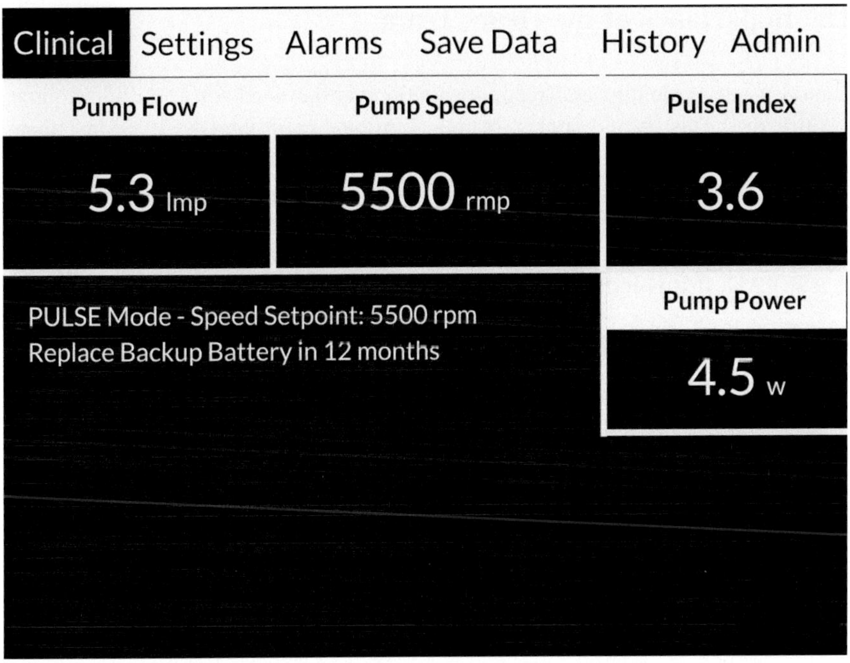

Fig. 3 A typical HeartMate 3 console display. Flow (l min^{-1}) is dependent upon pump speed and gradient across the pump. Devices are preload dependent and afterload sensitive. Pump flows are calculated from pump speed and power use, with higher pump speeds and power resulting in higher displayed flows. Flows are an estimated (derived) value and are not directly measured. Speed (rpm) can be adjusted with aid of echocardiography to allow adequate left ventricular filling. Power (W) is related linearly with flow. Increases in left ventricular preload and high pump speed increases flow and power consumption. The presence of aortic regurgitation necessitates increased power consumption to generate increased flow. An abrupt increase in power output may indicate pump thrombosis. Reductions in power consumption are usually because of reduced preload with reduced pump speed. They can also occur with inflow cannula obstruction. Pulsatility index is a dimensionless measure of the extent of left ventricular pulsatility. It is inversely related to the amount of assistance provided by the pump. A low pulsatility index typically indicates either low intravascular volume or minimal native cardiac function. Factors which affect pulsatility index include preload, native left ventricular contractility, afterload, heart rate and rhythm and pump speed

There are no black and white rules and each decision for each patient is taken following a full discussion amongst the multidisciplinary team and with a thorough clinical and echocardiographic assessment. That said, some have described weaning and explanting criteria [23].

The Importance of the Heart Team

Central to all guidelines and recommendations is the need for a multidisciplinary 'heart team'. This should consist of: interventional cardiologists; surgeons; anaesthetists; physiotherapists; speech and language therapists; psychologists; a structural heart disease expert; and radiologists, amongst others. The process of referral from distant hospitals for patients with acute heart failure should be clear, as should be the process through which such patients get access to emergency support, such as a BiVAD, if it is indicated at any time of the day or week.

Acknowledgements No external funding and no conflicts of interest.

Recommended Readings

1. Ponikowski P, Voors AA, Anker SD, et al. 2016 ESC Guidelines for the diagnosis and treatment of acute and chronic heart failure: the task force for the diagnosis and treatment of acute and chronic heart failure of the European society of cardiology (ESC) developed with the special contribution of the heart failure association (HFA) of the ESC. Eur Heart J. 2016;37:2129–200.
2. Charlesworth M, Ashworth AD, Barker JM. Decision-making in response to respiratory veno-venous extracorporeal membrane oxygenation referrals: is current practice precise enough? Anaesthesia. 2018;73:154–9.
3. Thiele H, Zeymer U, Neumann F-J, et al. Intraaortic balloon support for myocardial infarction with cardiogenic shock. NEJM. 2012;367:1287–96.
4. Seyfarth M, Sibbing D, Bauer I, et al. A randomized clinical trial to evaluate the safety and efficacy of a percutaneous left ventricular assist device versus intra-aortic balloon pumping for treatment of cardiogenic shock caused by myocardial infarction. J Am Coll Cardiol. 2008;52:1584–8.
5. Ouweneel DM, Eriksen E, Sjauw KD, et al. Percutaneous mechanical circulatory support versus intra-aortic balloon pump in cardiogenic shock after acute myocardial infarction. J Am Coll Cardiol. 2017;69:278–87.
6. Thiele H, Jobs A, Ouweneel DM, et al. Percutaneous short-term active mechanical support devices in cardiogenic shock: a systematic review and collaborative meta-analysis of randomized trials. Eur Heart J. 2017;38:3523–31.
7. Thiele H, Sick P, Boudriot E, et al. Randomized comparison of intra-aortic balloon support with a percutaneous left ventricular assist device in patients with revascularized acute myocardial infarction complicated by cardiogenic shock. Eur Heart J. 2005;26:1276–83.
8. Kar B, Gregoric ID, Basra SS, Idelchik GM, Loyalka P. The percutaneous ventricular assist device in severe refractory cardiogenic shock. J Am Coll Cardiol. 2011;57:688–96.

References

9. Stub D, Bernard S, Pellegrino V, et al. Refractory cardiac arrest treated with mechanical CPR, hypothermia, ECMO and early reperfusion (the CHEER trial). Resuscitation. 2015;86:88–94.
10. Charlesworth M, Barker JM, Greenhalgh D, Ashworth AD. Perioperative extracorporeal cardiopulmonary resuscitation: the defibrillator of the 21st century? a case report. A&A Practice. 2018;11:87.
11. Rao Prashant, Khalpey Zain, Smith Richard, Burkhoff Daniel, Kociol Robb D. Venoarterial extracorporeal membrane oxygenation for cardiogenic shock and cardiac arrest. Circ: Heart Fail. 2018;11:e004905.
12. Charlesworth M, Garcia M, Head L, et al. Venoarterial extracorporeal membrane oxygenation for postcardiotomy cardiogenic shock—A six-year service evaluation. Artif Organs. 2020;44:709–16.
13. Distelmaier K, Schrutka L, Binder C, et al. Cardiac arrest does not affect survival in post-operative cardiovascular surgery patients undergoing extracorporeal membrane oxygenation. Resuscitation. 2016;104:24–7.
14. Fux T, Holm M, Corbascio M, Lund LH, van der Linden J. Venoarterial extracorporeal membrane oxygenation for postcardiotomy shock: Risk factors for mortality. J. Thorac Cardiovasc Surg. 2018;156:1894–1902.e3.
15. Liden H, Wiklund L, Haraldsson A, Berglin E, Hultman J, Dellgren G. Temporary circulatory support with extra corporeal membrane oxygenation in adults with refractory cardiogenic shock. Scandinavian cardiovascular journal: SCJ. 2009;43: 226–32.
16. Loforte A, Marinelli G, Musumeci F, et al. Extracorporeal membrane oxygenation support in refractory cardiogenic shock: treatment strategies and analysis of risk factors. Artif Organs. 2014;38:E129–141.
17. Luo X, Wang W, Hu S, et al. Extracorporeal membrane oxygenation for treatment of cardiac failure in adult patients. Interact Cardiovasc Thorac Surg. 2009;9:296–300.
18. Mikus E, Tripodi A, Calvi S, Giglio MD, Cavallucci A, Lamarra M. CentriMag venoarterial extracorporeal membrane oxygenation support as treatment for patients with refractory postcardiotomy cardiogenic shock. ASAIO J (American Society for Artificial Internal Organs: 1992). 2013;59:18–23.
19. Wang L, Han J, Jia Y, et al. Early and intermediate results of rescue extracorporeal membrane oxygenation in adult cardiogenic shock. Ann Thorac Surg. 2009;88:1897–903.
20. Yang F, Jia Z, Xing J, et al. Effects of intra-aortic balloon pump on cerebral blood flow during peripheral venoarterial extracorporeal membrane oxygenation support. J Transl Med. 2014;12:106.
21. Lang SA, O'Neill B, Waterworth P, Bilal H. Can the temporary use of right ventricular assist devices bridge patients with acute right ventricular failure after cardiac surgery to recovery? Interact Cardiovasc Thorac Surg. 2014;18:499–510.
22. Hayes T, Charlesworth M, Garcia M. Patients with left ventricle assist devices presenting for thoracic surgery and lung resection: tips, tricks and evidence. Curr Opin Anesthesiol. 2020;33:17–26.
23. Dandel M, Hetzer R. Myocardial recovery during mechanical circulatory support: weaning and explantation criteria. Heart, Lung and Vessels. 2015;7:280–8.
24. Holmes DR, Rich JB, Zoghbi WA, Mack MJ. The heart team of cardiovascular care. J Am Coll Cardiol. 2013;61:903–7.

Postoperative Management of Heart Transplantation

Nicholas James Lees

Heart transplantation remains the definitive treatment for eligible patients with end-stage heart failure refractory to medical management and currently around 4000 are performed each year with a good one-year survival of >80%. The most common aetiologies are idiopathic dilated cardiomyopathy, ischaemic cardiomyopathy and congenital heart disease. As a result of donor shortage and thanks to improving technology and safety, more patients are being bridged to transplant with mechanical circulatory support (MCS) in the form of durable, implantable ventricular assist devices. Acutely deteriorating patients on transplant lists may also be supported with veno-arterial (VA) ECMO or other short-term MCS device. As such the patients presenting for heart transplantation are diverse, either coming from home or as inpatients, with or without MCS devices, with different considerations and associated risks.

Once the heart transplantation surgery has been completed and the patient has been transferred to the intensive care unit, care must be taken to preserve the function of the graft which is acutely susceptible to changes in the early post-operative period and is at risk of deterioration, in particular from right ventricular (RV) failure and ensuing cardiogenic shock. Early identification and management of this remains the main focus for the clinician, but heart transplantation has other important systemic considerations additional to those affecting cardiac function. In this chapter the approach to managing a heart transplant recipient in intensive care will be discussed systematically.

N. J. Lees (✉)
Royal Brompton and Harefield Hospitals, London, UK
e-mail: n.lees@rbht.nhs.uk

M. Vives and A. Hernandez (eds.), *Cardiac Anesthesia and Postoperative Care in the 21st Century*, https://doi.org/10.1007/978-3-030-79721-8_30

Monitoring

Cardiovascular monitoring should be already in place from the operating room and includes as a minimum arterial and central venous pressure (CVP) monitoring, a pulmonary artery (PA) catheter, a cardiac output monitor and continuous ECG. At the author's institution the PA catheter is connected to a continuous cardiac output monitor and oximetry displaying mixed venous oxygen saturation (SvO_2). The CVP although not a sensitive indicator of volume status is very useful in assessing trends and a rising CVP should be seen as a marker of increasing right atrial preload and worsening RV function. The PA catheter although used less commonly now in general intensive care is an important tool to assess RV afterload from the measured PA pressures and to calculate pulmonary vascular resistance (PVR). The pulmonary capillary wedge pressure represents left atrial pressure (occasionally also transduced directly with a monitoring line placed during surgery) and in turn left ventricular end-diastolic pressure. Intermittent or continuous cardiac output monitoring is essential to be able to track changes in function and titrate inotropic and fluid therapy. Echocardiography is performed often, with trans-oesophageal echocardiography (TOE) the most appropriate modality in the early post-operative phase as it allows better views. TOE should be performed routinely and early in event of any concern to evaluate ventricular dysfunction or presence of collections/tamponade.

Monitoring of other systems is similar to any other high risk post-surgical critical care patient including urine output and fluid balance with careful note of chest tube drainage, ventilation parameters and core temperature.

Cardiovascular

One should be aware of the changes in the newly transplanted heart which have implications for management. It is surgically denervated of its parasympathetic and sympathetic connections which leads to a number of physiological changes (Table 1). The heart rate is higher, typically over 90 bpm and the chronotropic

Table 1 Changes in the transplanted heart

Higher resting heart rate
Reduced heart rate variability
Slower and reduced chronotropic response to exercise/stress such as hypovolaemia
Impaired baroreceptor reflex
Cardiac output 'preload dependent'
Impaired chemoreceptor reflex (cardiac sympathetic response to hypoxia, hypercapnia, acidosis)
Altered conduction (arrythmia risk)
Altered response to cardiovascular drugs
Diastolic dysfunction

response to stress or exercise is slower with a lower peak maximum rate and a longer time to normalise afterwards compared to a non-transplanted heart.

There is a dependence on circulating catecholamines or administered inotropes to increase cardiac output which, as the heart rate component is relatively fixed, therefore relies more on adequate preload (venous return). There is an altered response to certain cardiovascular medications. Transplanted hearts tend to have a degree of diastolic dysfunction, with elevated left and right atrial pressures and reduced ventricular compliance. As such the normal response to changes in preload such is altered.

Drugs with parasympathetic nervous system effects such as atropine and digoxin will be ineffective whereas agents that act directly on the heart such as catecholamines will work. The normal compensatory heart rate response to drugs acting on afterload such as nitrates will be absent, so patients would be more sensitive to these drugs.

Haemodynamic aims early post-transplant are to have a MAP >65, CVP 6–12 mmHg, HR 90–100, PAOP (or LA pressure) 6–12 mmHg, CI >2.2 L min m^{-2} and SvO_2 >65%.

The rate should be kept around 90 bpm, and chronotropic agents such as isoprenaline may be used. Usually this is achieved by using the temporary epicardial pacemaker. Any tachyarryhthmias should be treated with direct current cardioversion or antiarrhythmic medication, with amiodarone usually being the most appropriate first-line choice. The early onset of AF or persistent atrial or ventricular arrythmias is often a sign of rejection and if suspected should be treated and investigated with angiography and endomyocardial biopsy.

Inotropic agents are used to maintain and augment contractility and cardiac output post-operatively, maintaining stability. The lowest effective doses should be used, with monitoring of their effect using cardiac output monitoring, clinical assessment and echocardiography. These drugs should usually be weaned off after a few days. Inotropes used include the catecholamines epinephrine, dobutamine and dopamine and phosphodiesterase-3 inhibitors milrinone and enoximone. Levosimendan is a calcium sensitizer that increases cardiac contractility and relaxation without increasing myocardial demand and can improve coronary perfusion and is used in some institutions. Choice of inotrope is usually down to institutional preference and familiarity.

It is common to need vasopressors to maintain the mean arterial pressure. The catecholamine norepinephrine is usually the first line agent with α and some β agonist activity. At lower doses, vasopressin acts on vascular smooth muscle V1 receptors and causes pulmonary vasodilatation via stimulation of endothelial nitric oxide, but at higher doses it has disadvantageous properties in the setting of RV failure, causing pulmonary and coronary artery vasoconstriction.

Escalating doses of inotropes/vasopressors or hypotension should trigger urgent echocardiography, as mechanical circulatory support (MCS) may be indicated.

Right Ventricular Failure

The RV is at risk of failure in the newly transplanted heart because of the direct myocardial injury associated with donor brain death, ischaemia–reperfusion injury, the effects of cardiopulmonary bypass and cardioplegia and having to adapt to changes in afterload (pulmonary vascular resistance) and volume such as transfusions. Owing to the difference in physiology of the RV, tolerance for these conditions is much less than that of the LV. Therefore acute RV failure can occur in response to increases in afterload, reductions in contractility, excessive preload or a combination of all three. RV failure manifests as low cardiac output state or cardiogenic shock, with low cardiac index, high CVP and worsening acidosis and end-organ function (Table 2). These patients are no longer preload responsive and in fact increasing preload worsens the haemodynamics. Increased filling pressures can also lead to ischaemia via coronary sinus congestion and reduced coronary blood flow. These patients will not be responsive to volume challenges and typically have CVP values 15–20 mmHg.

Echocardiography will show impaired RV systolic function, with RV dilatation and tricuspid regurgitation.

Through ventricular interdependence, abnormal ventricular septal motion and reduced LV filling, leads to a drop in stroke volume and cardiac output. Management principles are reducing preload, augmenting RV contractility and reducing PVR. Arrythmias should be treated and ventilation optimised to avoid excessive intrathoracic pressures (Fig. 1). Preload reduction can be achieved with loop diuretics or in more severe cases, especially if associated acidosis, by using renal replacement therapy. CVP should be targeted between 8 and 12 mmHg.

Table 2 Features of RV failure

Monitoring:
CVP > 15 mmHg CI < 2 L min m^{-2} Hypotension Low pulse pressure Acidosis, raised serum lactate Evidence of organ dysfunction (e.g. oliguria, AKI, rise in liver enzymes)
Echocardiography:
TAPSE < 17 mm FAC < 35% S' < 10 cms^{-1} RV dilatation (base > 42 mm, mid-point > 35 mm) RV:LV size ratio increased (RV equal or more size to LV apex) Tricuspid regurgitation Dilated RA Dilated, fixed IVC Flattened or D-shaped interventricular septum 'Underfilled' (small cavity) LV

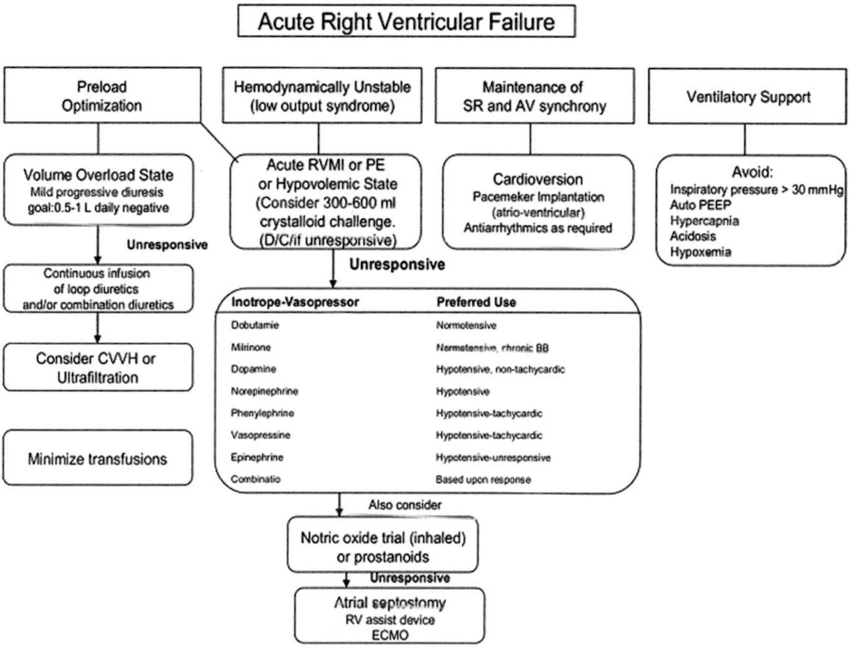

Fig. 1 Management of RV failure. Reprinted from *The International Society of Heart and Lung Transplantation Guidelines for the care of heart transplant recipients, Maria Rosa Costanzo* et al., *The Journal of Heart and Lung Transplantation Vol 29 edition 8, Page 918, Figure 1, Copyright 2010*, with permission from Elsevier

Contractility is augmented by inotropic agents, the phosphodiesterase inhibitors milrinone/enoximone are popular choices as they tend to reduce afterload (in odilators) and act at different pathways to the catecholamine adrenergic agonists therefore in combination may be additive. Compared with dobutamine, milrinone causes less tachycardia and greater reductions in RV and LV end-diastolic pressure but is associated with more hypotension and the half-life is longer, so vasopressors are often needed to maintain perfusion as a result. The author's institution uses a combination of milrinone and epinephrine as first line inotropic therapy for cases of RV failure. Afterload (PVR) is reduced with inhaled nitric oxide which requires a specialised delivery/monitoring system, or prostacyclin which can be nebulised. If despite all these measures, with escalating inotropic and vasoconstrictor dosages improvement is not being seen clinically, then this is a strong indication for urgent MCS such as VA ECMO.

Primary Graft Dysfunction

Primary graft dysfunction (PGD) occurs within 24 hours of implantation and may affect the LV or RV, or both. It is characterised by a drop in ejection fraction, cardiac index, rise in filling pressures (Table 3) and hypotension. It is a separate condition from secondary graft dysfunction due to e.g. overtransfusion.

Risk factors for the development of PGD are associated with the donor, such as age, ischaemic time and size mismatch; the recipient, such as age, pulmonary hypertension, medical co-morbidities, pre-operative requirement for inotropes or mechanical ventilation and perioperative factors such as ischaemic time, being on an LVAD pre-transplant and multiple transfusions. There is overlap with isolated RV failure as described above, and treatment is the same with inotropes, inhaled pulmonary vasodilators and MCS. Re-transplantation for severe PGD may be indicated in select patients but this is very uncommon as the patient will be extremely high-risk. The risk of PGD can be reduced by good donor care and selection, careful donor heart preservation and surgical technique, careful anaesthetic and early post-operative care. If deterioration is suspected, acting early (especially by instituting MCS early) can prevent worsening organ function and death.

Mechanical Circulatory Support

MCS after heart transplant is usually required because of RV failure refractory to medical management, typically with worsening end-organ function and metabolic state with high levels of pharmacological support. LV or biventricular failure may also be present though. MCS devices that may be used are venoarterial (VA) ECMO and short-term ventricular assist devices such as the CentriMag™ system (Abbott) and Impella® (Abiomed). VA ECMO is usually the quickest and most straightforward modality to implement either femorally (or centrally if placed in the OR) and will be a bridge to recovery in many cases, weaned off after a few days once recovery has been seen both on echocardiography and clinically with

Table 3 PGD

	Clinical features	Severe features
PGD–LV (LV primarily affected)	CI < 2.0 L min m^{-2} EF < 40% CVP > 15 mmHg PAOP > 20 mmHg	High inotropes Need for IABP Need for ECMO or other MCS device
PGD–RV (RV primarily affected)	CI < 2.1 L min m^{-2} CVP > 15 mmHg PAOP < 15 mmHg PA < 50 mmHg, TPG < 15 mmHg	High inotropes Need for ECMO or other MCS device

improving organ function, improved pulsatility and improvement in other end-organ dysfunction. Note that although of benefit to the RV and for 'circulatory support' in the form of organ perfusion; VA ECMO via the femoral artery will increase afterload and is not advantageous to a failing LV. In this situation a left-sided Impella is an option.

Respiratory

Patients will remain sedated, intubated and mechanically ventilated in the early postoperative period until cardiovascular, respiratory and metabolic stability is achieved. Care should be taken not to generate excessive intrathoracic pressures with mechanical ventilation, which may worsen RV function. Once stability is achieved, i.e. monitored haemodynamic parameters are acceptable, inotropes at low doses, nitric oxide weaned off, acidosis resolving, bleeding has stopped then patients can be weaned from the ventilator and extubated, typically in the first 24–48 hours.

Renal

Care in the postoperative period should be taken with excessive filling (volume) because of diastolic dysfunction and the risk of fluid overload and RV failure. Filling pressures need to be adequate for sufficient preload, but not too high. In practice the CVP should be kept on the lower side, between 8 and 12 mmHg. Fluid administration should be in small aliquots and may be guided by CVP and PAOP values but should be ceased if the filling pressures become elevated. Furosemide by bolus or infusion may be used to promote a diuresis if filling pressures are high or the patient has a positive fluid balance. The incidence of acute kidney injury (AKI) is around a third post-transplant, with risk factors including multiple blood transfusion, bleeding and surgical complexity. Heart transplantation is currently contraindicated if the preoperative recipient has a GFR of <30 ml/kg/1.73 m^2. Renal replacement therapy is used in the case of AKI or if volume management is required.

Bleeding

The risk of bleeding is increased in cases of re-sternotomy or previous thoracic surgery such as LVAD explant. Recipients may be taking anticoagulant or antiplatelet medication pre-operatively making transfusion more likely. Monitoring for bleeding should involve checking chest drain output and laboratory investigations. Tamponade should be suspected in both bleeding and non-bleeding patients with hypotension, elevated CVP and a drop in cardiac index and TOE should be performed as the patient may require urgent re-exploration. Often these signs are associated with other problems such as RV failure or primary graft dysfunction. In general transfusion should be minimised and point of care testing such as thromboelastography (TEG) is helpful to guide management. The use of clotting factor concentrates such as prothrombin complex concentrates and fibrinogen concentrate is advantageous as the administered volumes are low. Transfusions should be restricted as much as possible prior to transplantation as exposure to multiple blood donations may cause alloimmunisation to human leucocyte antigen (HLA) antigens and a reduced chance of receiving a cross-match negative graft; 30% of patients with LVADs develop HLA antibodies. Primary heart transplant without prior cardiac surgery poses a low risk however of alloimmunisation toward HLA or red cell antigens. Blood products should be cross-matched and leucocyte-reduced. CMV seronegative patients receiving seronegative organs should receive CMV-safe blood products. In general blood does not need irradiating prior to transfusion.

Infections, Immunosuppression and Rejection

Prophylactic broad-spectrum antibiotics are used perioperatively and continued if the patient leaves the operating room with risk factors for infection (e.g. infected LVAD driveline extracted during surgery or open chest). Immunosuppression is started at the time of transplant with methylprednisolone and most transplant centres commence immunosuppressive T-cell induction therapy early post-operatively. Immunosuppression is then maintained with a combination of corticosteroids, antiproliferative drugs (e.g. mycophenolate mofetil and calcineurin inhibitors (e.g. tacrolimus). These drugs have important considerations particularly as their levels can be affected by other medications and they have side effects such as nephrotoxicity and marrow suppression. Close involvement with a specialist pharmacist is recommended.

Hyperacute rejection due to preformed donor antibodies is rare nowadays but acute rejection still occurs in up to a fifth of heart transplants and is a significant cause of early mortality. The clinical picture varies with severity, but a fall in cardiac function is seen. Acute rejection is caused by acute cellular rejection (ACR), antibody-mediated rejection (AMR), or a mixed pattern, with most episodes due to ACR. Initial treatment is supportive care i.e. inotropes, vasopressors or MCS if required as detailed above and with pulse dose corticosteroids e.g. intravenous methylprednisolone 1g. Diagnosis is by endomyocardial biopsy (EMB), but treatment is not delayed for this. In the case of AMR, presentation is similar but unlike in ACR there is a lack of inflammatory cell infiltrates on EMB. Treatment includes additional immunosuppression, plasmaphoresis and IVIG. Additional antimicrobial prophylaxis against infections including antifungals is necessary whilst immunosuppression is enhanced. Re-transplantation in refractory cases has a high mortality.

Conclusion

The early postoperative course is a crucial time as the newly transplanted heart undergoes a number of physiological stresses and behaves differently to a non-transplanted heart. Standard evidence-based general intensive care principles are still important in the management of these patients but additional expertise is required in recognising and managing specific concerns relevant to heart transplant. As such, there is more monitoring and the need for immediate access to echocardiography and other members of the specialist multi-disciplinary team. Important complications to recognise are RV failure and PGD. It is important to recognise when medical therapy is no longer effective and MCS is required.

Recommended Readings

1. The international society of heart and lung transplantation guidelines for the care of heart transplant recipients. J Heart Lung Transp. 2010;29(8).
2. The reader is advised to check other International society of heart and lung transplantation guidelines at: https://ishlt.org/publications-resources/professional-resources/standards-guidelines/professional-guidelines-and-consensus-documents.

Infections and Management After Cardiac Surgery

F. J. González Moraga, P. Bono, J. M. Barrio, J. Casanova, and J. Hortal

Introduction

Patients undergoing major heart surgery (MHS) represent a special subpopulation at risk for nosocomial infections because they are usually older than other ICU patients, need long surgical procedures, and suffer frequent invasive manoeuvres during the perioperative period, including the cardiopulmonary bypass (CPB) pump and ischemia-reperfusion injury, that may increase the endothelial permeability and release endotoxins to the bloodstream. Postoperative infection is the main non-cardiac complication after MHS and has been clearly related to increased morbidity, use of hospital resources and mortality.

Data from an European multicenter observational cohort study, led by our group, on nosocomial infections prevalence in MHS (Fig. 1) are the following: Ventilator-acquired pneumonia (VAP) was the most frequent nosocomial infection following MHS (median 3.8%; IQR 1.8–4.9), followed by surgical wound infection (median 1.6%; IQR 0.8–3), catheter-related bloodstream infection (median 1.3%; IQR 0.8–2.1), mediastinitis (median 1.1%; IQR 0.4–1.6), urinary tract infection (median 0.6%; IQR 0.4–1.4) and nosocomial endocarditis (median 0.2%; IQR 0.0–0.9).

F. J. G. Moraga (✉) · P. Bono · J. M. Barrio · J. Casanova · J. Hortal
Department of Anesthesiology in Cardiovascular Surgery, Gregorio Marañón Universitary General Hospital, Doctor Esquerdo street, 46, 28007 Madrid, Spain

M. Vives and A. Hernandez (eds.), *Cardiac Anesthesia and Postoperative Care in the 21st Century*, https://doi.org/10.1007/978-3-030-79721-8_31

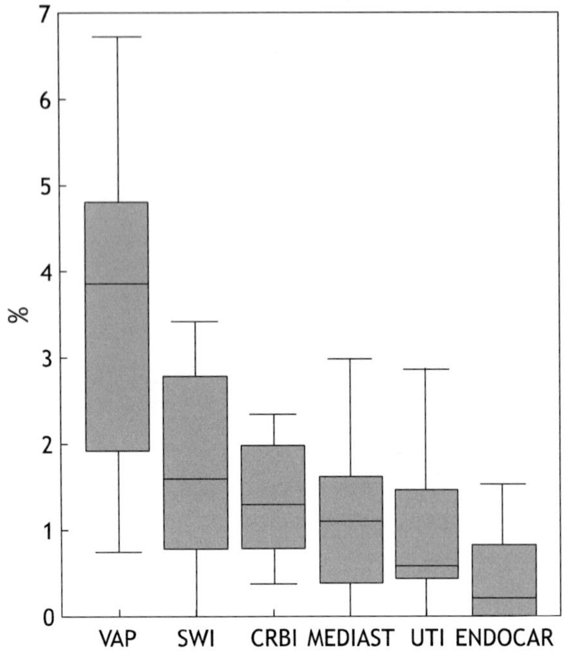

Fig. 1 Incidence of infections. The horizontal line inside the box is the median. The Box denotes 25–75th percentiles, and the outer bars denote 10 and 90% confidence limits. VAP, ventilator-associated pneumonia; SWI, surgical wound infection; CRBI, catheler-related bloodstream infection; MEDIAST, mediastinitis; UTI urinary treat infection; ENDOCAR, nosocomial endocarditis

Different Types

Pneumonia

Pneumonia is defined as the presence of new lung infiltrate plus clinical evidence of its infectious origin, which includes the new onset of fever > 38°C or leukocytosis/leukopenia or impaired mental status and two of the following: new purulent sputum or tachypnea/dyspnea/cough or decline in oxygenation. VAP is defined as pneumonia occurring more than 48 h after endotracheal intubation. Several risk factors for VAP have been identified (Table 1). VAP is the most frequent infection after MHS, with incidence rates ranging from 5.7 to 21.6%, although incidence can reach 46% in high-risk patients, requiring mechanical ventilation (MV) for more

Table 1 VAP risk factors

Age
Woman
Chronic obstructive pulmonary disease (COPD)
Heart failure
Prolonged surgery and time of CPB
Prolonged mechanical ventilation
Re-orotraqueal intubation
Politransfusion
Emergent surgery
Use of transesophageal echocardiography

than 48 h. Its incidence densities ranges from 22.2/1,000 days to 34.5/1,000 days of MV in all patients undergoing surgery.

Overall, 32.8% of VAP were caused by *Enterobacteriaceae*, 28.6% were caused by *Pseudomonas aeruginosa*, and 27.1% by *Staphylococcus* aureus (65.8% of them were *methicillin-resistant staphylococcus aureus* -MRSA-). VAP was polymicrobial in 13.5% of the cases.

It is recommended noninvasive sampling (endotracheal aspiration) with semi-quantitative cultures to diagnose VAP. There is no evidence that invasive microbiological sampling with quantitative cultures improves clinical outcomes. Non-invasive sampling can be done more rapidly than invasive sampling, with fewer complications and resources. Approximately 15% of patients with VAP are associated with bacteremia.

In patients with suspected VAP, it is recommended including coverage for *S. aureus*, *P. aeruginosa*, and other gram-negative bacilli in all empiric regimens. It is also recommended that empiric treatment regimens be informed by the local distribution of pathogens associated with VAP and their antimicrobial susceptibilities. It is suggested including an agent active against MRSA for the empiric treatment of suspected VAP, either vancomycin or linezolid, only in patients with any of the following: a risk factor for antimicrobial resistance, patients being treated in units where > 10–20% of *S. aureus* isolates are MRSA, and patients in units where the prevalence of MRSA is not known. When empiric treatment that includes coverage for *Methicillin-susceptible staphylococcus aureus* MSSA (and not MRSA) is indicated, it is suggested a regimen including piperacillin-tazobactam, cefepime, levofloxacin, imipenem, or meropenem. Oxacillin, nafcillin, or cefazolin are preferred agents for treatment of proven MSSA but are not necessary for the empiric treatment of VAP if one of the above agents is used. It is suggested prescribing 2 antipseudomonal antibiotics of different classes for the empiric treatment of suspected VAP only in patients with any of the following: a risk factor for antimicrobial resistance, patients in units where >10% of gram-negative isolates are resistant to an agent being considered for monotherapy, and patients in an ICU where local antimicrobial susceptibility rates are not available.

Data from local performance of strategies for the prevention of VAP from international guidelines have been recently published with excellent results, which include the following: education programs, systematic aspiration of subglottic secretions by using special endotracheal tubes, devices to facilitate the semi-recumbent position, oral care with clorhexidin or the use of selective digestive tract decontamination measures.

Surgical Site Infections (SSIs)

Superficial sternal wound infections (SSWIs) involve the skin, subcutaneous tissue and pectoralis fascia, with an incidence of 0.5% to 8%. Deep sternal wound infections (DSWIs) involve the sternal bone, the substernal space and the mediastinum. However, this last complication can be potentially lethal, increasing mortality twofold, when present in some series of patients. As defined by the Centers for Disease Control and Prevention, DSWI requires the presence of one of the following criteria: (1) an organism isolated from culture of mediastinal tissue or fluid; (2) evidence of mediastinitis seen during operation; or (3) presence of either chest pain, sternal instability, or fever (>38ºC), and purulent drainage from the mediastinum, or isolation of an organism present in a blood culture or a culture of the mediastinal area. There are many risk factors associated to the development of postoperative SSIs and mediastinitis (Table 2).

Computed tomography (CT) scanning is very sensitive in the diagnosis of DSWI, but its specificity is low within 21 days of surgery (39 vs 85% after 21

Table 2 Risk factors for sternal wound infection and mediastinitis

Patient Specific or Preoperative Risk Factors	Surgery or Situation Specific intra- and postoperative Risk Factors
• Obesity	• Prolonged operation and perfusion times
• Diabetes	• Use of internal mammary artery grafts
• Prior Cardiac Surgery	• Open sternum postoperatively
• Tobacco use	• Heart transplant
• Osteoporosis	• Need for reoperation in early postoperative period
• Peripheral vascular disease	• Postoperative hyperglycemia
• Preoperative Chest deformities	• Length of stay in hospital > 5 days before surgery
• Malnutrition	• Prolonged postoperative intensive care unit course and mechanical ventilation
• Immunocompromised status	
• Stroke	• Improper timing of antibiotic prophylaxis
• Heart failure	• Pedicled internal thoracic artery
• Advanced age	• Postoperative hemorrhage and blood transfusion
• Myocardial infarction	• Emergency surgery
• Cardiogenic shock	• Steroids
• Renal failure	• Use of intra-aortic counterpulsation devices
• Atrial fibrillation	• Redo surgery
• Peripheral vascular disease	

Table 3 More representative measures in our centre for Mediastinitis

	Recommendations
Prevention	Optimize perioperative levels in diabetic patients with high levels of HbA1c (> 6,5–7%)
	Mantain glucose perioperative levels below 180 mg/dL with insulin drip
	Give up smoking at least 30 days before surgery
	Nutritional supplies in patients with poor nutritional state. Albumin < 2,5–3gr/dl
	Dose adjustment of prophylactic antimicrobials, exhaustive surgical field preparation and reasssurement of a stable closure of the sternal wound to avoid dehiscence
	In overweight patients, systematic use of a vacuum assisted closure
	PCR techniques are recommended when a quick identification is needed, due to its high negative predictive value
Surgical treatment	The use of surgical steel wires to close the sternum is better than other techniques to reduce the incidence of mediastinitis
	In high risk patients, prophylactic therapy with negative pressure on the wound may reduce the risk of infection
	We recommend the use of postoperative sternal vest is every patient undergoing MHS
Medical treatment	In a patient with signs and symptoms of severe acute infection, start empirical antimicrobial treatment as soon as possible if mediastinitis is suspected
	In the adult patient with subacute mediastinitis, empirical treatment must not be started and must be directed regarding the laboratory findings in surgical samples
	To include coverage against SAMR and gram-negative bacilli in the treatment of acute mediastinitis
	We recommend an average treatment of 4 to 6 weeks in bacterial mediastinitis
	In sternal osteomielitis and/or fungal mediastinitis, a prolonged treatment is advised (months)

days). This issue can be solved by using Positron Emission Tomography/Computed Tomography (PET/CT). *S. aureus* is detected in bloodstream in 75% of the cases of DSWIs.

Regarding prevention and treatment of DWSI, we follow several standardized recommendations in our centre, which are summarized in Table 3.

Access and Monitoring Device Infections

The rate of infection of central venous catheter (CVC) represents 4,7% of all the perioperative infections in cardiac surgery, with a 5,twofold increase of SSI. The most frequently isolated microorganisms are coagulase-negative *Staphyloccus* followed by gram-negative bacteria and *S.aureus*. Although it has not been proven that the site of device placement may cause an increase risk of infection rate, femoral site is still avoided as the first choice, especially in obese patients. Following the clinical practice guidelines for the management and catheterization of CVCs has decreased the incidence of Central Line-associated bloodstream infections (CLABSI). These measures include: the use of ultrasound guidance to CVC cannulation, the use of chlorhexidine impregnated CVCs dressings or the use of disinfection caps that avoid the need of scrubbing prior to infusions or draws. The antiseptic impregnated catheters or sutures securement devices are other tools that can be used to reduce CLABSI.

Related to Ventricular Assist Device (VADs), infection is one of the most important complications, with a mortality rate up to 20%. In short-term and intermediate-term VADs (ECMO, Levitronix) infections are similar to other patients in cardiac surgery, although microorganisms that produce biofilm should be taken into account. In long-term VADs (as bridge to transplantation or as a destination therapy) infection is produced by the migration of bacteria from the skin through the driveline. In 85% of the cases, driveline infection occurs 30 days after the VAD implant, with an average of 6 months. Diagnosis is achieved through ultrasonography or CT scan and microbial isolation with blood cultures. Most of those infections are produced by *Staphylococcus, Enterococcus, Candida* or gram-negative bacteria. Patients with infection may be presented with clinical worsening secondary to sepsis or, less frequently, a device malfunction and septic embolism.

Prosthetic Valve Endocarditis

The risk is much higher within the first 3 months after surgery, considered as nosocomial if it appears within two months after the procedure, due to a direct contamination during the intraoperative period or to bacteraemia secondary to infection in other sites. Most common pathogens are *S. aureus and coagulase-negative staphylococci*, followed by gram-negative bacteria, *enterococcus and Candida.* Regarding the pathophysiology of the late prosthetic valve endocarditis, it is similar to native valve endocarditis, as a result of a transient bacteriemia in outpatients, being streptococcus, *staphylococcus* and *enterococcus* the most common causes. It should be emphasized that any positive blood culture in the postoperative period of a patient with a prosthetic valve, must be considered as potential infective endocarditis (IE). For the diagnosis, we use the Duke Criteria, needing the echocardiographic finding of vegetation or secondary valve destruction. Transoesophageal echocardiography (TOE) has higher sensitivity (90% vs 40%) than transthoracic echocardiography (TTE). However, it may be negative if it is performed within the first seven days. At least six weeks of antibiotic therapy will be needed. Surgical indications are the presence of an abscess, prosthetic valve dehiscence, valvular obstruction or regurgitation (Picture 1), and the persistence of bacteriemia or septic embolisms despite a correct antibiotic treatment.

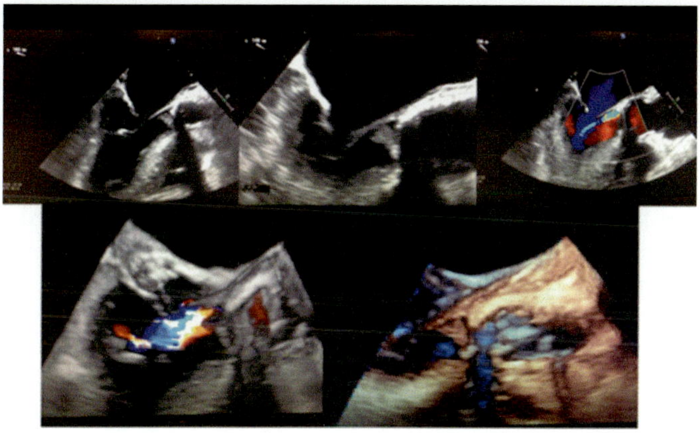

Picture 1 Transoesophageal echocardiography images (2D/3D). Native aortic valve infective endocarditis. We can observe aortic valve regurgitation and abscess

Diagnostic

Nosocomial infections after cardiac surgery usually appear within 48–72 h post-operatively (see Table 4). Fever within the first 24–48 h has a low sensibility as an infection sign, presenting in up to 70–80% of patients due to systemic inflammatory response syndrome (SIRS) produced by cardiovascular surgery, being caused directly by an underlying infection in only 13–15% of the cases.

Table 4 Major infectious causes of fever in Postoperative Cardiac Surgery Patients

Before 48–72 h	Community-acquired infection present before surgery, nosocomial infections in patients hospitalized prior to surgery, or infections that prompt surgery (e.g., endocarditis)
After 48–72 h	Sternal wound infection and mediastinitis (usually presents at 1 week) Pneumonia or aspiration (VAP, ventilator-associated pneumonia) Urinary tract infection Intravascular catheter-related infection Bloodstream infection secondary to any of the above ± prosthetic endovascular infection Endocarditis Acute cholecystitis Pancreatitis Clostridium difficile-associated diarrhea Leg wound cellulitis (at site of vein harvest) Sinusitis Infected hematoma Empyema Thoracic aortic graft infection Left ventricular assist device pocket infection (usually within 1 month) or driveline infection (usually after 1 month)

Performing multiple tests simultaneously does not necessarily produce better results. It has been demonstrated that isolated blood cultures, leukocytosis or leukopenia, urine cultures and/or chest radiographs have low yield for identifiying the source of infection. Only 6% of blood cultures, 8% of urine cultures and 46% of respiratory cultures will be positive. Leukocytosis, with a plasmatic peak in the first 3 days after surgery, is considered normal after cardiac surgery. However, when this elevated leukocyte count is persistent or increasing after the third day, especially if accompanied by an increase in neutrophils and immature cells, it highly suggests infection.

Cultures

When fever presents within the first 48–72 h after surgery, 2 sets of blood cultures must be drawn (in our centre, 3 sets are drawn according to our protocol), one of those from peripheral blood. If the results are negative, they should be interpreted in the context of prophylaxis or antibiotic treatment administered preoperatively, that may result in false negatives. Although there are commensal microorganisms like *coagulase-negative Staphylococcus* that may give false positive results or contamination, we must take into account that they also have a great pathogenic potential in patients undergoing valvular replacement surgery. Isolation of the same microorganism in several blood cultures increases the probability of infection or bacteriemia.

If any sign of local infection is observed in the surgical wound or adjacent to the puncture site of arterial or venous catheters, a sample should be drawn and cultured. If respiratory tract infection or VAP is suspected, a tracheal aspirate for culture and gram stain, should be urgently performed. Broncho alveolar lavage should be considered in immunocompromised patients, since they are in greater risk of infection caused by more unusual pathogens. Urinalysis and urine culture should be drawn in patients presenting with symptoms of urinary infection and/ or fever in patients with communication issues (under mechanical ventilation, sedated…), being difficult to distinguish infection of colonization in a urethral catheterized patient. Any new onset diarrhea in febrile patients after surgery should be evaluated and infection secondary to *Clostridium difficile* should be ruled out.

Biomarkers and Molecular Diagnostics Tools

C-reactive protein (CRP) and procalcitonin (PCT). We must take on account its limitations in surgical patients, since surgery itself increases those acute phase proteins. Furthermore, an increase in CRP after surgery has been observed, even in the absence of infection. However, a persistent elevation of CRP greater than 100 mg/dl during 4 days after major surgery like MHS, suggests an underlying infection. Regarding PCT, cardiac surgery and CPB provoke a plasmatic peak during the first postoperative day, returning to normal levels in the third day, with 85% sensitivity and 95% specificity below 1 ng/ml. Values above 10 ng/ml of PCT are highly suggestive of infection after surgery and its seriation can help us to choose the best antibiotic treatment.

Imaging Tests

Positron Emission Tomography/Computed Tomography (PET/CT): Important tool in the detection of infection, useful for the diagnosis of our patients with prosthetic valve endocarditis, intravascular devices or endovascular prosthesis. Moreover, it can detect septic emboli in cases of endocarditis. Given that it provides useful anatomic information, it may guide us in cases of surgical reintervention. Its use is limited by its high cost, the lack of availability in every hospital, the hemodynamic status of the patient, that sometimes prevents him from being carried to the radiology room, and the higher probability of false positives in 18F-fluorodeoxyglucose (18F-FDG) PET within the first 4 weeks after surgery.

Echocardiography: Especially indicated in patients presenting persistent fever (lasting more than seven days) undergoing valvular repair or valvular/ vascular prosthetic replacement surgery, with a poor nutritional status and that do not respond properly to the antibiotic treatment. TEE is superior to TTE to assess valvular prosthesis (>90% vs > 40% sensitivity). TEE provides a more reliable evaluation of complications such as abscesses, fistulas, perforation or periprosthetic regurgitation.

Lung ultrasound: Compared to chest X ray, it allows us to assess with higher sensitivity and specificity the presence of pleural effusions, pneumothorax, haemothorax, atelectasis and/or consolidations.

Prevention

We have already seen different preventive measures to reduce the incidence of the different infections after cardiac surgery. Now, we are going to explain some of the more extended ones.

Intranasal mupirocin: In our centre, it is a standard measure to apply intranasal mupirocin ointment to every patient undergoing cardiac surgery, once the nasal exudate sample has been taken. The treatment is kept for five days in positive *Staphylococcus aureus* carriers and removed in case of a negative result in the nasal exudate. Recent data suggest that the rapid test polymerase chain reaction (PCR) to diagnose *S. Aureus* colonization, along with mupirocin treatment in carriers and chlorhexidine 2% body washings reduces significatively the risk of DSWI.

Antibiotic prophylaxis: Selection of antibiotics is based on the activity against gran positive bacteria, since they cause the 80% of SSI, being cefazoline (first generation cephalosporin) the recommended one by the Thoracic Surgeons Society and the European Association of Cardiothoracic Anaesthesia and Intensive Care (EACTAIC) guidelines. In populations with high incidence of Methicillin-resistant *S. Aureus (MRSA)*, vancomycin is the mainstay, alone or in combination with cefazoline. The antibiotic must be administered at least 60 min before the surgery to obtain the optimal peak levels, and the dose must be repeated every two half-lives intraoperatively (92 min for cefazoline). Coverage for more than 48 h is not recommended and the most common practice is to give antibiotic 24 h postoperatively.

Antibiotic management: When infection is suspected, empirical broad-spectrum antibiotic treatment is started once cultures are drawn (blood, urine and respiratory) being suspended once 48 h have passed, the source of the infection has not been identified and the hemodynamic situation of the patient has improved. Selection of the agent must take into account the prevalence of different microorganisms in each hospital, the most common regimens are vancomycin added to a beta-lactam, such as cefepime or piperacillin/tazobactam, keeping antifungal therapy for high-risk cases for Candida infection, such as immunocompromised patients (cardiac transplant), CVCs or vascular devices lasting more than five to seven days (even less if they are in the femoral region), receiving parenteral nutrition or with high colonization of Candida identified in skin samples. Furthermore, it is advisable in patients with high suspicion of mediastinitis or with VADs. In these cases, we recommend an echinocandin (anidulafungin) as the mainstay, due to the high risk of resistances to fluconazole (Picture 2).

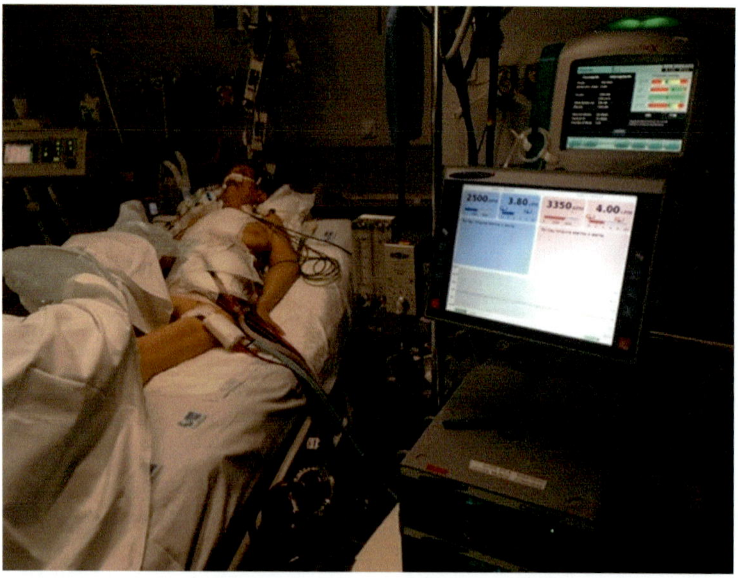

Picture 2 High-risk of infection patients, with VAD, hemofiltration, mechanical ventilation, CVCs Management

Recommended Readings

1. Cove ME, Spelman DW, MacLaren G. Infectious complications of cardiac surgery: a clinical review. J Cardiothorac Vasc Anesth. 2012;26(6):1094–100.
2. Paternoster G, Guarracino F. Sepsis After Cardiac Surgery: From Pathophysiology to Management. J Cardiothorac Vasc Anesth. 2016;30(3):773–80. Review.
3. Gelijns AC, Moskowitz AJ, Acker MA, et al. Management practices and major infections after cardiac surgery. J Am Coll Cardiol. 2014;64:372–81.
4. Rhee C, Sax PE. Evaluation of fever and infections in cardiac surgery patients. Semin Cardiothorac Vasc Anesth. 2015 Jun;19(2):143–53. Review.
5. Hortal J, Giannella M, Pérez MJ, Barrio JM, Desco M, Bouza E, Muñoz P. Incidence and risk factors for ventilator-associated pneumonia after major heart surgery XE "Major heart surgery" . Intensive Care Med. 2009;35(9):1518–25.

Enhanced Recovery for Cardiac Surgery

Alexander J. Gregory, Michael C. Grant, and Nick Fletcher

Enhanced Recovery and Quality Improvement Initiatives in Cardiac Surgery

Enhanced recovery programs aim to reduce complications, improved the patient experience, and promote efficient use of health care resources. Since its inception, guidelines and associated Enhanced Recovery After Surgery (ERAS) protocols have been developed for a multitude of non-cardiac surgical sub-specialties. The cardiac surgical community has a robust history of developing multidisciplinary (surgery, anesthesiology, and critical care) quality improvement initiatives. Cardiac surgery "fast-track" was the first such initiative, promoting early extubation through a balanced anesthesia technique: lower doses of opioids, increased utilization of volatile anesthetics, and avoidance of long-acting hypnotics. Now considered standard of care, it remains an important turning point in the modernization of cardiac-surgical perioperative care. Subsequent efforts include:

A. J. Gregory (✉)
Department of Anesthesiology, Perioperative and Pain Medicine,
Cumming School of Medicine, University of Calgary, Calgary, AB, Canada
e-mail: alex.gregory@ahs.ca

Libin Cardiovascular Institute, Cumming School of Medicine,
University of Calgary, Calgary, AB, Canada

M. C. Grant
Department of Anesthesiology and Critical Care Medicine,
Johns Hopkins University School of Medicine, Baltimore, USA

N. Fletcher
Institute of Anaesthesia and Critical Care, St Georges University Hospital,
London, UK

Cleveland Clinic London, London, UK

M. Vives and A. Hernandez (eds.), *Cardiac Anesthesia and Postoperative Care in the 21st Century*, https://doi.org/10.1007/978-3-030-79721-8_32

- Creation risk stratification models, such as the European System for Cardiac Operative Risk Evaluation (EuroSCORE) and STS Adult Cardiac Surgery Risk Score, for identification of high-risk patients, facilitate informed decision-making on appropriate therapeutic options, and direct resources to those who will benefit most.
- Large multi-national outcome repositories, including the European Association for Cardio-Thoracic Surgery (EACTS), STS, and the International Registry of Acute Aortic Dissection (IRAD) databases promote measuring and reporting of key outcomes, as well tracking inter- and intra-institutional performance.
- Multidisciplinary collaboration, initiated through international multi-society quality improvement committees, has led to the publication of several best-practice guidelines.
- Standardized application of care bundles previously demonstrated with the advent of cardiac surgical clinical pathways.

Society for Enhanced Recovery After Cardiac Surgery (ERAS® Cardiac) Guidelines

In 2017 the Society for Enhanced Recovery After Cardiac Surgery (ERAS® Cardiac) was established [www.erascardiac.org]. In accordance with the recommendations of the Institute of Medicine for developing clinical practice guidelines, a multidisciplinary group of experts was assembled to formulate key questions, perform a systematic review of existing literature, appraise available evidence, and complete a delphi process in order to obtain consensus on recommendations for inclusion in the Guidelines for Perioperative Care in Cardiac Surgery.

Each recommendation was then graded for Class of Recommendation (COR; Strength) and Level of Evidence (LOE; Quality), following the recommendations of the American College of Cardiology, American Heart Association, The American Association for Thoracic Surgery, and the Society of Thoracic Surgeons position statements on developing and grading clinical practice documents. The resulting guidelines are composed of 22 recommendations, covering the spectrum of the perioperative period, based on the best-available current evidence (Table 1).

Alcohol and Smoking Cessation

Tobacco smoking and excessive alcohol consumption have been identified as lifestyle risk factors which can lead to lung, wound, bleeding, metabolic and infectious complications. Cessation of smoking and alcohol consumption 4-weeks prior to surgery can reduced these complications.

Table 1 Summary of the recommendations of targeted interventions for implementation in a cardiac enhanced recovery program, from the Society for Enhanced Recovery After Cardiac Surgery. The Class of Recommendation (COR): strong (I), moderate (IIa), weak (IIb), or no benefit/harm (III). Level of Evidence (LOE): A, B-R (randomized), B-NR (non-randomized), C-LD (limited data), of C-EO (expert opinion). Abbreviations: CPB, cardiopulmonary bypass; EAA, epsilon aminocaproic acid; LD, limited data; NR, non-randomized; R, randomized; TXA, tranexamic acid

COR	LOE	Recommendations
I	A	TXA or EAA is recommended during on pump cardiac surgical procedures
I	B-R	Perioperative glycemic control is recommended
I	B-R	A care bundle of evidence-based best practices is recommended to reduce surgical site infections
I	B-R	Goal-directed fluid therapy is recommended to reduce postoperative complications
I	B-NR	A multimodal, opioid sparing, pain management plan is recommended
I	B-NR	Persistent hypothermia after CPB should be avoided in the early postoperative period
I	B-NR	Maintenance of chesty patency is recommended to prevent retained blood
I	B-NR	Postoperative systematic delirium screening is recommended at least once per nursing shift
I	C-LD	Smoking and hazardous alcohol consumption should be stopped 4-weeks before elective surgery
IIa	B-R	Early detection of kidney stress and interventions to avoid acute kidney injury are recommended following surgery
IIa	B-R	Rigid external fixation can be useful to improve/accelerate sternal healing and reduce mediastinal wound complications
IIa	B-NR	Prehabilitation is recommended for patients undergoing elective surgery with multiple comorbidities or significant deconditioning
IIa	B-NR	An insulin infusion is recommended to treat hyperglycemia and all patients postoperatively
IIa	B-NR	Strategies to ensure excavation within 6 hours of surgery are recommended
IIa	C-LD	Patient engagement tools, including online/application-based systems to promote education, compliance, and patient-reported outcomes are recommended
IIa	C-LD	Chemical thromboprophylaxis is recommended following surgery
IIa	C-LD	Preoperative measurement of hemoglobin A1c is recommended to assist with risk stratification
IIa	C-LD	Preoperative correction of nutritional deficiency is recommended when feasible
IIb	C-LD	Clear fluids may be continued up until 2–4 hours before general anaesthesia
IIb	C-LD	Preoperative carbohydrate loading may be considered before surgery
III	A	Stripping or breaking the sterile field of chest tubes to remove clot is not recommended
III	B-R	Hyperthermia (>37.9 °C) while rewarming on cardiopulmonary bypass is potentially harmful and should be avoided

Antifibrinolytics

Tranexamic acid (TXA) or epsilon aminocaproic acid (EAA) reduce bleeding by inhibiting the lysis of polymerized fibrin, reversibly blocking the lysine binding site of plasminogen. Evidence from large randomized controlled trials has shown a reduction in blood product transfusion in patients given intra-operative TXA. Higher doses of TXA have been associated with an increased risk of post-operative seizure. Therefore, it is recommended to avoid TXA doses in excess of 4–6 g (or 100 mg/kg) when possible—especially in patients with advanced-age or renal dysfunction.

Biomarkers for Acute Kidney Injury

Two novel urinary renal biomarkers, insulin-like growth factor-binding protein 7 (IGFBP7) and tissue inhibitor of metalloproteinases-2 (TIMP-2) can identify patients with normal glomerular filtration, serum creatinine, and urine output who remain at risk of postoperative acute kidney in jury (AKI). Studies have demonstrated that interventions, guided by urinary biomarkers, and directed towards renal protection (ex: avoidance of nephrotoxic agents) and optimizing hemodynamic parameters can decrease the incidence of AKI.

Chest Drain Management

Chest tubes evacuate shed mediastinal blood, but may occlude as clot accumulates. Retained mediastinal blood can lead to mechanical compression of the heart or lungs, resulting in the need for re-interventions, and is a risk for post-operative atrial fibrillation, increased transfusion, AKI, and length of stay Milking or stripping tubes has been shown to be time consuming, ineffective, and potentially harmful due to the impact of significant negative intrathoracic pressure created by the maneuver. Active tube clearance may prevent chest tube occlusion, eliminate the need for stripping tubes, and reduce the incidence of the retained blood, and the complications associated with it, in cardiac surgery patients.

Delirium Screening

Delirium in critically ill patients is a major public health problem issue, occurring in a substantial number of cardiac surgery patients, and increasing costs of healthcare. The occurrence of delirium after cardiac surgery has been associated with reduced in-hospital and long-term survival, higher hospital readmission rates, and poorer cognitive and functional recovery. Finding an optimal balance of management strategies for analgesia, sedation, and anxiety, while minimizing interruptions in normal sleep, wakefulness, and physical activity patterns are critical in the prevention of delirium. Regular screening is key for early detection and timely intervention in post-operative delirium.

Early Extubation

Prolonged mechanical ventilation after cardiac surgery is associated with higher morbidity, mortality, and increased costs. Extubation within 6 hours is safe and can be facilitated by time directed protocols and reduced use of opioids and long-acting sedatives. The use of balanced, short-acting anesthetics that lessen the reliance upon high dose benzodiazepines and opioids has been repeatedly shown to reduce time to postoperative extubation. In addition, instituting standardized pathways for early extubation have been shown to safely result in reduced ventilator time and ICU length of stay. Appropriate overnight staffing levels in smaller units to ensure day-night continuity is important to achieve this outcome.

Glycemic Control

Perioperative hyperglycemia has been associated with poor clinical outcomes, likely resulting from direct glucose toxicity, increased oxidative stress, inflammation, and induction of a prothrombotic state. Perioperative glycemic control is recommended based on prospective randomized data in non-cardiac surgical patients, and supported by observational studies in patients undergoing cardiac procedures. An insulin infusion is the most effective way to maintain optimal glycemic control.

Goal-Directed Therapy

Goal-directed therapy (GDT) is an algorithm-based approach to perioperative resuscitation that involves tailoring of fluids and vasoactive therapy to several selected physiological parameters. The goal is to maintain optimal patient physiology, guide intervention, and avoid the harmful effects of excessive fluid or vasopressor administration. The overall result is a cycle of assessment and therapeutic response guided by modern cardiac monitoring, providing the physiologic substrate for effective patient recovery. Post-operative GDT in cardiac surgery patients has demonstrated reduced hospital length of stay. A reduction in complications has also been shown but is an inconsistent finding across all studies. Additional investigation is necessary to determine the optimal parameters and/or GDT algorithm.

Hemoglobin A1c and Correction of Nutritional Deficiency

Pre-operative serum hemoglobin A1c (HbA1c) <6.5% is associated with decreased complications, including sternal wound infection and myocardial ischemia. Additional studies are needed to determine if delaying non-urgent procedures to improve glycemic control will lead to improved outcomes. Intensive nutrition supplementation for 5–7 days prior to surgery may improve outcomes in patients with a pre-operative serum albumin <3.0 g/dL.

Hyperthermia

Cerebral hyperthermia following cardiac surgery is associated with neurologic injury, increased rates of mediastinitis, and postoperative acute renal failure. Limiting the maximum arterial outflow temperature ($\leq$37.0 °C), avoiding rapid rates of rewarming ($\leq$0.5 °C/min), and maintaining an arterial-venous gradient ($\leq$4.0 °C) during re-warming are recommended to avoid hyperthermia.

Hypothermia

Active measures of rewarming and maintaining warmth are required to avoid hypothermia during chest closure, transport, and admission to the ICU. Hypothermia <36 °C is associated with coagulopathy, increased incidence of wound infection, prolonged hospital stay and death. Large registry observational studies suggest that if hypothermia is prevented or treated, outcomes can be improved. Hypothermia can be reduced by using forced-air warming blankets, and by warming irrigation and IV fluids.

Infection Reduction Bundle

Surgical site infections, including sternal and vein harvest incisions, are a major contributor to patient morbidity and increased healthcare costs. Infection-reduction bundles have successfully reduced the incidence of infectious complications in the critical care setting, providing an ideal framework for adoption of similar practices in cardiac surgery. An infection-reduction care bundle is composed of multiple evidence-based interventions, performed together, and consistent applied—yielding superior results than if performed individually in a non-structured fashion. Examples of interventions for consideration, in addition to timely administration of prophylactic antibiotic dosing and sterile skin preparation before incision, includes pre-operative shower with chlorhexidine, chlorhexidine oral swish, and use of wound protective bandaging.

Multimodal Analgesia

Effective perioperative pain control improves the patient experience, reduces the negative physiologic effects of pain, facilitates mobilization, and accelerates the process of recovering normal function and quality of life. Inadequately treated acute pain can contribute to the development of chronic pain in 20% of patients. Adequate analgesia should be achieved with the minimum reliance on opioids as possible. Opioids are associated with the undesirable side effects of sedation, respiratory, depression, nausea, vomiting, and ileus. Increased postoperative reliance on opioids has been associated with an increase in new persistent post operative opioid use. Multimodal opioid-sparing analgesia is an essential component of a cardiac ERAS program. It has been shown to be feasible, reduce opioid use proportionately to number of adjuncts employed, and achievable without an increase in reported pain scores.

Optimization of Sternal Closure

Most non-cardiac surgeons repair fractures/osteotomies while adhering to the principles of approximation, compression, and stabilization of the bone with rigid fixation. Wire cerclage for sternotomy closure has remained the standard of care in cardiac surgery due to the perceived low rate of sternal wound complications and the low cost of wires. However, this lack of rigid fixation commits patients to a period of "sternal precautions" to promote bone healing, limiting postoperative mobilization. Internationally, there is wide variation in approaches to sternal closure. Emerging data has shown that sternotomy closure with rigid plate fixation resulted in better sternal healing, fewer sternal complications, improved patient reported outcomes, and no additional cost at 6 months after surgery when compared to wire cerclage. Patients who may particularly benefit from this approach include elevated body mass index, prior chest wall radiation, severe lung disease, or chronic steroid use.

Patient Engagement Technology

Enhanced recovery is a patient-centered paradigm. Numerous e-health innovations have emerged aimed at increasing patient and care-giver engagement. These technologic advancements provide a user-friendly tool to promote patient engagement, education, communication, as well as facilitate the collection of patient-reported outcomes. Caregivers should consistently communicate that all efforts are directed towards a good recovery and that it is a partnership rather than a dependency. This message is empowering and truly places the patient at the centre of their own care. Increased patient activation, in addition to improving their perioperative experience, also results in improved delivery of surgical care.

Prehabilitation

Frailty, cardiopulmonary deconditioning, malnutrition, sarcopenia, and socioeconomic factors are often present in the cardiac surgical population and are barriers to optimal recovery. Prehabilitation is a comprehensive approach that includes screening for areas of concern and implementing protocols to ameliorate the patent's exercise, nutritional, and psychological status prior to surgery. Prehabilitation has been shown to improve preoperative exercise capacity, resulting in faster postoperative recovery and shorter lengths of stay.

Prolonged Fasting

Prolonged preoperative fasting may contribute to postoperative insulin resistance. Additionally, administration of a carbohydrate drink within 2–4 hours of surgery has been shown to reduce insulin resistance and tissue glycosylation, with corresponding improvements in postoperative glucose control, earlier return of gut function, and reduced length of stay. Maintenance of a clear liquid diet until 2–4 hours before surgery, as well as a preoperative carbohydrate load, have been a mainstay of non-cardiac ERAS protocols. The data for cardiac surgery patients is less robust, hence this recommendation's low LOE grading.

Thromboprophylaxis

Vascular thrombotic events (VTE) include both deep venous thrombosis and pulmonary embolism. They occur at a high incidence compared to other non-cardiac surgical patients and are a preventable cause of morbidity and mortality.

Pharmacologic prophylaxis after cardiac surgery can reduce the risk of VTE without increasing the risk of bleeding or cardiac tamponade. It is recommended that pharmacological prophylaxis is initiated once satisfactory hemostasis has been achieved, in addition to the use of mechanical prophylaxis with intermittent pneumatic compression devices.

Implementation

Knowledge of the current existing evidence supporting clinical interventions to promote enhanced recovery is only one step in the process. Without a comprehensive and inclusive implementation plan, a cardiac enhanced recovery program will not achieve its maximum potential for improving patient care. Implementation strategies have been previously described in detail and can be summarized as a 6-step iterative cycle (Fig. 1). Building a team is best accomplished through a bottom-up approach, with early input from all stakeholders, and identification of "champions". The team will require membership from a broad group of individuals to maximize the benefits of diversity in perspective, expertise, and experience (Table 2). Following establishment of the team, the process of education, self-assessment, goal-prioritization, discussion, protocol/bundles development, and program planning can commence. Founded in science, successful implementation

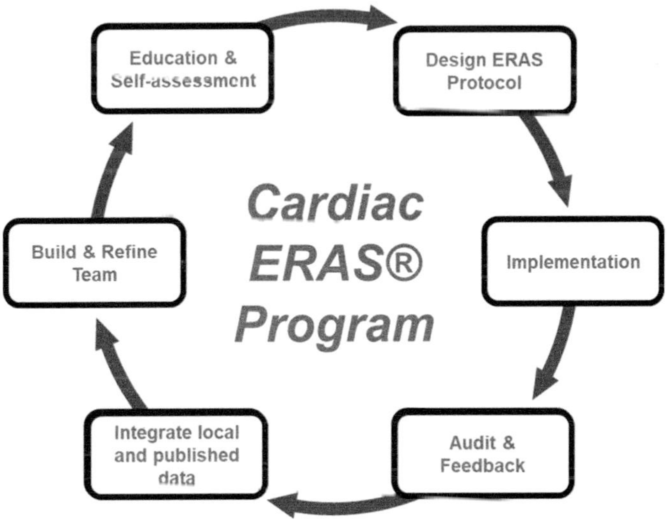

Fig. 1 A summary of the 6-step iterative cycle the describes the basic components for successful development and implementation of a cardiac surgery enhanced recovery program. Adapted from Salenger et al. "Cardiac Enhanced Recovery After Surgery: A Guide to Team Building and Successful Implementation"; Semin Thorac Cardiovasc Surg 32(2) 2020

Table 2 List of members, including general role in providing medical care, for consideration when building an ERAS Cardiac team

Role	Team member
Physician	Anesthesiologist
	Cardiologist
	Cardiothoracic surgeon
	Critical care physician
Non-physician Care Provider	Advanced medical practitioners
	Dietician
	Nursing
	Perfusionist
	Pharmacist
	Physiotherapist
	Pre-admission clinic
	Respiratory therapist
	Social worker
Administration	Clinical educators
	Hospital administration
	Information technology
	Operating room managers
	Ward managers
Patient Advocates	Family members
	Former patients (cardiac)
	Former patients (non-cardiac)
	Other care providers
	Patient advocacy groups

incorporates the individual and group psychology of change, strong two-way communication, inter-personal and inter-system dynamics, knowledge translation, and feedback loop strategies (Table 3). Many of these concepts require knowledge, network building, and experience in enacting organizational change that are not common areas of expertise for most clinicians- further highlighting the importance of multidisciplinary collaboration and self-education. It is imperative to have an open, accessible, and convenient communication platform to direct comments, suggestions, and questions to the ERAS team. While feedback is important, a formal audit process is critical to the creation and sustainability of an ERAS program. Audit allows for standardized quantification of key-outcomes (including patient-reported), post-implementation improvements, and protocol adherence. Measuring and reporting protocol adherence is particularly important, as increased adherence rates are correlated with improved outcomes related to the ERAS protocol.

Table 3 Summary of the key phases, steps, or components of 3 well-studied frameworks for successfully implementing change within healthcare systems: Knowledge-to-Action (KTA), Quality Enhancement Research Initiative (QUERI), and Theoretical Domains Framework (TDF)

	KTA	QUERI	TDF
Key steps	Identify problem that needs addressing	Identify high-risk/ volume diseases or problems	Who needs to do what differently to adopt best practice?
	Review, and select knowledge or research relevant to the problem	Identify best practices	What barriers and enablers need to be addressed?
	Adapt identified knowledge or research to local context	Define existing practice patterns and outcomes	Which interventions can be employed to overcome these barriers?
	Assess barriers to using the knowledge	Implement interventions to promote best practices	Which interventions can enhance enablers to uptake best practice?
	Tailor and implement interventions to promote use of knowledge	Document that best practices improve outcomes	What is the best method measure and understand behavior change?
	Monitor knowledge use	Document outcomes that are associated with improved health	
	Evaluate outcomes of knowledge utilization		
	Sustain ongoing knowledge use		

Published Results from Cardiac Enhanced Recovery Programs

Prior to publication by Fleming et al. of one of the first formal cardiac enhanced recovery programs, there had already been publications on the benefits of colorectal ERAS programs in entire healthcare systems, large multinational registries, and meta-analyses. Since this time, additional publications have highlighted benefits achieved in the perioperative care of cardiac surgical patients. This includes one of the only prospective randomized trials, within all surgical subspecialties, demonstrating the benefits of implementing an enhanced recovery program. Though incongruent in study design, interventions, outcome measures, and reported benefits, the results from existing publications in cardiac surgery populations highlight the benefits of enhanced recovery (Table 4). To build on our current level of knowledge, both of the ERAS Cardiac Guidelines and the reported benefits of program implementation, further study is warranted.

Table 4 Summary of existing publications on results from cardiac surgery enhanced recovery programs, including Digital Object Identifier (DOI). Abbreviations: ICU, intensive care unit; LOS, length of stay

Author	Year	DOI	Country	Study design	Number of patients	Reported outcome benefits
Fleming	2016	10.1053/j.jvca.2016.01.017	UK	Prospective Non-randomized	105	Analgesia Complications Opioid use
Li	2018	10.1093/ejcts/ezy100	China	Prospective Randomized	226	Bowel function Complications Cost ICU LOS Intubation time Vasoactive support
Grant	2019	10.1016/j.jtcvs.2019.05.035	USA	Retrospective Propensity-matched	451	Hospital LOS Intubation time
Williams	2019	10.1016/j.jtcvs.2018.10.164	USA	Prospective Non-randomized	932	Bowel function Hospital LOS ICU LOS Opioid use
Zaouter	2019	10.1053/j.jvca.2019.05.006	France	Prospective Non-randomized	46	Analgesia Hospital LOS ICU LOS

Conclusion

The enhanced recovery paradigm has fundamentally shifted our perspective on patient-centered, quality-driven perioperative surgical care. The rich tradition of multidisciplinary quality improvement initiatives facilitated the rapid adoption and implementation of enhanced recovery protocols in cardiac surgery. The foundation of the Society for Enhanced Recovery After Cardiac Surgery and publication of its guidelines were crucial towards initiating development and implementation of protocols to improve outcomes in this high-risk population. Early evidence of the benefits of enhanced recovery show that it is a promising concept. However, additional research into the current recommended practices, as well areas of future growth, will be vital for cardiac enhanced recovery to reach its maximum potential.

Recommended Readings

1. Engelman DT, Ben Ali W, Williams JB, et al. Guidelines for perioperative care in cardiac surgery: enhanced recovery after surgery society recommendations. JAMA Surg. 2019;154:755–66.
2. Gregory AJ, Engelman DT, Williams JB, Arora RC, Boyle EM. Cardiac surgery ERAS. In: Ljungqvist O, Francis NKK, Urman RD, editors. Enhanced recovery after surgery: a complete guide to optimizing outcomes. 1st ed. Switzerland: Springer International Publishing; 2020. p. 497–505.
3. Noss C, Prusinkiewicz C, Nelson G, Patel PA, Augoustides JG, Gregory AJ. Enhanced recovery for cardiac surgery. J Cardiothorac Vasc Anesth. 2018;32:2760–70.
4. Ljungqvist O, Scott M, Fearon KC. Enhanced recovery after surgery: a review. JAMA Surg. 2017;152:292–8.
5. Salenger R, Morton-Bailey V, Grant M, Gregory A, Williams JB, Engelman DT. Cardiac enhanced recovery after surgery: a guide to team building and successful implementation. Semin Thorac Cardiovasc Surg. 2020;32(2):187–96.
6. Gramlich LM, Sheppard CE, Wasylak T, et al. Implementation of enhanced recovery after surgery: a strategy to transform surgical care across a health system. Implement Sci. 2017;12:67.

Correction to: Valvular Surgery

Matias Caceres Quinones and Jacobo Moreno Garijo

Correction to:
Chapter “Valvular Surgery” in:
M. Vives and A. Hernandez (eds.), *Cardiac Anesthesia and Postoperative Care in the 21st Century*, https://doi.org/10.1007/978-3-030-79721-8_16

In the original version of chapter 16, the title of Chapter has been changed from “Cardiac Anaesthesia and Postoperative Care in the Twenty-First Century” to “Valvular Surgery”. The correction chapter and the book has been updated with the change.

The updated version of this chapter can be found at
https://doi.org/10.1007/978-3-030-79721-8_16

M. Vives and A. Hernandez (eds.), *Cardiac Anesthesia and Postoperative Care in the 21st Century*, https://doi.org/10.1007/978-3-030-79721-8_33

Index

M. Vives and A. Hernandez (eds.), *Cardiac Anesthesia and Postoperative Care in the 21st Century*, https://doi.org/10.1007/978-3-030-79721-8

GPSR Compliance

The European Union's (EU) General Product Safety Regulation (GPSR) is a set of rules that requires consumer products to be safe and our obligations to ensure this.

If you have any concerns about our products, you can contact us on ProductSafety@springernature.com

In case Publisher is established outside the EU, the EU authorized representative is:

Springer Nature Customer Service Center GmbH
Europaplatz 3
69115 Heidelberg, Germany

Batch number: 08999478

Printed by Printforce, the Netherlands